American Medi
Physicians dedicated to the

Controversies & Conversations in Cutaneous Laser Surgery

Kenneth A. Arndt, MD
Jeffrey S. Dover, MD, FRCPC
Editors

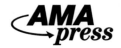

Controversies and Conversations in Cutaneous Laser Surgery

Additional copies of this book may be ordered by calling 800-621-8335.
Secure online orders can be taken at www.ama-assn.org/catalog.
Mention product number OP120501.

ISBN 1-57947-261-3
BP58:02-P-034:8/02

CONTENTS

PART ONE   WILL LASER SKIN RESURFACING EVER
RETURN TO ITS GLORY DAYS?   1

1 Carbon Dioxide vs Erbium:YAG Laser in Laser Skin Resurfacing   3
Christopher B. Zachary, MBBS, FRCP

2 The Quest for Reliable Results After Laser Resurfacing   7
Javier Ruiz-Esparza, MD

3 Ideal Tissue Effects of Laser Resurfacing   9
Richard E. Fitzpatrick, MD

4 Efficacy of Laser Skin Resurfacing   13
Suzanne L. Kilmer, MD

Discussion Part One   20
Jeffrey S. Dover, MD, FRCPC, Moderator

PART TWO   POSTOPERATIVE CARE AFTER LASER
RESURFACING: WHAT IS THE OPTIMAL
APPROACH?   27

5 Wound Care and Prophylaxis After Laser Resurfacing   29
George J. Hruza, MD

6 Nonocclusive Wound Care After Laser Resurfacing   37
Christian Raulin, MD

7 Improved Reepithelialization After Laser Resurfacing   39
Mitchel P. Goldman, MD

8 Postoperative Care After Laser Resurfacing: Review of the Literature   43
A. Jay Burns, MD

Discussion Part Two   49

Kenneth A. Arndt, MD, Moderator

PART THREE   PHOTOREJUVENATION AND SUBSURFACE
RESURFACING: DO THEY REALLY
WORK?   55

9   Quantitative Evidence of Benefits of Subsurface
Resurfacing   57

Roy Geronemus, MD

10   Photorejuvenation With the Pulsed Dye Laser:
Biochemical and Clinical Findings   61

Peter Bjerring, MD, PhD

11   Nonablative Dermal Remodeling and
Photorejuvenation: Clinical and Histologic
Findings   65

Brian D. Zelickson, MD

12   Nonablative Laser Resurfacing   73

David J. Goldberg, MD

13   Photorejuvenation and Subsurface Resurfacing   77

Robert A. Weiss, MD

Discussion Part Three   82

Jeffrey S. Dover, MD, FRCPC, Moderator

PART FOUR   NOVEL APPROACHES TO SKIN
REJUVENATION (EXCLUDING
PHOTOREJUVENATION)   91

14   A Novel Radiofrequency Technology   93

Michael S. Kaminer, MD

15   A New Nonablative Radiofrequency Device:
Preliminary Results   95

Suzanne L. Kilmer, MD

16   Volumetric Heating of Skin Using Radiofrequency:
Preliminary Findings   101

Javier Ruiz-Esparza, MD

17 Nonlaser Methods for Dermal Therapy   111
Jerome M. Garden, MD

Discussion Part Four   113
Kenneth A. Arndt, MD, Moderator

PART FIVE   HOW HAVE MILLISECOND-DOMAIN
LASERS CHANGED THE APPROACH TO
TREATMENT OF VASCULAR ANOMALIES
AND ECTASIAS?   **117**

18 Improved Results in the Treatment of Facial Vascular
Lesions Using Millisecond-Duration Lasers   119
Arielle N. B. Kauvar, MD

19 Treatment With Millisecond-Domain Lasers of Port-
wine Stains and Facial Telangiectasia   125
Pablo Boixeda, MD, PhD

20 Influence of Varying Pulse Durations, Different
Types of Lasers, and Intense Pulsed Light on
Vascular Anomalies and Ectasias   145
Christian Raulin, MD

21 Role of Millisecond-Domain Lasers and Intense
Pulsed Light in the Treatment of Vascular Anomalies
and Ectasias   149
Mark S. Nestor, MD, PhD

22 Effect of Pulse Duration on Laser Therapy for
Cutaneous Vascular Lesions   153
Jerome M. Garden, MD

Discussion Part Five   157
Kenneth A. Arndt, MD, Moderator

PART SIX   ADVANCES IN THE USE OF LASERS AND
LIGHT SOURCES IN THE TREATMENT OF LEG
VEINS   **163**

23 Role of Lasers in the Treatment of Leg Veins   165
Arielle N. B. Kauvar, MD

24   Photothermal Treatment of Leg Telangiectasia   171
Mitchel P. Goldman, MD

25   Treatment of Leg Veins With Lasers and Intense
Pulsed Light   175
Robert A. Weiss, MD

26   Clinical and Histologic Findings of Leg Veins
Treated With Laser   181
Robert M. Adrian, MD

Discussion Part Six   191
Jeffrey S. Dover, MD, FRCPC, Moderator

PART SEVEN   LASER, SCALPEL, DIAMOND KNIFE,
SHAW SCALPEL—AND THE WINNER
IS . . . ?   195

27   Incisional Laser Surgery   197
Brian S. Biesman, MD

28   Advantages and Disadvantages of the Laser, Scalpel,
and Diamond Knife in Cutaneous Surgery   201
Roland Kaufmann, MD

29   Thermal Scalpel in Incisional Surgery   205
Milton Waner, MD

Discussion Part Seven   207
R. Rox Anderson, MD, Moderator

PART EIGHT   IS SKIN COOLING A BUNCH OF
HOT AIR?   211

30   Thermal Imaging and Theoretical Modeling in
Skin Cooling   213
Peter Bjerring, MD, PhD

31   Practical Implementation of Skin Cooling   219
J. Stuart Nelson, MD, PhD

32   Is Skin Cooling a Bunch of Hot Air?   223
R. Rox Anderson, MD

33   Efficacy and Safety of Skin-Cooling Devices   227
Brian S. Biesman, MD

Discussion Part Eight   231

Kenneth A. Arndt, MD, Moderator

PART NINE   LASERS AND LIGHTS AS DIAGNOSTIC TOOLS:
WHERE ARE WE NOW?   235

34   Confocal Scanning Laser Microscopy and Optical
Coherence Tomography   237

Thomas E. Rohrer, MD

35   Noninvasive Diagnostic Tools for Characterization of
Port-wine Stains   247

J. Stuart Nelson, MD, PhD

36   New Electro-optic Imaging Tools   249

R. Rox Anderson, MD

Discussion Part Nine   253

Kenneth A. Arndt, MD, Moderator

PART TEN   LASERS AND PSORIASIS: AN ILLUMINATING
COMBINATION   255

37   Rationale for Vascular-Specific Laser Treatment of
Psoriasis   257

Brian D. Zelickson, MD

38   Treatment of Psoriasis With the 308-nm Excimer
Laser   263

Roy Geronemus, MD

39   Comparison of Lasers Used in Treatment of
Psoriasis   265

Richard E. Fitzpatrick, MD

Discussion Part Ten   269

Jeffrey S. Dover, MD, FRCPC, Moderator

PART ELEVEN   THE ROLE OF LASERS IN THE TREATMENT
OF SCARS, HYPOPIGMENTATION, AND
DEPIGMENTATION   273

40   Acne Scars: Classification and Treatment   279

Michael S. Kaminer, MD

41 Laser Treatment of Hypertrophic Scars 281
Whitney D. Tope, MPhil, MD

42 Laser Treatment of Scars 285
George J. Hruza, MD

43 Excimer Laser for Repigmentation of Laser-Induced and Surgically Induced Depigmentation 291
Roy Geronemus, MD

Discussion Part Eleven 295
Jeffrey S. Dover, MD, FRCPC, Moderator

PART TWELVE LASERS IN THE TREATMENT OF TATTOOS AND DERMAL PIGMENT: WHAT'S NEW AND WHAT'S NEXT? 301

44 Resistance of Tattoos to the Q-switched Laser 303
Whitney D. Tope, MPhil, MD

45 Removal of Dermal Pigment and Tattoos: Can't We Do Better? 309
E. Victor Ross, Jr, MD

46 Tattoos 317
R. Rox Anderson, MD

Discussion Part Twelve 319
Kenneth A. Arndt, MD, Moderator

PART THIRTEEN LASERS AND LIGHT SOURCES FOR HAIR REMOVAL 327

47 Hair Removal by Light: Accomplishments and Challenges 329
Christine C. Dierickx, MD

48 Laser Hair Removal: Optimal Parameters 333
Eliot F. Battle, Jr, MD

49 Current Practice and Experience in Laser Hair Removal 337
Melanie C. Grossman, MD

Discussion Part Thirteen 341
Jeffrey S. Dover, MD, FRCPC, Moderator

Index 347

CONTRIBUTORS

Robert M. Adrian, MD
Clinical Associate Professor, Georgetown University School of Medicine,
    Washington, DC
Director, Center for Laser Surgery, Washington, DC

R. Rox Anderson, MD
Associate Professor of Dermatology, Harvard Medical School and Massachusetts
    General Hospital, Boston, Mass
Wellman Laboratories of Photomedicine, Boston, Mass

Kenneth A. Arndt, MD
SkinCare Physicians of Chestnut Hill, Chestnut Hill, Mass
Clinical Professor of Dermatology, Section of Dermatologic Surgery and
    Oncology, Department of Dermatology, Yale University School of Medicine,
    New Haven, Conn
Adjunct Professor of Medicine (Dermatology), Dartmouth Medical School,
    Hanover, NH
Clinical Professor of Dermatology, Harvard Medical School, Boston, Mass

Eliot F. Battle, Jr, MD
Instructor in Dermatology, Harvard Medical School and Massachusetts General
    Hospital, Boston, Mass
Wellman Laboratories of Photomedicine, Boston, Mass

Brian S. Biesman, MD
Associate Clinical Professor of Ophthalmology, University of Tennessee Health
    Sciences Center, Nashville, Tenn

Peter Bjerring, MD, PhD
Professor of Dermatology, Manselisborg Hospital, Aarhus, Denmark

Pablo Boixeda, MD
Professor of Dermatology, University of Alcal<, Laser Unit, Hospital Ram\n y
    Cajal, Madrid, Spain

A. Jay Burns, MD
Assistant Professor and Laser Medical Director, University of Texas Southwestern
    Medical School, Dallas, Tex

Christine C. Dierickx, MD
Visiting Scientist, Harvard Medical School, Boston, Mass
Consultant, Department of Dermatology, University Hospital Ghent, Ghent,
    Belgium
Director, Laser Clinic, Boom, Belgium

Jeffrey S. Dover, MD, FRCPC
SkinCare Physicians of Chestnut Hill, Chestnut Hill, Mass
Associate Clinical Professor of Dermatology, Section of Dermatologic Surgery
   and Oncology, Department of Dermatology, Yale University School of
   Medicine, New Haven, Conn
Adjunct Professor of Medicine (Dermatology), Dartmouth Medical School,
   Hanover, NH

Richard E. Fitzpatrick, MD
Dermatology Associates of San Diego County Inc, San Diego, Calif
Associate Clinical Professor, Division of Dermatology, University of California,
   San Diego

Jerome M. Garden, MD
Associate Professor of Clinical Dermatology and Biomedical Engineering,
   Northwestern University Medical School, Chicago, Ill

Roy Geronemus, MD
Director, Laser & Skin Surgery Center of New York, New York, NY
Clinical Professor of Dermatology, New York University Medical Center, New
   York, NY

David J. Goldberg, MD
Director, Skin Laser & Surgery Specialists of New York and New Jersey,
   Westwood, NJ
Clinical Professor and Director of Laser Research, Mt Sinai School of Medicine,
   New York, NY

Mitchel P. Goldman, MD
Associate Clinical Professor of Dermatology, University of California, San Diego
Medical Director, Laser & Skin Surgery Center of La Jolla, La Jolla, Calif

Melanie C. Grossman, MD
Associate in Clinical Dermatology, Department of Dermatology, Columbia
   University, New York, NY

George J. Hruza, MD
Clinical Associate Professor of Dermatology and Otolaryngology/Head and Neck
   Surgery, St Louis University, St Louis, Mo
Laser & Dermatologic Surgery Center, St Louis, Mo

Michael S. Kaminer, MD
SkinCare Physicians of Chestnut Hill, Chestnut Hill, Mass
Assistant Clinical Professor of Dermatology, Section of Dermatologic Surgery and
   Oncology, Department of Dermatology, Yale University School of Medicine,
   New Haven, Conn.
Adjunct Assistant Professor of Medicine (Dermatology), Dartmouth Medical
   School, Hanover, NH

Roland Kaufmann, MD
Professor and Chair, Department of Dermatology, J. W. Goethe University,
   Frankfurt am Main, Germany

Arielle N. B. Kauvar, MD
Laser & Skin Surgery Center of New York, New York, NY
Clinical Associate Professor of Dermatology, New York University School of
    Medicine, New York, NY

Suzanne L. Kilmer, MD
Laser & Skin Surgery Center of Northern California, Sacramento, Calif

J. Stuart Nelson, MD, PhD
Professor of Surgery and Biomedical Engineering, Beckman Laser Institute and
    Medical Clinic, University of California-Irvine

Mark S. Nestor, MD, PhD
Center for Cosmetic Enhancement, Aventura, Fla
University of Miami School of Medicine, Miami, Fla

Christian Raulin, MD
Laserklinik Karlsruhe, Karlsruhe, Germany

Thomas E. Rohrer, MD
SkinCare Physicians of Chestnut Hill, Chestnut Hill, Mass
Associate Professor of Dermatology and Surgery, Boston University Medical
    Center, Boston, Mass

E. Victor Ross, Jr, MD
Residency Medical Director, Naval Medical Center, San Diego, Calif
Assistant Clinical Professor of Dermatology, University of California-San Diego

Javier Ruiz-Esparza, MD
Associate Clinical Professor of Dermatology, University of California-San Diego

Whitney D. Tope, MPhil, MD
Associate Professor of Dermatology, University of Minnesota, Minneapolis, Minn

Milton Waner, MD
Arkansas Children's Hospital, Little Rock, Ark

Robert A. Weiss, MD
Assistant Professor of Dermatology, Johns Hopkins University School of
    Medicine, Baltimore, Md
Director, Maryland Laser, Skin and Vein Institute, Baltimore, Md

Christopher B. Zachary, MBBS, FRCP
Clinical Professor of Dermatology, University of California-San Francisco

Brian D. Zelickson, MD
Assistant Professor of Dermatology, University of Minnesota, Minneapolis
Director, The Abbott Northwestern Cutaneous Laser Center, Minneapolis, Minn

PREFACE

The concept for the Controversies and Conversations in Cutaneous Laser Surgery symposium originated with Milton Waner, MD. Dr Waner assembled a group of physicians to talk objectively about cutaneous laser surgery and to present claims and counterclaims and pros and cons in a totally candid, if not provocative, manner. This symposium continues with the same philosophy that Dr Waner initially espoused. It is not designed to be a course. It is a discussion among colleagues—some from the podium, some from the audience—about what is going on in the field of cutaneous laser surgery. We encourage controversy, conversation, opinions, and arguments that are put forth in kind terms.

In addition, we invite representatives of the medical laser industry to participate fully, not just in the exhibit hall but also during the discussions. There is an enormous amount of talent in that group. Many of the ideas discussed at this conference will lead to an enhancement of existing lasers and development of new systems to meet yet unanswered needs.

This past year more people from the laser industry attended than ever before, and we had the largest number of participants this annual meeting has drawn. The popularity of the meeting speaks to the fact that there is a lot going on in this field that is interesting and exciting. We are very pleased that participants come from all over the world.

This is our favorite medical meeting of the year, because we learn a great deal and find it more intellectually stimulating every year. At the 2001 symposium, we discussed the newest information in laser resurfacing, photorejuvenation, treatment of vascular anomalies and leg veins, laser compared with the scalpel and diamond knife, skin cooling, lasers as diagnostic tools, and treatment of psoriasis and scars. Also included were discussions of the removal of tattoos, dermal pigment, and hair by lasers and light sources as well as novel approaches to skin rejuvenation.

The format of the meeting is a series of short discussions on a topic by several speakers, followed by 15 to 20 minutes for open discussion among everyone in attendance. We serve as directors of the symposium and moderators of the panel discussions. R. Rox Anderson, MD, is the associate director. Without him, much of what goes on at the symposium and in the field of cutaneous laser surgery would not happen. Dr Anderson also moderated the panel discussions.

This is the first year that the conference proceedings are being published. We are excited that the AMA Press agreed to publish the entire proceedings so that a wider audience can benefit from the knowledge and opinions voiced at the symposium.

Finally, we want to thank the participants and the presenters of this symposium, without whom there would have been no discussion.

Kenneth A. Arndt, MD
Jeffrey S. Dover, MD, FRCPC

Will Laser Skin Resurfacing Ever Return to Its Glory Days?

Carbon Dioxide vs Erbium:YAG Laser in Laser Skin Resurfacing

Christopher B. Zachary, MBBS, FRCP

I believe that interest in laser skin resurfacing has peaked, and its use has now flattened out to a more reasonable level, similar to what happened with dermabrasion and chemical peel. Despite this change, standard laser resurfacing has its place in the armamentarium of skin rejuvenation techniques. It has several benefits. Tissue tightening and debulking can be achieved with laser resurfacing, as can improvements in elastosis, photodamage, and effects of natural aging.

The purpose of this presentation is to compare the carbon dioxide (CO_2) and erbium (Er):YAG lasers for use in skin resurfacing in terms of results, postoperative complications, and safety. During this presentation, I will make 4 statements, and I want to survey whether symposium attendees agree with these statements.

COMPARISON OF CLINICAL OUTCOMES

The first statement is: *There is no difference in results between the CO_2 laser and the Er:YAG laser; it's all a question of technical expertise, good judgment, and luck.* Who agrees with that statement? Who disagrees? There is a good amount of disagreement—I like that.

Common thought is that the CO_2 laser is more effective for skin resurfacing and better able to cause tissue tightening than is the Er:YAG laser. However, it is also considered that the Er:YAG laser causes permanent hypopigmentation less often than does the CO_2. Both laser systems can be associated with slow healing, persistent redness, scarring, and other complications. Sequential use of the CO_2 followed by the Er:YAG laser may reduce certain complications and speed healing by reducing thermal injury. When I refer to Er:YAG, I am talking about "hot" Er:YAG lasers, not about the "cold," or early, Er:YAG lasers. There are 3 hot Er:YAG lasers in use today: Derma K (Lumenis, Santa Clara, Calif), CO_3 laser (Cynosure, Chelmsford, Mass), and Contour (Sciton Inc, Palo Alto, Calif).

Let's further compare the results of the new modulated or "hot" Er:YAG lasers with the CO_2 lasers.

In my opinion, the Cadillac of CO_2 lasers is the UltraPulse CO_2 laser (Lumenis), although any of the other high-energy short-pulsed CO_2 can be used to achieve similar results. With this device, one can regularly expect a number of benefits, including reduced photodamage and variable tissue tightening, depending on the parameters used. These changes would be visualized as a diminution of solar keratoses, lentigines, and telangiectases, associated with tissue contraction and a reduction in fine, medium, and coarse rhytids. One could often rejuvenate the face by anywhere from 2 to 10 years in appearance, depending on the aggressiveness of the laser resurfacing procedure, and the degree of photodamage and natural aging before the procedure.

Today CO_2 laser resurfacing tends toward a less aggressive approach, where the expectations are less, but so, too, are the potential complications. One of the main problems with CO_2 laser resurfacing pertained to the high likelihood of delayed-onset permanent hypopigmentation. This phenomenon is probably related to the degree of residual thermal damage and depth of vaporization.

My experience with the Er:YAG resurfacing lasers is that permanent hypopigmentation is much less common, occurring in approximately 5% of patients postoperatively compared with about 20% after CO_2 resurfacing. This is one of the main reasons to change from the CO_2 to the Er:YAG for laser rejuvenation of photodamaged and aging skin. Clearly, superficial lentigines, keratoses, and superficial telangiectases can be effectively removed with the Er:YAG laser. The real question here is, Can one achieve equivalent tightening with the Er:YAG laser as compared with the CO_2? In my experience, excellent tightening can be achieved with the new modulated or "hot" Er:YAG lasers. Remember that patients will see continued tightening for up to a year after laser resurfacing and that the early changes should be interpreted cautiously.

The second statement in my instant survey is: *Persistent redness is beneficial and likely to result in increased tightening of the skin.* Agree or disagree? Those who disagree with this statement appear to be in the majority.

Patients hate erythema. However, my opinion is "no redness, no result." Persistent redness is likely to allow more time for collagen deposition and wound remodeling. At 2 months, a patient treated with the Er:YAG laser (Sciton Contour) had good results, but her skin was still quite red (Fig 1-1).[1] Her photograph at 6 months indicates an excellent result, with good tissue tightening and little residual redness. Those patients who have no residual erythema at 1 month are less likely to have the same benefit.

In my discussion above, I am, of course, speaking about the erythema that is confluent, flat, and waning. Any patients with angulated or linear redness with associated skin thickening has incipient scarring and should be treated aggressively with the pulsed dye laser, steroids, and possibly intralesional 5-fluorouracil injections.

The third statement in my survey is: *Permanent hypopigmentation after laser skin resurfacing is mainly a problem in patients with skin types I and II.* Who would agree with that? Who would disagree? Everyone disagrees!

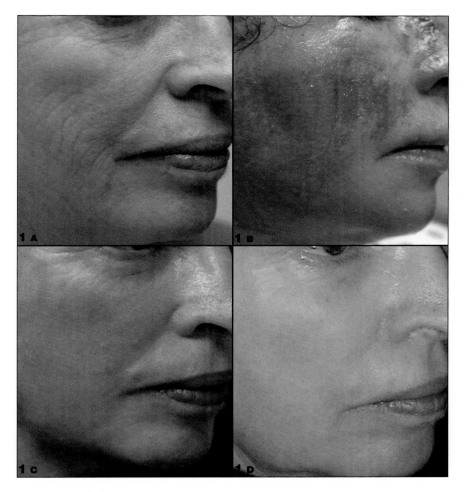

FIGURE 1.1

1A, Moderate photodamage and aging changes with significant rhytid formation before laser skin resurfacing. 1B, Immedite post erbium YAG. 1C, Two months after erbium:YAG laser resurfacing, there is good skin tightening, but erythema remains. 1D, Two years after erbium:YAG laser resurfacing, erythema has resolved, with good results. Reprinted from Zachary and Greken[1] with permission from LaserNews.net, a subsidiary of MDWeb News, Inc., San Francisco, Calif.

Well, you are all wrong! This statement is absolutely true. I have never seen delayed-onset permanent hypopigmentation in darker skin types, and I have treated many Hispanic, Asian, and African-American patients. As a rule, dark-skinned patients typically have good results from laser skin resurfacing and, apart from the inevitable transient postoperative hyperpigmentation, have very little permanent hyperpigmentation or hypopigmentation.

Another question here relates to the need to perform full-face laser abrasions in patients with skin types IV and higher. Anatomical boundaries in this group are often meaningless because of the absence of actinic bronzing in these racial groups. A white person with actinic bronzing will be left with a definite "tide mark" after laser resurfacing. The same is not true in patients with skin type IV or higher. Furthermore, these racial groups generally present for treatment of acne scarring of the central cheeks and do not require full-face resurfacing. I still perform careful feathering of the borders in these cases.

The forth statement in my survey is: *Rejuvenation of the neck may be performed safely with laser skin resurfacing.* Who agrees? Who disagrees?

There is a lot of hedging here. Most of those with an opinion disagree. That is probably the wise response in this case. Clearly, the neck can be resurfaced using either the CO_2 or the Er:YAG laser, but anything more than the lightest approach might result in an unsatisfactory outcome. Drs Suzanne Kilmer and Richard Fitzpatrick will show in Chapters 3 and 4 that rejuvenation of the neck can be performed safely, but only with great care. Dr Kilmer copiously applies a eutectic mixture of lidocaine and prilocaine (EMLA) several hours before surgery. The effect is to produce a protective superhydration of the epidermis, which limits the heat applied to the superficial dermis. Dr Fitzpatrick is careful to remove only a partial thickness of epidermis, again protecting the superficial dermis from excessive heat.

Every laser surgeon has a preference as to whether the CO_2 or Er:YAG laser is better for skin resurfacing. In actuality, most laser systems produce good results when used appropriately. Laser surgery creates a degree of tissue contraction not possible with dermabrasion. Consequently, laser resurfacing will continue to be used as a tool to modify the shape, texture, and appearance of the skin.

REFERENCE

1. Zachary CB, Greken RC. Dual mode Er:YAG laser systems for skin resurfacing [News & Views]. LaserNews.net. January 2000;1(1):1. Available from: http://www.lasernews.net.

The Quest for Reliable Results After Laser Resurfacing

Javier Ruiz-Esparza, MD

Years ago, Sigmund Freud asked himself the question, "What does a woman want?" Like Freud, I don't know that we can answer this question. However, we can easily guess at what women do not want. They do not want to look like a burn victim. Women, and men for that matter, do not want to look like that even for a short time. They wonder if they will ever look normal again. These days, patients' expectations have changed. Patients want minimally invasive procedures with minimal risk, and they want no pain and no downtime. They would prefer, if at all possible, that none of their friends know they had cosmetic surgery.

Expectations also were high at the time that lasers were introduced as skin resurfacing tools. The notion of a high-tech device capable of producing great results time after time resulted partly from seeing "lasers" at work in the *Star Wars* movie series. For the general public, expectations of laser skin resurfacing did not match reality. Laser resurfacing fell from its pedestal for one reason; it failed to deliver its implicit advantage over older resurfacing methods: predictable results.

UNMET EXPECTATIONS

What went wrong with laser resurfacing? Plenty. Postoperative complications, poor training of many of the physicians who were performing it, overaggressive use of resurfacing lasers, lack of standardization of postoperative care, and media coverage of horror stories in which patients had bad outcomes. Too many prospective patients knew somebody who had laser resurfacing and whose skin was red for months. In the eyes of the public, the long, unpredictable healing period after aggressive laser resurfacing was the worst enemy of this procedure.

IMPROVEMENTS

Most laser surgeons, however, still believe that resurfacing is a great procedure to rejuvenate skin. It can be safe and rewarding, when performed by capable, experienced surgeons. Patients need to know this. Laser surgeons must inform them. We have to reinvent our approach to laser resurfacing, and we must also let other physicians know that we can make this a kinder, gentler procedure. We must adapt to the times and give our patients what they want. We need to be able to show our patients that they are going to look a certain way on postoperative days 1, 2, 3, 4, 5, and 6, every time.

How can we make resurfacing less invasive and its results more predictable? In my opinion, the carbon dioxide (CO_2) laser produces fine results as long as the surgeon does a single pass, with no wiping and no irritants used before or after resurfacing.

THREE-STAGE RESURFACING

In my practice, we do erbium:YAG fractionate resurfacing in 3 stages, one pass each time, and delivering anywhere from 2 to 24 J/cm^2 each time. This is a 10-minute procedure, so it takes less of the surgeon's time and there is less cost to the patient. It can be performed every month for 3 consecutive months, with good results and less risk. There is a rapid recovery, usually several days. Patients can have the procedure on Thursday and go back to work on Monday. They do not have to wait 3 or 4 months to look better. In a week they look better. They look like themselves, not as if they had been operated on. When the procedure is repeated, patients continue to improve in appearance. Even immediately after the procedure, patients do not have severe erythema. For any type of skin, I would recommend skin resurfacing performed in 3 sessions with the scanning erbium:YAG laser, applied in a single pass with at least 2 J/cm^2, and with no manipulation of the tissue or wiping.

Will laser skin resurfacing ever return to its glory days? It will, when we have successfully shown our patients that it can, in fact, deliver predictable results.

chapter 3

Ideal Tissue Effects of Laser Resurfacing

Richard E. Fitzpatrick, MD

Will laser skin resurfacing ever return to its glory days? It will never return to the glory days it once had, because there will never be the hype surrounding it that there was previously. However, I think that laser resurfacing is a necessary procedure if skin rejuvenation is desired. Many of the people who are getting superficial facial rejuvenation procedures or nonablative laser resurfacing will, I believe, want to have ablative resurfacing in the future.

Nevertheless, laser resurfacing has its problems. In considering what's wrong with the procedure, I ask: Do we need a better laser?

IDEAL TISSUE EFFECTS OF RESURFACING

There are several different ways of looking at the ideal tissue effects of resurfacing. First, I think that ablation of 50 to 100 mm of tissue per pass is perfect. Thermal necrosis of approximately 50 mm is nearly ideal, because that will seal off the capillaries. In studies of tissue tightening, my coworkers and I found that delivery of approximately 7 J/cm^2 of laser energy achieves excellent collagen contraction.[1] In addition, I think that having soft edges to the laser beam where the collagen distribution is located is far easier to work with than is a flat-top beam. It greatly minimizes the risk of making holes in tissue. Also, the ability to separate ablation and coagulation features is ideal. Therefore, we actually have lasers that have all these capabilities.

If we have an ideal laser, why don't we have an ideal resurfacing procedure? The reason is the procedure itself. There are intrinsic problems that occur with ablation of the skin. First, there is always a contrast between untreated, sun-damaged skin and laser-treated skin. Somewhere, whether in the middle of the face, on the neck, or on the chest, that contrast is going to be present, and that is not something you can change. It is part of the procedure itself.

ADVERSE REACTIONS

The second problem with laser resurfacing is that, as with any ablative procedure, there is the potential of wound healing complications. These complications include hyperpigmentation, prolonged erythema, acne, hypopigmentation, and scarring. Is there some way to decrease the risk of any of these complications? Hyperpigmentation is either postinflammatory, which is related to the preexisting level of natural pigmentation, or it is related to melasma or is sun-induced. Clearly, the only prevention of sun-induced hyperpigmentation is for patients to avoid sun exposure.

Regarding prolonged erythema, I agree with Dr Christopher Zachary that erythema reflects wound healing and new collagen formation (Chapter 1). However, when erythema lasts too long, usually it is either related to the depth of resurfacing or due to excessive thermal injury or postoperative complications such as infection or allergic contact dermatitis. Thus, factors leading to erythema can be controlled to some extent.

Acne and milia commonly occur in patients who have a past history of acne, but they also seem to be partly related to thermal effects. Physicians usually attribute these problems to occlusive therapy, but I do not believe that occlusive therapy is a major factor. I think the cause is more likely some intrinsic factors and disruption of the sebaceous gland as well as some thermal effects. Thus, there may be things that can be done to prevent the postoperative occurrence of acne and milia, by controlling acne with antibiotics and by controlling the amount of heat delivered to tissue.

Hypopigmentation occurs because of replacement of the photodamaged skin with skin that is not photodamaged. There may be an inability of severely photodamaged skin to repigment adequately, and this occurs primarily in skin types I and II. I also agree with Dr Zachary that I never see hypopigmentation in skin types IV and V and very rarely, if ever, in type III. However, true hypopigmentation also can result when resurfacing is too deep, and there is a lot about this phenomenon that we do not understand. It appears that inactive melanocytes are present but are not functioning properly. This has been found to be the case when biopsies of hypopigmented areas have been performed. There is a problem in transferring pigment to the epidermis.

Scarring is related to poor technique or secondary effects that extend the wound deeper than intended, such as infection or allergic or irritant contact dermatitis, or there may be abnormal intrinsic factors.

In summary, the most common adverse effects of resurfacing have varied causes; some cases are related to depth of the procedure, some are thermally induced, some are related to intrinsic factors, and some occur postoperatively. Thus, to improve results, we need to control the overall depth of tissue destruction, the heat delivered to tissue, and the type of care provided in the postoperative phase. The potential use of growth factors and antioxidants, I think, can really change the postoperative phase by enhancing wound healing and decreasing postoperative complications. Intraoperatively, the safest skin rejuvenation procedure would be to leave the epidermal debris intact. Once the epidermal debris is removed—whether you do 1, 3, or 10 passes—the potential exists for wound healing problems. I do not think that a single pass with removal of the epidermal debris is any safer than 10 passes. Finally, I recommend avoiding unintended injuries by the following: avoid pulse stacking, consider decreasing fluence on the second or third pass, leave epidermal debris from a single pass intact at the periphery of the face, and avoid resurfacing too deeply when using the erbium:YAG laser as a sculpting, ablative modality in conjunction with the carbon dioxide (CO_2) laser.

REFERENCE

1. Fitzpatrick RE, Rostan EF, Munchell N. Collagen tightening induced by carbon dioxide laser versus erbium:YAG laser. *Lasers Surg Med.* 2000;27:395–403.

chapter 4

Efficacy of Laser Skin Resurfacing

Suzanne L. Kilmer, MD

My answer to the question of whether laser skin resurfacing will ever return to its glory days is that it never left them. At my facility, we are performing more laser resurfacing procedures than ever. Each week we perform an average of 9 resurfacing procedures, and I do most of them. The number of these procedures that we perform is increasing each year. Why? Because resurfacing rules.

EFFICACY

There is no question in my mind that laser resurfacing has the best efficacy among the skin rejuvenation procedures, especially for improving wrinkles and acne scars. Other than in patients who have skin sagging and need a face-lift, laser skin resurfacing will rejuvenate the skin much better than either chemical peels or nonablative lasers. With resurfacing, the solar-induced epidermal damage, including lentigines, seborrheic keratoses, and actinic keratoses, are removed in one fell swoop, in a single treatment. It also smoothes fine wrinkles, sebaceous hyperplasia, nevi, and other growths. In addition, the risk of side effects is low.

Laser resurfacing offers far better improvement in epidermal changes than do nonablative procedures. When I talk to patients about whether they should have laser resurfacing vs nonablative treatment, I tell them that with laser resurfacing they likely will have an improvement in their epidermal changes of 50% to 60%, maybe even 70%, depending on the extent of the epidermal changes. With nonablative treatment, the best improvement they are probably going to have, after 3 to 6 treatments, is 25% to 35%. Laser resurfacing offers immediate, substantial improvement. The tissue tightening is visible by the end of 1 week, as opposed to 6 months with the nonablative procedures. In addition, similar to nonablative procedures, the skin tightening is still evident 6 months after resurfacing.

For resurfacing, I use a carbon dioxide (CO_2) laser (UltraPulse 5000C, Lumenis, Santa Clara, Calif). I participated in the original clinical trials conducted by the manufacturer years ago. Many of my patients who underwent resurfacing of facial skin had numerous actinic keratoses and a history of basal cell carcinoma. I still follow up most of those patients, and they hardly ever have facial lesions requiring cryotherapy, but the non–laser-treated skin on the rest of their body frequently has lesions that must be removed. Laser skin resurfacing can reliably remove all the solar-induced damage. In addition, it can eliminate fine wrinkling and smooth out other epidermal and some dermal changes. Even some fine vessels are improved after resurfacing.

Patients who undergo multiple nonablative procedures have increased cost, and although they have no downtime, they probably spend more time in the physician's office. Whereas nonablative laser surgery requires multiple procedures, laser resurfacing has substantial benefits with a single procedure for most patients. For some patients with severe scars or deeper wrinkles, I may perform a second (or even a third) treatment 6 or more months after the procedure.

SIDE EFFECTS

The side effect profile of laser resurfacing need not be as poor as has been reported. Of the approximately 2000 resurfacing procedures that my associates and I have performed, only 9 patients experienced hypopigmentation, an incidence of less than 0.5%. Eight of the 9 patients have skin types I and II, and 1 patient has type III. I have performed resurfacing in many patients with skin type IV or higher, and I have never observed hypopigmentation in any of them.

Hyperpigmentation can be a problem after resurfacing. However, it is not as severe with use of zinc oxide sunscreen. I think that intraoperative hydration also decreases the amount of hyperpigmentation, probably because it helps mediate the thermal effect.

Reepithelialization is complete 6 to 7 days after laser resurfacing. Almost all of my female patients who undergo resurfacing are able to wear makeup at 1 week postoperatively.

Figures 4-1 and 4-2 demonstrate the effects of hydration with laser resurfacing using the CO_2 laser (UltraPulse). Each patient had 3 fairly deep passes with the CO_2 laser. In Figure 4-1, a nevus is seen in the middle of the patient's forehead (left); postoperatively it was removed. In another patient, vessels that were seen preoperatively improved months after resurfacing (Fig 4-2). A moderate amount of skin tightening can be observed after laser resurfacing (Fig 4-3).

Sometimes I use the erbium:YAG laser after CO_2 laser resurfacing in an attempt to further smooth out some of the deeper lines and acne scars. Also, I now perform subcutaneous incisionless (Subcision) surgery,[1] to help lift up the acne scars.

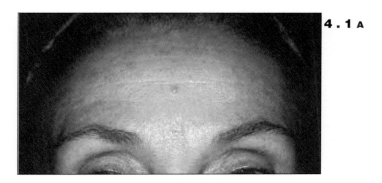

4.1A

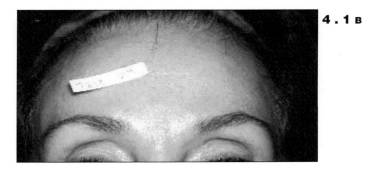

4.1B

FIGURE 4.1

Preoperatively, a nevus is seen in the middle of the patient's forehead (4.1a); postoperatively, it was removed (4.1b).

HYDRATION

Before laser resurfacing, I hydrate all patients with a eutectic mixture of lidocaine and prilocaine (EMLA Cream), which also serves as an anesthetic.[2] By leaving the cream on the skin for more than an hour, we achieve hydration of both the epidermis and the upper dermis. Hydration alters the effects of CO_2 laser-induced thermal damage and, in our opinion, increases the safety of resurfacing.

The neck skin can be resurfaced, but hydration must be used. Wiping cannot be done on the neck. In Fig 4-4, the patient had smoothing out of the skin

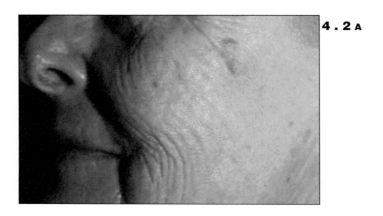

4.2A

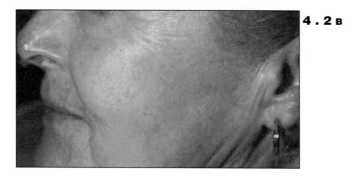

4.2B

FIGURE 4.2

Vessels seen preoperatively (4.2a) improved months after resurfacing (4.2b).

crinkling and improvement in some of the pigmentary changes. This patient had single-pass CO_2 laser treatment of the neck, with no wiping, and a density of 6 at the jaw line, gradually decreasing to a density of 1 further down the neck.

The histologic findings from this patient show single-pass resurfacing with no wiping, with and without EMLA Cream (Fig 4-5). With the use of EMLA Cream, there was much less thermal damage, with a thinner zone of thermal necrosis at the surface and a splotchier zone of thermal damage underneath. I think that the areas with less thermal damage to dermal collagen permit better and faster dermal regeneration and reepithelialization.

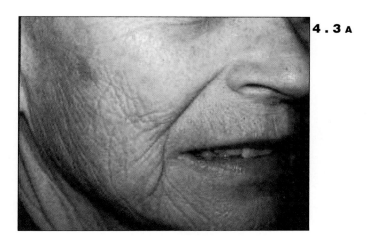

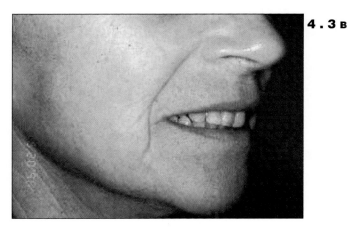

FIGURE 4.3

Before laser resurfacing (4.3a); skin tightening after laser resurfacing (4.3b).

In summary, laser skin resurfacing can be very safe. It is, in my opinion, made safer and more tolerable using hydration with EMLA Cream.

REFERENCES

1. Orentreich DS, Orentreich N. Subcutaneous incisionless (Subcision) surgery for the correction of depressed scars and wrinkles. *Dermatol Surg.* 1995;21:543–549.
2. Kilmer SL, Chotzen V, Calkin J, Silva S, McClaren M. Full face laser resurfacing utilizing topical anesthesia alone [abstract]. *Lasers Surg Med.* 1999(suppl 11):30.

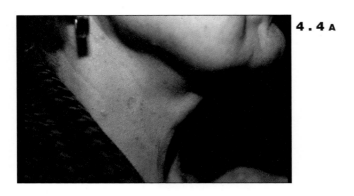

4.4A

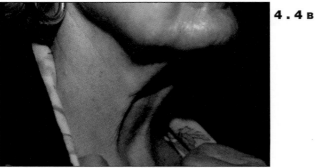

4.4B

FIGURE 4.4

Before treatment (4.4a); after treatment the patient had smoothing out of skin crinkling and pigmentary change improvement (4.4b).

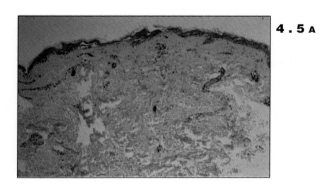

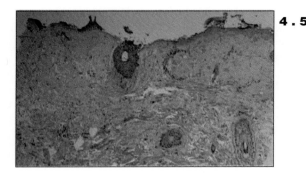

FIGURE 4.5

With use of EMLA cream (4.5a); without use of EMLA cream (4.5b).

PART ONE DISCUSSION

Jeffrey S. Dover, MD, FRCPC, *Moderator*

David J. Goldberg, MD: There are probably very few people here who would argue about the benefits of ablative laser skin resurfacing. I think the press has done an enormous disservice to ablative laser resurfacing, and I would like to hear other people's thoughts about that.

Roy Geronemus, MD: I just had a couple of comments for Dr Christopher Zachary regarding his presentation. I think that persistent skin redness is usually predictive of depigmentation that will occur over the long term. I agree with Dr Richard Fitzpatrick that redness is often related to depth of thermal injury. I think persistent redness is not necessarily good, although it may suggest that the patient will have a better result in terms of removal of lines and improvement of skin tone. Over the long term, however, I think one will see loss of pigmentation in increased incidence.

The other concern I had about your presentation, Dr Zachary, was when you showed the regional resurfacing in a patient with dark skin. I think you should have shown a long-term follow-up of at least 6 to 12 months in this case. In my experience, one is more likely to see changes in pigmentation at that time period rather than early in the postoperative period, when pigmentary changes are not likely.

Christopher B. Zachary, MBBS, FRCP: Are you talking about *hyper*pigmentation or *hypo*pigmentation?

Dr Geronemus: Hypopigmentation. I am not worried about hyperpigmentation, as that fades.

Dr Zachary: I totally disagree with you. I think the problems of hypopigmentation in Asians or darker skin types are going to occur early in the postoperative period. If they occur, it is because the laser surgeon has been too aggressive and has induced scarring. Regarding your question about persistent redness, what is your definition of persistent redness? Do you mean redness that persists at 1 month or 3, 6, or 10 months?

Dr Geronemus: Three months and beyond.

I would like to return to the question of this panel discussion as to why laser skin resurfacing is no longer widely accepted. I think the challenge is on us, the physicians who teach other physicians and nonphysicians to use lasers and the manufacturers who promote these devices to people who are not necessarily qualified to do the procedures. In my state, many of the complications I have seen have occurred in the hands of professionals who had inadequate training. They did not understand the laser technology or proper postoperative wound care. It is the problems resulting from this lack of knowledge that the media publicized, so I do not think the press was wrong. Experienced physicians who frequently perform resurfacing do not see many complications from this procedure. I think there is a degree of legitimacy to this issue of safety, but we have to look at what our responsibility is, and not just in resurfacing. These issues go far beyond resurfacing. We must be very careful about who we are teaching and who has accessibility to lasers. If we do not, we are going to have problems over the long term, not only with resurfacing lasers but also with nonablative laser techniques.

Dr Dover: Before we continue, let me ask for a show of hands of how many of you who perform laser skin resurfacing have seen a decrease in the last 5 years in the number of cases you do annually? How many have seen no decrease in the number of cases you have done in the last 5 years? So, about 4 or 5 physicians have seen no decrease or maybe an increase in resurfacing cases, and about 70 people have seen a decrease. In my practice, we have seen a decrease. I think the declining popularity of this procedure is a tremendous disadvantage to patients because, as Dr Suzanne Kilmer said in her presentation, laser resurfacing rules. The results with resurfacing done properly are much better than what can be achieved with nonablative techniques. Although the 2 techniques cannot be compared with each other, because 1 targets primarily epidermis and the other targets dermis, some products are approved based on comparisons between photorejuvenation and laser skin resurfacing. We have a lot of patients who are excellent candidates for laser skin resurfacing but do not have the procedure because they are frightened by the negative comments of their friends or what they saw on television. It seems that the weekly television news magazine shows air the same bad stories about resurfacing complications over and over again, because they apparently get high ratings when they run those pieces.

Richard E. Fitzpatrick, MD: I want to comment on what was just said. I think it is important to teach not only the proper ways of performing the laser procedure but also wound care. Anyone performing ablative resurfacing really has to be an expert in wound healing, and that is one component that is often missing in the training.

I want to raise another point. I hear of a number of legal cases that are based on problems with resurfacing in patients receiving isotretinoin (Accutane). Supposedly, isotretinoin decreases fibroblast production of collagenase and therefore may cause excessive collagen buildup. However, studies done in animals showed no difference in wound healing between those receiving isotretinoin and those that did not receive the drug. In the literature, there also are 50 cases of patients who have been treated with resurfacing either while they were still receiving isotretinoin therapy or within 6 months of taking the drug and who healed totally normally. We do not even know what the incidence of abnormal wound healing is, yet the literature recommends no laser therapy for patients within 6 months to 2 years of treatment with isotretinoin. Do people here think that isotretinoin use is a problem in patients undergoing laser resurfacing, or is this just hype?

Kenneth A. Arndt, MD: Let me make 2 comments. First, I think a lot of people are responding to resurfacing as it once was. The way resurfacing is done now, with different dressings, somewhat different techniques, and often 2 different lasers used, it is quite a different procedure. Patients have 7 to 10 days of mild erythema, compared with several months when laser resurfacing was in its infancy. I think that the perception of healing after resurfacing has not caught up to the reality. The reality is that laser resurfacing is a much more benign procedure than it once was, and although fewer physicians are performing it, in general, they are more skilled.

Second, I was on a panel last weekend with Dr James Leyden, who also commented on the fallacy of isotretinoin being a contraindication for laser resurfacing. He strongly believes that use of this drug has been overemphasized as a cause of adverse events after surgical procedures.

Jerome M. Garden, MD: On another topic, I was a bit concerned about the message that may be perceived regarding resurfacing darkly pigmented patients. We know that darkly pigmented patients do have hypopigmentation problems, and I cannot believe that the resurfacing procedure somehow magically stops hypopigmentation in these patients. It may be that the patients who have skin type I or II are indeed more susceptible to hypopigmentation. Maybe there is a greater deposition of melanocytes in the higher skin types, and perhaps that somehow protects them from hypopigmentation. However, I have a patient, a Latino woman in her late 20s, who was referred to me after resurfacing of acne scars. More than 2 years after the procedure, she has permanent hypopigmentation and must wear makeup to cover the pigmentary problem. When I hear a panel of experts say they do not see hypopigmentation in dark-skinned patients, I believe they do not see it because they are experts and not patients. Dark-skinned patients, in my opinion, will have hypopigmentation if their skin receives enough thermal energy.

Javier Ruiz-Esparza, MD: I agree with that. I treat many Hispanic patients, and I have seen 2 patients who have been referred to me for treatment of hypopigmentation.

Henry H. Chan, MD: When we see patients with hypopigmentation, they tend to also have scarring, so the laser procedure was performed using inappropriate parameters. Certainly I have seen cases of hypopigmentation that turned out to be a medicolegal issue. However, I agree that most dark-skinned patients do not have much of a problem with hypopigmentation after resurfacing.

Jo S. Bohannon, MD: What percentage drop in carbon dioxide (CO_2) resurfacing procedures have the practitioners at the major universities seen since the heyday of laser resurfacing, which I think was 1995 to 1997? I am a solo practitioner, with more than 75% of my practice composed of cosmetic procedures. I started performing CO_2 resurfacing procedures in 1995 but have not done a CO_2 resurfacing since 1999 because of negative publicity from the media. Patients are intolerant of the long-term erythema. Despite giving informed consent and receiving follow-up care, if a patient has long-lasting skin redness—perhaps 3 to 6 months—there might be the threat of a personal injury lawsuit. That is why I do not perform laser resurfacing anymore; I don't want the risk of a lawsuit.

Dr Zachary: This litigious society can put practitioners at a real disadvantage. That is why I think it is helpful to have panelists and experts around the country talking about the fact that the problem with isotretinoin is overblown, talking about the fact that persistent redness may actually be beneficial, and so forth. Maybe this group should disseminate some guidelines about laser resurfacing to support those of us who feel somewhat threatened by potential legal action.

Milton Waner, MD: I have a question for Dr Fitzpatrick. Could the hypopigmentation sometimes seen after resurfacing be related to the fact that one is altering the subepidermal layer? Is perhaps a microscopic or histologic scar being caused to a certain extent? One is affecting the collagen layer, so the light reflecting off that surface is altered. In other words, is the melanocyte count or the melanin concentration the same, or is it just the light-tissue reaction?

Dr Fitzpatrick: No, it is clearly melanin. You can see it in different lighting.

Dr Waner: So the concentration of melanin is altered?

Dr Fitzpatrick: Correct.

Dr Waner: Another comment I want to make is that I have often performed resurfacing in children with atrophic scarring resulting from hemangiomas. In fact, nearly every hemangioma that involutes leaves an area of atrophic scarring. In patients with diffuse or segmental hemangiomas—very large lesions—that have ulcerated and who have a tremendous amount of atrophic scarring, I have resurfaced these lesions and obtained some very good results. I know that there are objections to performing resurfacing in young children because of the sebaceous gland activity, but the procedure seems to work. So far we have not had any catastrophes.

Christine C. Dierickx, MD: I have a question for the panel. What is your approach toward patients who have had filler substances placed into wrinkles? I refer not to transient filler substances but to more permanent dermal fillers, such as expanded polytetrafluoroethylene (Gore-Tex). Would you resurface the skin of these patients, and do you think that wound healing will be influenced by those components in the skin?

Dr Fitzpatrick: I have performed resurfacing in such patients without any problem. One must be aware of where the filler is, but as long as the resurfacing is not too deep, the laser treatment is not going to interfere with the filler. I have not seen wound healing problems secondary to resurfacing over dermal fillers.

Dr Dover: Has anybody here ever seen a problem in resurfacing a patient who has had soft-tissue augmentation of the face with either liquid injectable silicone or Gore-Tex?

Dr Geronemus: I resurface over silicone filler quite often. I use resurfacing to remove some of the silicone granulomas that we commonly see, and there are no problems at all. It is actually an excellent treatment.

Dr Fitzpatrick: We have seen a couple of patients who have had silicone granulomas, and they have responded reasonably well to resurfacing.

Whitney D. Tope, MPhil, MD: I agree with the comments that resurfacing as we practice it now is completely different from the days when it began, in the early to mid-1990s. I think that the complications we are seeing are far different as well, in particular, their incidence. The only way to rejuvenate the popularity of laser skin resurfacing is to conduct prospective studies of its complications and publish the results, showing a lower rate of problems. This would especially be effective if the results came from the same groups that already have published about complications of laser resurfacing.

Dr Arndt: We have come a long way since we first started talking about laser skin resurfacing years ago. Questions that we discussed at previous meetings and in other forums included: How do we take care of patients who undergo laser resurfacing? What should we use for treatment before resurfacing: topical tretinoin (Retin-A), a-hydroxy acid, oral antibiotics, or antiviral agents? Do we continue any of these treatments after resurfacing? What kinds of dressings are used? Some of those questions have been resolved, and the preoperative and postoperative approach for resurfacing is quite different than what we employed previously. This new approach, I believe, has made a major difference in the final result that is being obtained with laser resurfacing today.

ADDENDUM

Dr Dover: One of the participants asked whether the panelists who spoke about resurfacing could describe the way they do the procedure. Would some of the panelists tell us your actual technique and the laser you use?

Dr Burns: I use the erbium:YAG from Sciton (Sciton Inc, Palo Alto, Calif) laser. I basically use the first pass with ablation, 100 μm and 25 to 50 μm coagulation. This is a total effective depth of 125 to 150 μm per pass. Therefore, 2 passes reach a total effective depth of 250 to 300 mm. I doubt the actual histologic depth is exactly 250 to 300 μm (as read from the control panel on the machine), but I know, from extensive clinical experience, that it is going to give me an effective result. Then I spot treat with 30 μm of ablation with *no* coagulation at all. At that point, I can evaluate clinical end points. Those end points include wrinkle ablation and dermal bleeding patterns. I get down to a level that I think is fairly safe in the lower papillary dermis and maybe the upper reticular dermis. I spot treat with no ablation at all, so I can observe true bleeding end points. It should be pointed out that I use coagulation on the first 2 phases to minimize bleeding.

Dr Ruiz-Esparza: These days I use mostly erbium:YAG lasers for resurfacing. I perform mostly superficial resurfacing. I resurface the skin of patients with active acne, and I obtain great improvement. I use an inert ointment (Aquaphor Healing Ointment) for only 2 days and no more, and I allow the patient to desquamate, after which I think the acne improves. When a patient with deep acne scarring comes to me for resurfacing, I do not hesitate to do multiple passes, but I am very gentle with the tissue. I do not rub hard when I use the CO_2 laser (UltraPulse), which is seldom now. With the erbium:YAG laser, one can apply 2 to 36 J/cm^2 per pass. I do up to 3 passes on the scarred areas at settings of 24 J/cm^2 and only 1 pass on the areas that are not scarred, just to achieve uniformity of skin tone. I think that the degree of erythema seen after 3 passes with the erbium:YAG laser is minimal, and the patients heal quickly. The reason is that I don't pretreat or post-treat; I just use the laser. Patients of any skin type can be treated. I can even treat regional areas, going very deep, and I don't get any difference in pigmentation in the postoperative follow-up, because I do not challenge the skin pharmacologically. I am very careful not to touch the tissue when doing the procedure.

The anesthesia I use is topical lidocaine without occlusion for 2 hours. Immediately before the procedure, the patient has to wash thoroughly—3 times—with soap and water. That washing is enough to degrease the skin and allow for better penetration and absorption of the anesthetic.

Dr Kilmer: The way I do laser resurfacing with a eutectic mixture of lidocaine and prilocaine (EMLA) is probably a bit different than how others are used to doing it. We ask patients to take a shower before they even come to our office, including hot, soapy soaks on their face to degrease the skin. After they dry off, they immediately apply an entire tube of EMLA and leave it on. They come into the office about 45 minutes before their surgery. At that point, we give them 60 mg of ketorolac tromethamine (Toradol); 10 mg of diazepam (Valium); and 2 narcotic analgesic drugs, such as hydrocodone bitartrate (Vicodin), propoxyphene napsylate-acetaminophen (Darvocet), or oxycodone (Percocet). Then, we apply a second tube of EMLA. As the patients recline in a chair, we apply the EMLA around the eyes and out to the edges of the face, and also on the neck if we are going to

resurface there. At this point, the patients probably have had the EMLA on for almost 2.5 hours. There was a study published about the depth of anesthesia with EMLA that reported it is possible to go 6 mm deep without pain after 2.5 hours, only
4 mm deep after 2 hours, and about 1 mm deep after only 1.5 hours. In any event, we have pretty good pain control. We offer all patients local injections of lidocaine and regional nerve blocks or additional anesthesia that they can have whenever they want. However, the EMLA almost always gives sufficient anesthesia and is especially great for the peripheral areas, which are difficult to block anyway. In a retrospective review, 4 of 100 patients requested additional anesthesia, injections that were already drawn up and on the tray, so they were easy to provide.

After administration of the anesthesia, we perform the laser procedure in quadrants. Typically I start on 1 side of the face, wipe off the cheek and under the eye, and do each of the 3 passes. I use the CO_2 laser (UltraPulse), 300 mJ, 60 W, at a density of 7. The density is increased a little because of the hydration. My second pass is usually at a density of 5. I typically do not do a second pass on the lateral one-third of the cheeks, because I think that is a treacherous area, especially in skin types I and II. I may do a second pass there in someone who has severe acne scarring that is spread out to the lateral cheeks. A third pass (density of 4 to 5) usually is done to the glabellar region, inner canthal areas, and periorbital regions.

I then treat the neck with only one pass. At the jaw line, I decrease the density from setting 6 to 1, one setting at a time, and feather into the surrounding skin. This really helps minimize any line of demarcation using this technique. I get excellent results using this technique. In treatment of the neck, it is important to not wipe on the neck. I stop wiping at the lateral aspect of the cheek in most cases and along the jaw line, because that is also a trouble area. Not wiping helps to blend the treated with the untreated areas. I then use the short-pulse erbium:YAG laser to any residual wrinkles or acne scars.

Robert M. Adrian, MD: I am now a medical expert in a lawsuit involving the case of a 20-year-old man who died of an anaphylactic reaction to tetracaine during a hair removal procedure. I caution everybody who plans to use the EMLA procedure, as Dr Kilmer described, to have defibrillators, oxygen, advanced cardiac life support, and other precautionary devices in the office. The combination of sedatives that Dr Kilmer described is a whopping cocktail. Before physicians try to do this procedure in their office, they should be prepared for an emergency that could arise.

PART 2

Postoperative Care After Laser Resurfacing: What Is the Optimal Approach?

Wound Care and Prophylaxis After Laser Resurfacing

George J. Hruza, MD

WOUND CARE

Most surgeons believe that moist wound care is needed after laser skin resurfacing. There is still some debate, however, on open wound care—whether to use occlusive dressings or nonocclusive dressings. In my practice, we use both types of dressings. We apply bio-occlusive dressings for the first 72 hours. Typically we use a silicone-polytetrafluoroethylene (Silon-TSR) dressing, which has openings in it to allow some drainage, or a Vigilon dressing if a partial-face procedure was performed. It is very important to check the patient at 1 and 3 days postoperatively.

Bio-occlusive dressings used in the first 2 to 3 days have been shown to speed reepithelialization after laser skin resurfacing, so that maximum benefits occur in 48 hours.[1] I think that the initial use of occlusive dressings also dramatically reduces pain. In the past, my patients needed narcotics, but now they almost never use any of their narcotic prescriptions. Bio-occlusive dressings used for relatively short periods clearly do not increase the risk of infection. I avoid opaque dressings, such as Flexzan, because they do not allow a view of how the wound is healing. Also during the first 24 hours, we apply ice packs around the patient's eyes to reduce the amount of swelling.

Figure 5-1 shows a patient before and immediately after laser skin resurfacing with the variable-pulse erbium:YAG (CO_3) laser. That chamois color may occur if the laser resurfacing goes very deep on someone with bad acne scars.

To apply the Silon-TSR dressing shown in Figure 5-2 usually requires 3 people. Optimally, 2 people stretch the dressing on both sides, and then the third person quickly opens up the breathing space, cutting out openings for the mouth and nose as well as the eyes. Otherwise, patients can quickly become claustrophobic during application. Once the dressing is in place, it should be secured as well as possible (Fig 5-3). Often a few areas of the dressing are difficult to secure, but if you can get the dressing the way it is shown in Figure 5-3, that

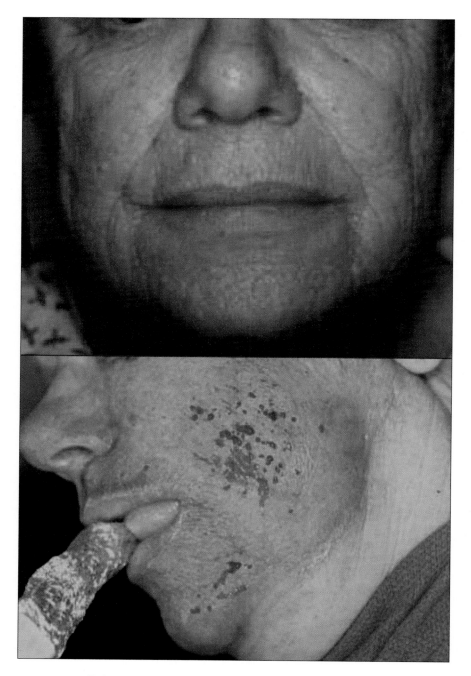

FIGURE 5.1

Patient with rhytids before (top) and immediately after (bottom) variable-pulse erbium:YAG (CO_3) laser resurfacing.

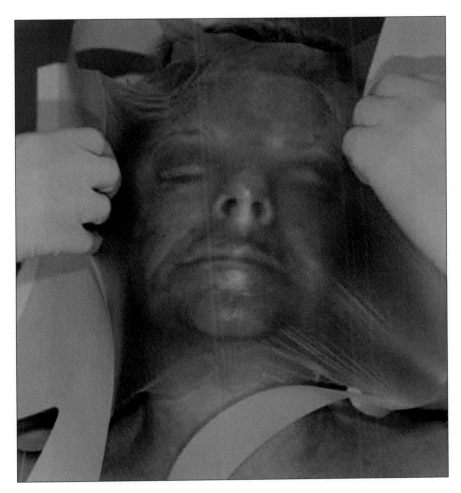

FIGURE   5.2

Silicone-polytetrafluoroethylene (Silon-TSR) dressing being applied.

is good. There is probably a bit more gauze than you need. We do not use as much now; the patient in this figure is one of the first patients in whom we used the Silon-TSR dressing. It is good to have a separate waiting room and exit for patients who must wear these dressings.

The patient in Figure 5-3 is shown 24 hours postoperatively in Figure 5-4. Note the difference in skin color where the dressing stayed in place; it is pink, not the yellow shade seen immediately after surgery. In the areas where the bandage dried out and pulled away from the skin, the skin does not appear as healthy and has begun to form scabs. So in any skin area that is not fully covered, we encourage moist wound healing by having the patient apply an occlusive ointment such as Aquaphor Healing Ointment.

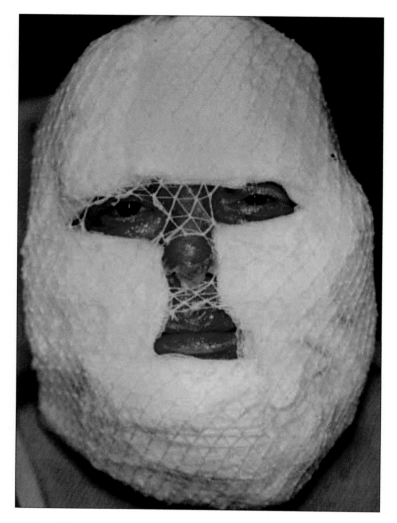

FIGURE 5.3

Silicone-polytetrafluoroethylene (Silon-TSR) dressing covered with absorbent material and secured with flexible netting.

I do not apply occlusive dressings long term because infection or other problems may occur if the same dressing is left on for a long time. After the first 3 postoperative days, I switch to open wound care using 0.25% acetic acid soaks, followed by application of Aquaphor Healing Ointment. This ointment maintains moist wound healing while effectively removing any of the exudate, so it keeps the bacterial count and colonization low. We avoid use of polymyxin B sulfate-bacitracin zinc (Polysporin), bacitracin, and polymyxin B sulfate-bacitracin zinc-neomycin (Neosporin) antibiotic ointments because of the risk of

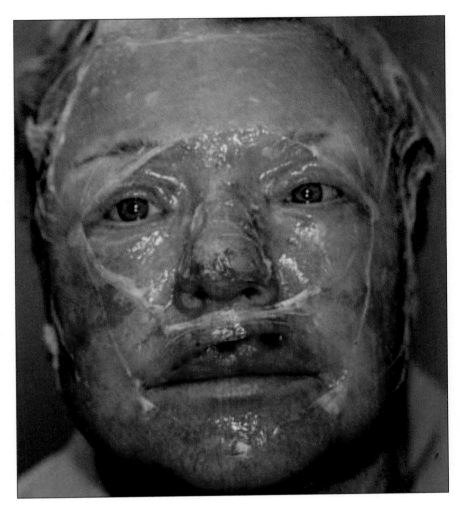

FIGURE 5.4

One day after resurfacing showing pink areas where Silon-TSR dressing stayed in place as well as early scabs and more pronounced redness in areas without dressing in place.

contact dermatitis.[2] Petrolatum is not recommended, because folliculitis may develop, especially if its use is not discontinued immediately after reepithelialization is completed.[3] After the seventh postoperative day and immediately after reepithelialization, we discontinue use of the Aquaphor Healing Ointment, to avoid folliculitis. I tell patients that when their skin is a dull pink on the surface to stop using the ointment.

I recommend that the laser surgeon see the patient at 7 days postoperatively. At 6 days after full-face resurfacing using 2 passes with the long-pulse

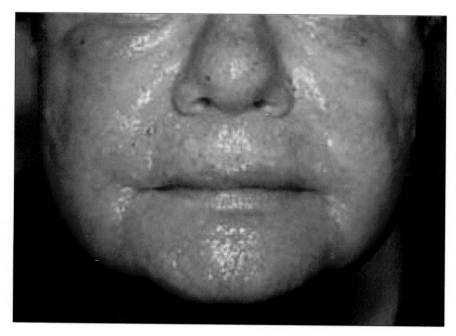

FIGURE 5.5

Six days after skin resurfacing with long-pulse erbium:YAG laser and after 72-hour application of bio-occlusive dressing.

erbium:YAG laser, the forehead skin does not appear pink anymore (Fig 5-5). After the first week, I follow up my patients monthly for at least 6 months until all the skin redness is gone and their appearance is back to normal. At 6 weeks, usually the redness has disappeared or the skin is only slightly pink.

Approximately 7 days after resurfacing, patients can start wearing camouflage cosmetics. Patients may find it helpful during the initial period of redness to work with an aesthetician, who can help them apply a concealer type of makeup such as green-tinted foundation. Usually patients need concealing makeup no longer than 6 weeks. In addition, I recommend that patients wear a broad-spectrum sunscreen containing transparent zinc oxide.

PROPHYLAXIS

In patients with a history of herpes labialis, laser resurfacing can trigger an outbreak that can spread to involve the entire denuded skin surface and cause increased pain, prolonged healing, and an increased risk of scarring. I have encountered several patients who denied any history of herpes labialis but who experienced severe herpes outbreaks after laser resurfacing. Therefore, all my patients who undergo resurfacing, regardless of whether they report a history of cold sores or fever blisters, prophylactically receive an antiviral agent up to 2 days before surgery and for at least 10 days after the procedure. A commonly prescribed antiviral drug after resurfacing is valacyclovir hydrochloride (Valtrex), 500 mg orally twice a day. Other oral antiviral treatment options include famciclovir (Famvir), 250 mg twice daily, and acyclovir (Zovirax), 400 mg 3 times a day. I ask patients to start taking the antiviral drug the morning of surgery, because many patients have a hard time remembering when to start an antiviral regimen after surgery.

After laser resurfacing, there is a layer of necrotic, thermally coagulated dermis that will slough over several days. This material serves as an ideal bacterial cultural medium, making infection a concern. Therefore, patients usually are given prophylactic antibiotics starting up to 1 day before surgery and continuing for 5 days.[3] I prefer narrow-spectrum antibiotics[4]; broad-spectrum antibiotics, I believe, may slightly increase the possibility of greater overgrowth of resistant organisms. A narrow-spectrum antibiotic, such as oral dicloxacillin sodium (500 mg twice a day), may be given. Penicillin-allergic individuals may be prescribed oral azithromycin (500 mg/d the first day followed by 250 mg/d on days 2 through 5).

A few laser surgeons recommend a dose of fluconazole on the day of resurfacing to reduce the risk of candidal infection in the treated area.[5,6] However, I rarely use antifungal agents, because most of my patients do not report having a problem with candidiasis.

Some laser surgeons prescribe a short course of oral corticosteroids perioperatively, in an attempt to reduce the substantial edema that usually occurs during the first 72 hours after the procedure. This therapy is controversial, and the data in the literature are conflicting as to whether it helps with swelling. Occasionally I prescribe corticosteroid therapy, because I find that it does greatly decrease swelling. I will prescribe steroids for patients receiving full-face resurfacing who have no contraindications. The patient in Figure 5-1, who had substantial swelling, did not receive corticosteroids.

I allow erythema to resolve spontaneously. I do not like to prescribe topical corticosteroid therapy, because milia and other problems can develop. Darker redness should be treated right away with topical corticosteroids, pulsed dye laser, and intralesional corticosteroids, because it can lead to incipient scarring. Milia may be treated with tretinoin (Retin-A) and selective extraction. Therapy for hyperpigmentation includes sun avoidance, transparent zinc oxide sunscreens, hydroquinone medications, and 0.05% tretinoin emollient cream (Renova). If treatment is begun early, hyperpigmentation usually resolves within 3 months.[3,7]

REFERENCES

1.   Batra RS, Ort RJ, Jacob C, Hobbs L, Arndt KA, Dover JS. Evaluation of a silicone occlusive dressing after laser skin resurfacing. *Arch Dermatol.* 2001;137:1317–1321.

2. Fitzpatrick RE, Williams B, Goldman MP. Preoperative anesthesia and postoperative considerations in laser resurfacing. *Semin Cutan Med Surg.* 1996;15:170–176.

3. Lowe NJ, Lask G, Griffin ME. Laser skin resurfacing: pre and posttreatment guidelines. *Dermatol Surg.* 1995;21:1017–1019.

4. Ross EV, Amesbury EC, Barile A, Proctor-Shipman L, Feldman BD. Incidence of postoperative infection or positive culture after facial laser resurfacing: a pilot study, a case report, and a proposal for a rational approach to antibiotic prophylaxis. *J Am Acad Dermatol.* 1998;39:975–981.

5. Fitzpatrick RE, Goldman MP, Satur NM, Tope WD. Pulsed carbon dioxide laser resurfacing of photo-aged facial skin. *Arch Dermatol.* 1996;132:395–402.

6. Sriprachya-Anunt S, Fitzpatrick RE, Goldman MP, Smith SR. Infections complicating pulsed carbon dioxide laser resurfacing for photoaged facial skin. *Dermatol Surg.* 1997;23:527–535.

7. Ho C, Nguyen Q, Lowe NJ, Griffin ME, Lask G. Laser resurfacing in pigmented skin. *Dermatol Surg.* 1995;21:1035–1037.

Nonocclusive Wound Care After Laser Resurfacing

Christian Raulin, MD

The effect of laser skin resurfacing with the carbon dioxide (CO_2) laser or erbium:YAG laser is equivalent to a second-degree burn. Secondary bacterial and viral infections in the postoperative phase can have a crucial influence on the cosmetic result. Thus far, no general recommendations for postoperative wound care have been developed. I therefore performed a study to evaluate nonocclusive wound care after laser resurfacing.

PATIENTS AND METHODS

Between April 1995 and December 2000, colleagues and I conducted a retrospective study of full-face or perioral laser resurfacing in 340 patients, with a follow-up of 2 weeks. We used a pulsed CO_2 laser or the erbium:YAG laser or a combination of both. The indications for resurfacing were facial wrinkles and acne scars. The patients ranged in age from 19 to 78 years (average, 57 years). Patients had skin types I to III and were not tanned.

Before laser treatment, 208 of the patients (61%) received tretinoin cream. All patients were advised to use sunblock and not to use bleaching cream due to the possibility of an allergic reaction. All patients received antiviral therapy starting the day before laser therapy. We used no locally or systemically administered steroids and no locally administered antibiotics. One patient received a prophylactic systemic administration of antibiotics because of a cardiac valvular defect.

Postoperatively, we used nonocclusive wound care. For the first 3 days, we used petrolatum ointment in combination with cold tea compresses and crushed ice. We did not manually remove the crusts. Persisting crusts were loosened after 3 to 5 days with chlortetracycline hydrochloride. After 3 or 4 postoperative days, we prescribed water-in-oil emulsions instead of petrolatum ointment, to avoid folliculitis. Patients were seen for wound control after 3 or 4 days and after 2 weeks. If needed, patients received oral analgesics and anti-inflammatory medications.

RESULTS

In this study, we had a low rate of complications. Eczema herpeticum developed in only 1 patient, and it healed with oral acyclovir treatment (800 mg 5 times a day) combined with topical acyclovir. Five patients had disseminated folliculitis, but without severe infection. In all 5 patients, the folliculitis healed with minocycline therapy (50 mg twice daily).

We also encountered 5 patients who had a severe burning sensation. There was no evidence of inflammation, and we found no reason for the burning. Perhaps alcoholism or use of tranquilizers can explain it.

COMMENT

In this study, occlusive lipid-containing ointments and moist open wound care made it possible to have a controllable healing process with a low rate of complications. In contrast to the occlusive method of wound care, this approach can be easily self-administered by the patient at home and is much cheaper.

In general, I suggest antiviral prophylaxis before laser resurfacing, as was done in this study. My colleagues and I do not systemically administer antibiotics to these patients except in the case of valvular defects or immunosuppression. After laser resurfacing, we always use cooling (compresses and ice) to reduce the side effects during the operation and postoperatively. If required, the patients receive oral analgesics and anti-inflammatory medication after the operation.

Patient compliance is a crucial factor in the healing process after laser resurfacing, and patients therefore must be well informed. The keys to successful skin resurfacing are also early diagnosis of complications and intervention by experienced dermatologists or laser experts.

I would like to thank Baerbel Greve, MD, who provided substantial research assistance with the study mentioned herein.

chapter 7

Improved Reepithelialization After Laser Resurfacing*

Mitchel P. Goldman, MD

Wound healing is critical in laser resurfacing. Laser skin resurfacing produces a thermal injury, and if the laser surgeon properly controls the different phases of wound healing, better healing will result. Reepithelialization occurs due to migration from the appendages, from the hair follicles and eccrine glands. If the ablation is too deep and destroys all these follicles and glands, delayed wound healing will occur. To obtain optimal wound healing, we need to facilitate 2 steps: cellular migration and keratinization. To optimize postoperative care, we need to manage the wound fluid, enhance cell regeneration, and establish the proper skin barrier.

Occlusive dressings have many benefits, including increasing the speed of epidermal wound healing by decreasing wound adherence, maintaining a moisture barrier, and allowing contact with healing factors.[1] One type of occlusive dressing contains a thin film of silicone and polytetrafluoroethylene (PTFE) blended into an interpenetrating polymer network (Silon-TSR). This dressing is very easy to apply and is pain-free. To create a wound healing mechanism that could potentially provide improvements in wound healing over that of the silicone-PTFE dressing, we developed and tested a resurfacing recovery system using a collagen-alginate dressing.[2]

MATERIALS AND METHODS

The resurfacing recovery system involves an absorbent collagen-alginate dressing (Fibracol) that is hemostatic and bacteriostatic, a hydrogel with retentive cover, and application of petrolatum ointment (Fig 7-1). The collagen-alginate dressing becomes a gel when it comes in contact with exudative fluid and then conforms to the face and neutralizes all bacteria. The hydrogel basically is composed of water and is a heat sink providing cooling and soothing relief. The newer types

*Adapted with permission from the *Journal of the American Academy of Dermatology* (2002;46:399–407).

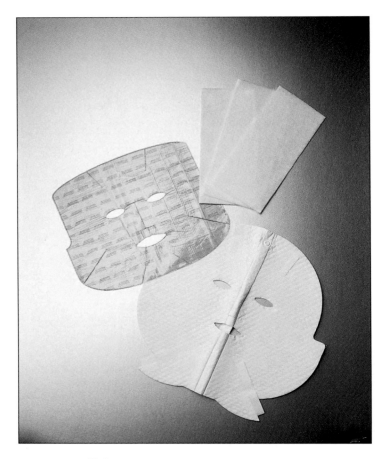

FIGURE 7.1

Resurfacing recovery system, which employs collagen-alginate dressing, hydrogel with retentive cover, and application of petrolatum ointment.

of hydrogel have an internal polyethylene mesh to support the polymer. The hydrogel is applied 3 days postoperatively for hydration.

We compared our resurfacing recovery system with the silicone-PTFE (Silon-TSR) dressing in a study of 42 patients who underwent laser skin resurfacing.[2] We performed laser resurfacing with the carbon dioxide (CO_2) laser (UltraPulse 5000C, Lumenis, Santa Clara, Calif) or Sciton (Contour, Sciton Inc, Palo Alto, Calif), and randomized the patients into 3 groups receiving different wound care. One group received the silicone-PTFE dressing, one group received occlusive ointment (Aquaphor Healing Ointment), and the other received the resurfacing recovery system.

RESULTS

Reepithelialization was faster with the resurfacing recovery system (Figs 7-1 and 7-2). Reepithelialization occurred in 7 days with either the silicone-PTFE dressing (Fig 7-3) or application of an occlusive ointment (Aquaphor Healing Ointment). The resurfacing recovery system produced reepithelialization in only 6 days.

Wound management with the resurfacing recovery system also was good compared with the silicone-PTFE dressing. Patients with the collagen-alginate dressing reported no pain associated with the dressing.

COMMENT

Because the resurfacing recovery system speeded reepithelialization in patients after laser resurfacing, we believe it provides an advance over the silicone-PTFE dressing. The collagen-alginate dressing used in the resurfacing recovery system requires a change at 2 to 3 days postoperatively, so patients are asked to return to the office in 2 days for a dressing change. It is painless as well as bacteriostatic.

One aspect of postoperative care not addressed in our study is the treatment of erythema. I believe it is important to decrease the erythema with topical corticosteroids. The key is to use a corticosteroid with no other preservatives or stabilizers in it. The only such topical corticosteroid on the market that I am aware of is 0.025% fluocinolone acetonide (Synalar) ointment. It is applied for 1 week at night, beginning at the seventh postoperative day. In my experience, this ointment dramatically decreases erythema after laser resurfacing.

I have tried giving topical vitamin C to decrease erythema but found that it caused skin irritation in some patients.

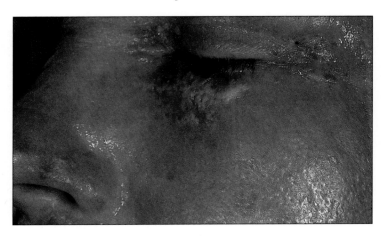

FIGURE 7.2

Six days after application of resurfacing recovery system in patient who underwent laser resurfacing.

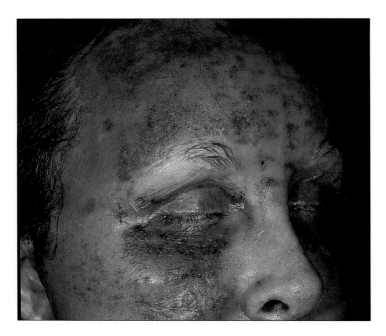

FIGURE 7.3

Six days after application of silicone-polytetrafluoroethylene (Silon-TSR) dressing in patient who underwent laser resurfacing.

REFERENCES

1. Weiss RA, Goldman MP. Interpenetrating polymer network wound dressing versus petrolatum following facial CO_2 laser resurfacing: a bilateral comparison. *Dermatol Surg.* 2001;27:449–451.
2. Goldman MP, Roberts TL, Skover G, Lettieri JT, Fitzpatrick RE. Optimizing wound healing in the face after laser abrasion. *J Am Acad Dermatol.* 2002;46:399–407.

chapter 8

Postoperative Care After Laser Resurfacing: Review of the Literature

A. Jay Burns, MD

For laser skin resurfacing, the goals of postoperative care should be to accelerate reepithelialization time; minimize morbidity, such as pain, infection, and erythema; and strive to obtain optimal results. There are 3 types of postoperative wound care. Dressing occlusion is occlusion with some type of dressing for as little as 24 hours up to the completion of reepithelialization at 10 to 14 days. Moist occlusion involves a petrolatum- or water-based ointment, often accompanied by water and/or vinegar soaks intermittently. The third option is dry wound management, which allows eschar to form.

In this presentation, I would like to review the literature on postoperative care in laser resurfacing.

REVIEW OF THE LITERATURE

A review of the literature leaves no question that maintenance of a moist wound environment optimizes healing and minimizes pain.[1-3] Using a porcine model, Davis et al1 showed that all groups receiving occlusive wound care had improved healing compared with those receiving dry wound management (eschar). A case report by Davis et al[1] described less erythema in patients in whom half the face was treated with an opaque occlusive dressing (Flexzan) compared with the other half of the face treated with an occlusive ointment (Aquaphor Healing Ointment). Improved histologic findings occurred at 19 days postoperatively on the side with the dressing, exemplified by more rete ridges, a thicker epidermis, and new collagen formation.

Comparison of dressings

Newman et al[2] compared wound dressings, including a clear film dressing impregnated with silicone gel and polytetrafluoroethylene (PTFE) (Silon-TSR), a closed dressing (RevitaDerm), a hydrogel dressing (Second Skin), a nonadherent dressing with woven silicone mesh (Mepitel), and Flexzan. The authors were most satisfied with the Mepitel dressing, which they reported was stable and easy to change. However, it imprints on the skin for 1 to 2 weeks. The authors found the Flexzan dressing to be adherent but requiring time-consuming dressing changes. All occlusive dressings have advantages and disadvantages, and are well outlined by Newman et al.[2] We all have biases and preferences; therefore, laser surgeons should continue using whatever dressing works well for them. The important principle to remember is that the postoperative method is variable based on personal style, although the maintenance of an occlusive, moist environment should not be compromised.

Infection

Once the method of occlusion is agreed upon, the issue of infection must be addressed. Bacterial colonization occurs under occlusive dressings but does not impair wound healing unless it reaches the critical mass (1×10^6 colony-forming units [CFU]) to convert that to a clinical infection.[4-6] With regard to infection rates after laser resurfacing, the literature varies. Sriprachya-Anunt and coworkers[7] reported a 20% infection rate using an occlusive dressing (Silon II), which prompted the authors to recommend a 10- or 14-day course of antibiotics. A multicenter trial by Manuskiatti et al[8] reported a 4.7% infection rate in 106 patients who received full-face laser resurfacing and occlusive dressings. A large study by Christian and colleagues[9] in 354 patients reported a 1.4% infection rate using an occlusive dressing (Flexzan). These large disparities in infection rates imply a multifactorial relationship. Another large study used Silon-TSR, and the infection rate was cut in half with use of antibiotics.[8] A 1.7% rate of yeast infection was unaffected by antibiotics (intranasal mupirocin) but was eliminated totally with prophylactic antifungal agents.[8]

In a study by my group, we looked at infection rates when we first started performing laser resurfacing, using open wound care (moist occlusion), and we had a 12% infection rate.[10] We encountered several cases of *Pseudomonas* and fungal infections. We later studied infection rates in 102 consecutive patients who underwent full-face laser resurfacing after we started using occlusive dressings (Flexzan). In this group, we reapplied the dressing on postoperative days 1 and 3 and removed it at day 5 or 6. We did a meticulous debridement and treated with cephalexin (250 mg 3 times a day) for 5 days and valacyclovir hydrochloride (Valtrex, 500 mg twice daily) for 10 days. The group with the dressings had no bacterial infections but had 2 herpetic infections, for a total infection rate of 2%. I believe that although antibiotics are helpful, as evidenced by several studies noted earlier, the most important element is meticulous and thorough debridement on a regular basis until reepithelialization is complete.

Antioxidants

Antioxidants can improve healing after laser resurfacing. Alster and West[11] demonstrated a marked reduction in erythema with use of 10% topical vitamin C. McDaniel et al[12] showed that antioxidants (4% tocopherol acetate, 4% pyruvic acid sodium salt, 6% lecithin, and fatty acids) improved epithelialization, erythema, swelling, and pain. Yet to be determined is which antioxidants are optimal and whether topical growth factors will play a role in the future. The obvious goal is to minimize recovery time while maintaining results. The articles cited[11,12] emphasize reduction of morbidity but do not relate it to long-term efficacy, which I believe is extremely important.

PERSONAL EXPERIENCE

I use occlusive dressings because they help decrease the pain to the patient, although they typically are more costly than moist occlusive techniques. In my patients, I apply occlusive dressings for 3 to 5 days postoperatively, then maintain moisture for the next few days, until reepithelialization is complete, with an occlusive ointment such as Aquaphor Healing Ointment. Once reepithelialization occurs, I discontinue therapy with the occlusive ointments. Natural moisturizers can then by resumed by the patient.

Among the occlusive dressings, I believe that Flexzan has some advantage with regard to the reepithelialization rate.[1] The disadvantage of Flexzan is the time required for dressing changes, but I believe it is time well spent. The dressing changes are performed by my nurse, who has been carefully trained in the meticulous debridement that is so critical.

The wound in Figure 8-1 (Fig 8-1a) looks fairly clean after careful removal of the occlusive dressing (Flexzan), but a closer view (Fig 8-1b) shows fibrinous debris. All the fibrinous debris must be removed, because if another dressing is immediately applied over it, there is a risk of high bacterial counts. I prescribe prophylactic antibiotics, but I do not think that antibiotic therapy is as critical as meticulous debridement. Good wound care, whether it is closed or open, should minimize problems with infection. Antiviral therapy is critical. I do not prescribe antifungal medications after laser resurfacing, although there is adequate evidence that they may be beneficial. Fungal infections simply have not been a major problem for my patients, but for any practice that sees this complication, I would recommend adding an antifungal agent to the patient's postoperative regimen.

I do recommend antioxidants postoperatively to my patients. They are to be used as tolerated.

We have some clear direction in wound care for laser resurfacing. I have tried to support my personal opinion based on a literature review and my own findings. The question that remains in my mind is the true role of inflammation. In trying to decrease inflammation, may we be inhibiting mediators that could

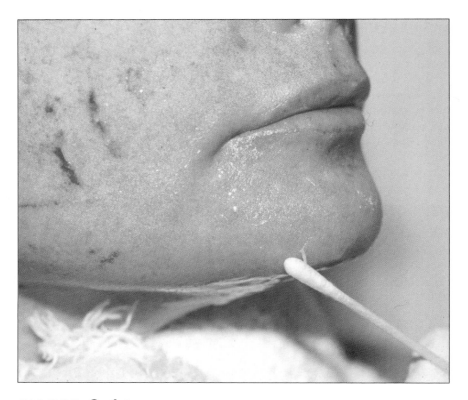

FIGURE 8.1a

Wound looks fairly clean after removal of occlusive dressing (Flexzan) (Fig8-1a); closer view shows fibrinous debris (Fig 8-1b).

produce a beneficial effect, such as new collagen formation? Until this question has been answered, it is unclear in my mind what role anti-inflammatory steroids play.

Antioxidants appear helpful, but I believe we should discover the most optimal antioxidants in a healing wound. Finally, it is unclear what role topical growth factors will have on a healing wound. One could certainly theorize that wound healing could be enhanced, but too much collagen deposition could result in keloidal scarring.

REFERENCES

1. Davis SC, Badiavas E, Rendon-Pellerano MI, Pardo RJ. Histologic comparison of postoperative wound care regimens: laser resurfacing in a porcine model. *Dermatol Surg.* 1999;2:387–391.

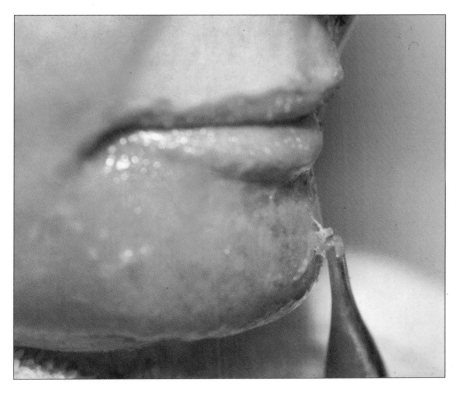

FIGURE 8.1b

2. Newman JP, Fitzgerald P, Koch RJ. Review of closed dressings after laser resurfacing. *Dermatol Surg.* 2000;26:562–571.
3. Collawn SS. Occlusion following laser resurfacing promotes reepithelialization and wound healing. *Plast Reconstr Surg.* 2000;105:2180–2189.
4. Alvarez OM, Mertz PM, Eaglstein WH. The effect of occlusive dressings on collagen synthesis and re-epithelialization in superficial wounds. *J Surg Res.* 1983;35:142–148.
5. Handfield-Jones SE, Grattan CE, Simpson RA, Kennedy CT. Comparison of a hydrocolloid dressing and paraffin gauze in the treatment of venous ulcers. *Br J Dermatol.* 1988;118:425–427.
6. Gilchrest BA. In vitro lessons for wound healing. *Clin Dermatol.* 1984;2:45–53.
7. Sriprachya-Anunt S, Fitzpatrick RE, Goldman MP, Smith SR. Infections complicating pulsed carbon dioxide laser resurfacing for photoaged facial skin. *Dermatol Surg.* 1997;23:527–535.
8. Manuskiatti W, Fitzpatrick RE, Goldman MP, Krejca-Papa N. Prophylactic antibiotics in patients undergoing laser resurfacing of the skin. *J Am Acad Dermatol.* 1999;40:77–84.
9. Christian MM, Behroozan DS, Moy RL. Delayed infection following full-face CO_2 laser resurfacing and occlusive dressing use. *Dermatol Surg.* 2000;26:32–36.

10. Schwartz RS, Burns AJ, Rohrich RJ, Barton FE, Byrd HS. Long-term assessment of CO_2 facial laser resurfacing: aesthetic results and complications. *Plast Reconstr Surg.* 1999;103:592–601.
11. Alster TS, West TB. Effect of topical vitamin C on postoperative carbon dioxide laser resurfacing erythema. *Dermatol Surg.* 1998;24:331–334.
12. McDaniel DH, Ash K, Lord J, Zukowski M. Accelerated laser resurfacing wound healing using a triad of topical antioxidants. *Dermatol Surg.* 1998;24:661–664.

PART TWO DISCUSSION

Kenneth A. Arndt, MD, *Moderator*

Dr Arndt: Let me ask the audience a few questions. There has been a discussion in the literature about the pros and cons of use of oral antibiotics for patients who undergo laser skin resurfacing. By a show of hands, how many *do not* prescribe oral antibiotics along with laser resurfacing? Only 4 of the approximately 150 individuals in the room do not, so we appear to be in agreement about the use of oral antibiotics.

How many prescribe antifungal agents after resurfacing? Approximately 18. My coworkers and I performed a study in 20 patients, to determine the presence of fungal organisms in the healing laser wound (Alam M, Pantanowitz L, Harton AM, Arndt KA, Dover JS. A prospective trial of *Candida* colonization after laser resurfacing of the face: correlation between culture positivity and symptoms of pruritus. Submitted for publication). We found yeast organisms in 3 of the patients, *Candida albicans* in 1, and a couple of other yeast organisms in a fifth patient. It was not clear whether the organisms were pathogens; they seemed to be; however, so we are still unsure about the need for antifungal agents after resurfacing.

How many in the audience use open dressings only? How many use closed dressings? The great majority use occlusive dressings. Several years ago, the numbers would have been reversed, so there has been a dramatic change.

The use of cold air intraoperatively is interesting. Dr Raulin, would you like to say more about that?

Christian Raulin, MD: During the operation, we exposed only 1 side of the face to cold air. On this side, we had a reduction of pain during the operation by about 70% to 80%. I think wound healing also improves somewhat by the use of cold air.

Dr Arndt: Do your patients receive topical or general anesthesia or conscious sedation?

Dr Raulin: It depends on the procedure. If I perform a full-face resurfacing, anesthesia is given. For resurfacing of the perioral region, I give just oral analgesic medications, and patients do not have a problem with pain.

Suzanne L. Kilmer, MD: We also use a cold fan during the procedure toward the end and for the next 15 minutes after resurfacing, and it dramatically reduces pain.

Cyrus Chess, MD: With regard to blowing cold air intraoperatively, I am concerned about what happens to the laser plume, which we are generally very careful about evacuating with suction. It strikes me that we need some kind of device that can cool the skin and still evacuate the plume effectively after treatment.

On another subject, I did not hear the speakers address the option of using low-fluence subpurpuric pulsed dye laser therapy for erythema that persists longer than the patient is willing to tolerate. A series of treatments generally works very well to accelerate fading of the erythema.

Richard E. Fitzpatrick, MD: Regarding antioxidants, I also have found that vitamin C is sometimes too irritating because of the pH. I have been applying tocotrienol ointment to laser-treated skin after the first 3 postoperative days. I apply a silicone-polytetrafluoroethylene dressing (Silon-TSR) and then instead of applying just petrolatum ointment, I use tocotrienol ointment.

Dr Arndt: What is that?

Dr Fitzpatrick: Tocotrienol is a vitamin E precursor. It is more bioactive than tocopherol, and I think it has had dramatic results in reducing inflammation. It is hard to know whether or not we want inflammation at that stage, but I have been using this ointment, and it does decrease erythema.

I also want to mention that growth factors may be an important component of postoperative wound care. I have been using a naturally occurring mix of growth factors from a biotechnology company starting at day 7 postoperatively and have seen a dramatic enhancement of wound healing. Therefore, I think that use of growth factors and free radical quenchers may be a big step forward in postoperative care after resurfacing.

Mitchel P. Goldman, MD: I would like to address the comment about inflammation. Probably everyone thinks that inflammation is important, and I do not know why. In a study I conducted, we resurfaced half of patients' faces with the carbon dioxide (CO_2) laser (UltraPulse 5000C, Lumenis, Santa Clara, Calif) alone and the other half with the same CO_2 laser followed by the erbium:YAG laser (Goldman MP, Manuskiatti W. Combined laser resurfacing with the 950-microsec pulsed CO_2 + Er:YAG lasers. *Dermatol Surg.* 1999;25:160–163). We found that the combination treatment decreased inflammation histopathologically. Results at 6 months showed that both types of laser treatment were equivalent. We now have 3-year results, and the 2 treatments were still totally equivalent. So, at least in my mind, it is clear that inflammation is not a necessary component to having efficacy. Also, for the last 3 or 4 years, I have prescribed 0.025% fluocinolone acetonide (Synalar) ointment for 1 week after resurfacing to decrease the inflammation. We have shown that we can get good results after resurfacing with no inflammation or erythema.

A. Jay Burns, MD: Was there no difference in efficacy or no difference in erythema?

Dr Goldman: The study that was published showed that erythema decreases if one decreases the inflammation with the CO_2 laser followed by the erbium:YAG laser. Now that many laser surgeons have started to use this combination treatment, we see less inflammation, less erythema, and equivalent efficacy.

Dr Burns: Not everybody agrees with that. Dr. Tina Alster and I, in separate experiences, saw no difference in erythema and inflammation in patients treated with CO_2 followed by erbium:YAG laser. Clearly, superficial treatments translate into less erythema and less efficacy. Deeper injuries and/or those with more residual thermal damage result in greater efficacy at the expense of more inflammation and erythema.

Whitney D. Tope, MPhil, MD: I have 2 comments. The first regards use of either systemically or topically administered steroids during the time that reepithelialization takes place. At another conference 2 years ago, there were case reports of large granulating wounds after Mohs microsurgical resection of tumors that reached a certain stage in healing and then stopped the healing by second intention. The investigators called it wound healing arrest. They showed that use of topical or oral steroids or the nonsteroidal anti-inflammatory drug indomethacin could reinitiate the wound healing process. With this treatment, the wounds healed. So it may be that these agents can promote reepithelialization.

Also, I'm curious why nobody is talking about low-level laser therapy as a way to promote wound healing after resurfacing.

Javier Ruiz-Esparza, MD: I want to comment on the issue of inflammation. I think that inflammation works against the healing process, especially when the patient has very delicate or sensitive skin, such as dark skin. With prolonged inflammation comes prolonged erythema, which can cause problems. In a previous presentation about aggressive resurfacing in Hispanics, I reported that by not driving hard on the skin between laser passes, the surgeon can decrease the degree of edema postoperatively. The results are exactly the same, but with less prolonged erythema.

Also, I appreciated hearing about Dr Arndt's study on *Candida* and wound healing. In my own patients with a wound that took longer than normal to heal, cultures often yield yeast organisms. One time I tried using nystatin (Mycostatin) topical powder on a patient's dimple wound that was not healing but had yeast present, and the wound started healing again. I prescribe fluconazole for all my patients who undergo resurfacing.

Jerome M. Garden, MD: I wish to comment on the method of using forced cold, refrigerated air during the procedure. I think it is wonderful in terms of reducing the patient's discomfort. Such systems, or a fan, also reduce the heat in the operating room. My concern is that if these forced, refrigerated air systems are used directly on the skin during the procedure, much of the plume may be escaping. We need special vacuum systems that have greater ability to capture the plume.

Dr Burns: I agree with that.

David B. Vasily, MD: I have 2 comments. Fluconazole may have effects on wound healing beyond killing yeast. An article I read stated that fluconazole has remarkable immune-stimulating effects, that is, neutrophil-enhancing effects.

My other comment is about management of postoperative erythema. I have found a camouflage foundation known as Custom Color (Topix Pharmaceuticals Inc, North Amityville, NY) to be very effective in covering skin redness. Preoperative readings of the patient's skin color are obtained with spectrophotometry, and the foundation is customized to that color. The level of coverage can be changed as the erythema decreases. Despite the erythema, the patient's skin color does not change postoperatively with use of this excellent camouflage foundation. I should note that I was a paid consultant when a large cosmetic company conducted the original studies of this makeup, but I highly recommend it.

Dr Kilmer: I agree with what was just said about the effects of fluconazole. I think that there is a lot of subclinical yeast that we do not appreciate in the wound. By starting a regimen of fluconazole (Diflucan), the clinician can decrease the skin redness and perhaps slightly speed reepithelialization.

I also agree that camouflage makeup is a good idea to cover erythema. The other thing that we should consider with erythema is that contactants or skin irritants may prolong redness. For example, fabric softener sheets for the dryer may cause a reaction on exposed laser-treated skin.

A physician: I have been using cold-air cooling intraoperatively for about $4\frac{1}{2}$ years, and it works well during laser hair removal. However, my results were not as good during laser resurfacing. In the 1 patient I tried it on, the side of the face that was exposed to cooling was redder than the other side. I reasoned that the cold air works with laser hair removal because we apply gel first, but cold air dries out the skin, so I think there is going to be more thermal damage using this approach. Whereas I think air cooling is a good idea after the procedure, I would be hesitant to use it before or during the procedure.

Henry C. Gasiorowski, MD: Dr Raulin mentioned 5 patients who complained of a severe burning sensation after resurfacing. I speculate that if he had given them a 200-mg fluconazole (Diflucan) tablet the day of the surgery and then another tablet 3 days later, much of the itching and burning would have been eliminated. I think the burning is secondary to infection with yeast that cannot be seen but would be present on a culture specimen.

Dr Arndt: In patients of yours who have burning postoperatively, have you actually obtained a culture to prove a yeast infection before you gave them the fluconazole?

Dr Gasiorowski: I have not.

Dr Arndt: It would be very helpful if you did, because then you could prove your theory. In our study of yeast, the data were not as clear-cut as I had hoped. The patients with burning or itching did have culture-proven *Candida* organisms more often than those who did not burn or itch, but it was not as pure as we had predicted.

Jeffrey S. Dover, MD, FRCPC: It would be helpful if several investigators performed a prospective study and obtained cultures from every patient, not necessarily every day, to determine whether a burning sensation after resurfacing correlates with candidal infection. There are many other reasons besides subclinical *Candida* infection that patients feel burning or itching after laser resurfacing.

Dr Goldman: I want to further comment on infection. I believe that some people are misquoting the articles that I coauthored with Manuskiatti et al (Manuskiatti W, Fitzpatrick RE, Goldman MP, Krejci-Papa N. Prophylactic antibiotics in patients undergoing laser resurfacing of the skin. *J Am Acad Dermatol.* 1999;40:77–84). In every one of our patients with infections who were described in the articles, the infection occurred after the antibiotic therapy was discontinued. All the infections occurred at day 8 or 9, and the antibiotic regimen was discontinued at day 7. Since we began to prolong antibiotic therapy to 14 days, we have yet to see a patient with an infection after resurfacing.

Dr Dover: It is interesting that Dr Raulin had a series of more than 300 patients and administered no antibiotics except in 1 patient with a valvular defect, yet he encountered only 1 herpes infection and no bacterial infections. His findings would suggest the accuracy of what Dr Burns said, that fastidious postoperative care is probably more important than whether the patients receive antibiotics. I would never perform resurfacing without putting the patient on a perioperative regimen of antibiotics, and our infection rate is approximately 0.01%, and we believe that low rate is because of what we do. Although Dr Raulin proved in his study that a lower infection rate was not associated with antibiotic use, other studies contradict his findings. Ross published a study with a smaller number of patients than in Dr Raulin's study. He showed that without antibiotics the infection rates after laser resurfacing were higher at his institution, and that has been my impression, too. An early study by Geronemus showed that infection rates after resurfacing decreased with use of antibiotics. The issue of whether to prescribe antibiotics is still not clear.

Dr Arndt: I'd like to invite Dr Anderson to conclude this discussion with some comments about low-level laser therapy and any thoughts about inflammation and wound healing.

R. Rox Anderson, MD: Low-level light therapy is very common in Europe. Many researchers around the world believe that a low level of light, usually in the visible spectrum, but sometimes near-infrared diode lasers are used, can stimulate wound healing. There have been some well-controlled clinical trials that suggest this treatment actually does work, but the mechanism is unclear. In my laboratory, we are finding that low-level visible light induces increases in blood flow. Maybe laser surgeons should explore whether we can use photons to alleviate wound healing problems.

In considering the topic of inflammation and wound healing, I wonder whether destruction of the epidermis is the best approach. Laser removal of the entire epidermis seems extreme, because it requires both a very long time for reepithelialization to occur and the skills of a wound healing expert. Perhaps there can be a technique to rejuvenate the skin that is a compromise between ablative and nonablative rejuvenation. Maybe laser surgeons can spare the epidermis partially. It is very interesting that researchers have not done much to understand what happens when a small amount of epidermis is left in place during resurfacing. I think there are some further improvements we can make that will perhaps return laser skin resurfacing to its glory days.

PART 3

Photorejuvenation and Subsurface Resurfacing: Do They Really Work?

Quantitative Evidence of Benefits of Subsurface Resurfacing

Roy Geronemus, MD

There clearly has been tremendous hype with nonablative laser procedures, and the question of whether the hype is justified remains to be answered. In my opinion and in the opinion of my patients, the benefits of this technology are great, but investigators have not found definitive proof of the benefits. Photorejuvenation and subsurface resurfacing using lasers have been reported to offer benefit in the treatment of fine lines, skin tone, skin texture, and acne scars.[1-4] Improvement can be seen without post-treatment downtime, wounding, or need for postoperative care. Unfortunately, to date most of the studies have been anecdotal or subjective, in which physicians evaluated results as excellent, good, fair, or poor. The subjective analysis is complicated by the fact that photographic documentation is often difficult with these techniques and does not represent the benefits seen by the many satisfied patients and their physicians.

I and others attempted to objectively evaluate the efficacy of at least 1 of these technologies, nonablative skin rejuvenation with the Q-switched neodymium: YAG (Nd: YAG) laser. The results of this study are reported here.[5]

PATIENTS AND METHODS

A study was performed at my institution in New York City, the Laser and Skin Surgery Center of New York, in conjunction with Johnson & Johnson, based in New Brunswick, NJ. The aim of the study was to objectively quantify the efficacy of nonablative skin rejuvenation with the Q-switched neodymium:YAG (Nd:YAG) laser using 3-dimensional (3-D) in vivo optical skin imaging and biomechanical characterization (measurement of elastic deformation of the skin).

Twenty-two patients (18 women and 4 men) with mild to moderate acne scarring or superficial, fine lines were entered into the study. We performed a series of 5 treatments with the Q-switched Nd:YAG laser (1064 nm) at 2- and 3-week intervals. Patients were followed up 1, 3, and 6 months after the initial treatment (3 weeks after the third treatment session and 1 and 3 months after the fifth treatment session). Follow-up included a clinical examination to determine the degree of improvement.

We quantitatively evaluated the topography of the patients' skin using a 3-D in vivo optical skin measuring device (Primos, G. F. Messtechnik, Teltow, Germany) before laser treatment (baseline) and at each of the follow-up visits. This device employs a complex camera and a phase shift analysis to provide in vivo measurement of skin. It is capable of determining changes over time in wrinkles and lines.

In addition, we performed biomechanical characterization of the skin using an infrared targeting laser with negative pressure (BTC 2000, Surgical Research Laboratories Inc Technologies, Nashville, Tenn). With this device, we evaluated physical properties of the skin—compliance and stiffness. We compared these physical properties on the different sides of each patient's face as well as compared differences in patients before and after treatment and differences in results between men and women.

RESULTS

The 3-D optical imaging revealed improvement in the skin topography in patients with acne scarring after 3 treatment sessions, with further improvements seen after 5 sessions. The improvement in skin topography after the final treatment session ranged from 14% to 64%.

In addition, biomechanical skin characterization performed with a dynamic analyzer (BTC 2000) revealed post-treatment improvement in skin tone in a subset of patients. We found that the laser-treated area was firmer and had a quantifiably higher degree of skin stiffness. Improvement in the stiffness of the skin was more dramatic in the men than the women. In terms of skin compliance, we found that the laser-treated skin had lower energy absorption, and this difference also could be quantified.

The differences during the course of treatments were evident in the surface area. Five weeks after the final laser treatment, 3-D images showed continued improvement in skin topography over that seen at 3 weeks. Biomechanical skin characterization using infrared imaging also showed improvement of stiffness of the skin, which continued after further treatments.

The quantitative analysis objectively confirmed improvement in skin that was subjectively reported. A patient told us that she had substantial improvement in her acne scars, but we were unable to quantify the difference in a photographic analysis. However, 3-D images showed marked differences in the depth of the pitted scars and the scars themselves after a series of 3 to 5 treatments (Fig 9-1).

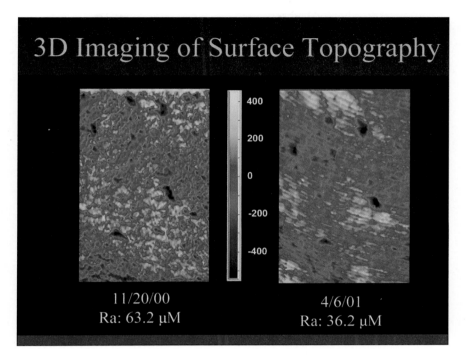

FIGURE 9.1

Three-dimensional imaging of surface topography measured in micrometers. Ra indicates arithmetic average of the absolute values of all points in the profile.

In the same patient, the infrared imaging analysis also demonstrated the differences in the acne scars (Fig 9-1). The blue color in this figure suggests a deeper involvement of the scars, and yellow and red show more superficial involvement of the scars; the increased amount of yellow and red seen in the post-treatment images suggests more superficial involvement after laser rejuvenation.

COMMENT

Quantitative analysis in this study demonstrated defined benefits of nonablative skin rejuvenation using the Q-switched Nd:YAG laser. Benefits seen with 3-D and infrared imaging included improvements in skin topography and elasticity, which continued over the course of treatment.

More dramatic changes were observed in the men, a finding suggesting that men and women may need to be treated differently with nonablative techniques.

Further comparative studies would be of value to determine differences in nonablative techniques and parameters.

REFERENCES

1. Zelickson BD, Kilmer SL, Bernstein E, et al. Pulsed dye laser for sun-damaged skin. *Lasers Surg Med.* 1999;25:229–236.
2. Goldberg DJ, Metzler C. Skin resurfacing utilizing a low fluence Nd:YAG laser. *J Cutan Laser Ther.* 1999;1:23–27.
3. Kelly K, Nelson J, Lask G, Geronemus R, Bernstein L. Cryogen spray cooling in combination with non-ablative laser treatment of facial wrinkles. *Arch Dermatol.* 1999;135:691–694.
4. Bitter PJ. Noninvasive rejuvenation of photoaged skin using serial, full-face intense pulsed light treatments. *Dermatol Surg.* 2000;26:835–843.
5. Friedman PM, Skover GR, Payonk G, Kauvar AN, Geronemus RG. 3D in-vivo optical skin imaging for topographical quantitative assessment of non-ablative laser technology. *Dermatologic Surgery.* 2002;28:199–204.

Photorejuvenation With the Pulsed Dye Laser: Biochemical and Clinical Findings*

Peter Bjerring, MD, PhD

In this chapter, I will discuss type II skin rejuvenation, which deals with wrinkle reduction and collagen remodeling, and I will focus on the pulsed dye laser. The pulsed dye laser technique was invented by Welsh researchers in 1996. My coworkers and I verified the effects biochemically and clinically,[1] which I will describe later, and the treatment was first launched in Europe in 1999. The proposed mode of action of the pulsed dye laser is that the vessels absorb the laser light. Consequently, fibroblast growth mediators are produced and released into the interstitium, which, in turn, stimulate fibroblast activity, and new collagen is then produced.

Wavelength, spatial profile, and energy stability of the laser beam are important parameters, but most important is the temporal profile of the laser beam, in order to cause only temporary damage to the vessels. In contrast to standard dye lasers, this pulsed dye laser targets normal capillaries, not large, dilated, abnormal vessels; the pulse duration is shorter and the rise time of the pulse has been changed.

BIOCHEMICAL EFFECTS

To show, by objective means, the effect of treatment with the pulsed dye laser, my colleagues and I chose to use a biochemical method. We created suction blisters in the skin after treating skin areas with the laser with 2 to 3 J/cm^2, and then we measured the concentration of procollagen molecules in the treated areas and the adjacent nontreated (control) areas. By measuring 1 of the terminal peptides of procollagen molecules, we were able to show an increase in collagen production of 84.6% after a single laser treatment compared with the production rate in

---

*Adapted with permission from *Journal of Cutaneous Laser Therapy* (2000;2:9–15).
Note: The journal is now titled *Journal of Cosmetic and Laser Therapy*
(www.dunitz.co.uk/JCLT.)

Collagen Production Rate

Increase in Collagen Production - 72hrs Post Treatment

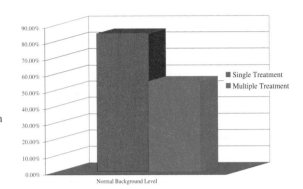

% Increase in
Collagen Production

FIGURE 10.1

Collagen production is increased after single treatment but less after multiple treatments.

NLite v Standard Dye Laser Pulse Form
Single Treatment

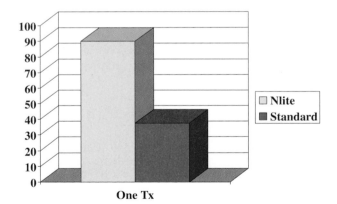

% Increase in
Collagen Production

FIGURE 10.2

The NLite pulsed dye laser appears to produce more collagen after a single treatment than the standard pulsed dye laser.

Collagen production rate:
585 nm dye laser compared with an IPL system
Double treatment - Two Weeks Treatment Interval

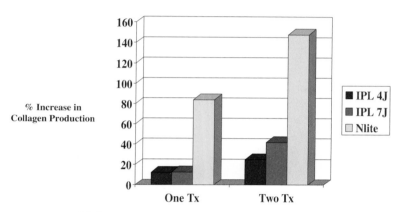

FIGURE 10.3

Comparison of collagen production between intense pulsed light at 7 J/cm² and pulsed dye laser at 2 to 3 J/cm² after 2 treatments at 2-week intervals.

the nontreated control area. It is important to realize that different combinations of wavelengths, energy level, pulse form, and pulse duration will greatly affect the skin collagen production. For instance, Figure 10-1 shows procollagen concentration after single-pass treatment and with 2 passes. A second pass immediately after the first is not appropriate.

Collagen production was much more increased after treatment (2 to 3 J/cm²) with this dye laser compared with an intense pulsed light (IPL) source at 7 J/cm2 (Fig 10-2). Two treatments with 2-week intervals further increased the collagen production induced by both the IPL and the pulsed dye laser (Fig 10-3).

Why not then use a standard dye laser? Whereas a 39% increase in collagen production was seen using a standard dye laser, we achieved an 85% increase in collagen production using this specially made pulsed dye laser.

CLINICAL RESULTS

The effects of this pulsed dye laser also were evaluated clinically. Wrinkle reduction 3 and 6 months after treatment has been demonstrated, and the effect seems to last for at least 9 months after treatment. Acne scars also respond favorably to treatment with the dye laser (Fig 10-4).

Acne Scarring – right cheek

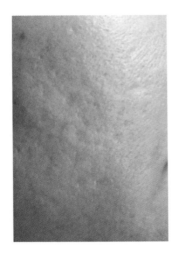

Pre Op   Post Op 30 days

FIGURE 10.4

Before (left) and 30 days after (right) treatment with pulsed dye laser of acne scars.

Wrinkle reduction with the pulsed dye laser is not as effective as with the carbon dioxide (CO_2) laser. A mathematical model comparison of the pulsed dye laser and the CO_2 laser indicates that the average score in reduction of wrinkles was 1.88 for the dye laser vs 2.25 with the CO_2 laser obtained by Fitzpatrick.[2] Thus, mathematically, the efficacy of the pulsed dye laser (NLite, ICN Pharmaceuticals Inc, Costa Mesa, Calif) is approximately 80% of that of the CO_2 laser.

However, as the results of my study[1] show, photorejuvenation with the pulsed dye laser is clearly effective in treating wrinkles and acne scars, and there has been no adverse pigmentary effects.

REFERENCES

1. Bjerring P, Clement M, Heickendorff L, Egevist H, Kiernan M. Selective non-ablative wrinkle reduction by laser. *J Cutan Laser Ther.* 2000;2:9–15.
2. Fitzpatrick RE, Goldman MP, Satur NM, Tope WD. Pulsed carbon dioxide laser resurfacing of photo-aged facial skin. *Arch Dermatol.* 1996;132:395–402.

Nonablative Dermal Remodeling and Photorejuvenation: Clinical and Histologic Findings

Brian D. Zelickson, MD

To answer the question of whether photorejuvenation and subsurface resurfacing really work, we must first understand each procedure and device and know the objective of treatment. There are 2 methods of photorejuvenation: (1) target collagen remodeling for treatment of wrinkles and scars and (2) target all signs of photodamage, including telangiectasia, irregular pigmentation, ectatic blood vessels, and wrinkles. Different devices address these issues. The pulsed dye laser supposedly can address some collagen remodeling, ectatic blood vessels, and some irregular pigmentation; an exception to treatment of the latter is the NLite brand of pulsed dye laser (ICN Pharmaceuticals Inc, Costa Mesa, Calif), because fluences used are too low to destroy the blood vessels (Fig 11-1). The intense pulsed light (IPL) device and the 532-nm potassium-titanyl-phosphate (KTP) laser can address irregular pigmentation, ectatic blood vessels, and collagen remodeling. The infrared lasers can accomplish collagen remodeling without any effect on ectatic blood vessels or irregular pigmentation.

In this chapter, I will discuss my experience with the pulsed dye laser compared with the IPL system, and then some preliminary experience with the long-pulse dye laser with integrated cryogen (Vbeam, Candela Corporation, Wayland, Mass).

PULSED DYE LASER VS IPL

This study was previously presented.[1] My coworkers and I compared results with the pulsed dye laser and the IPL system, 2 treatments 6 weeks apart. The pulsed dye laser had a duration of 0.45 milliseconds and a fluence of 4.5 J/cm^2 on the right side and 3.5 J/cm^2 on the other side. With the IPL system, we used high fluences of approximately 42 J/cm^2 and 38 J/cm^2 on the right and left sides, respectively (pulse durations of 10 and 20 milliseconds, respectively).

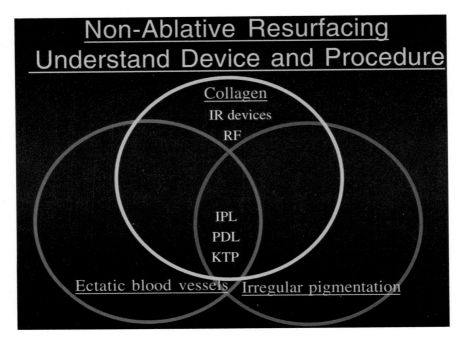

FIGURE 11.1

Schematic of which laser devices address collagen remodeling, ectatic blood vessels, and irregular pigmentation.

Each treatment group was composed of 10 women with mild to moderate wrinkling and pigmentation. The group undergoing treatment with the pulsed dye laser ranged in age from 44 to 68 years (average, 59 years), and the IPL group had an age range of 36 to 60 years (average, 48 years).

Follow-up was conducted at 6 and 12 weeks after treatment. Photographs were taken before and after treatment. Four double-blinded investigators independently rated the pretreatment and 12-week post-treatment photographs on a scale of 0 to 4, with 0 indicating no wrinkling or pigmentation and 4, severe wrinkling or pigmentation. Scores were averaged for each group. In addition, patients were asked to complete a patient satisfaction survey 12 weeks after the second treatment.

Eight subjects from the IPL group and 7 subjects from the other group completed the study. Twelve weeks after completion of 2 treatments, both techniques produced improved results, as observed clinically (Figs 11-2 and 11-3). The

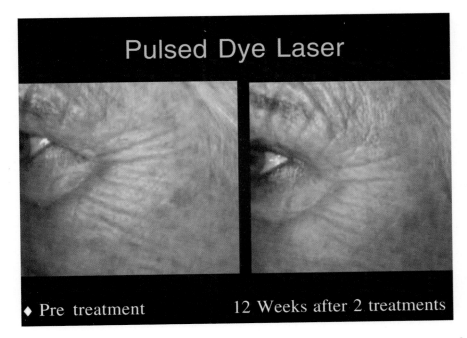

FIGURE 11.2

Before and 12 weeks after 2 treatments with pulsed dye laser.

pulsed dye laser produced approximately 7% improvement in the fine lines and wrinkles and 2% improvement in pigmentation. With the IPL system, there was approximately 19% improvement in wrinkles and 27% improvement in pigmentation.

Fourteen patients responded to the patient satisfaction questionnaire. In the pulsed dye laser group, 4 (67%) of 6 patients reported that they noticed improvement in their skin tone and texture. Seven (88%) of 8 patients noted improvement with IPL. Survey respondents rated the percentage of improvement as 35% to 45% on all treatment sites. Of the respondents who stated that their relatives noticed an improvement in the patients' skin tone and texture, 4 (67%) were in the pulsed dye laser group and 4 (50%) were from the IPL group. Five patients (83%) in the pulsed dye laser group and 6 (75%) in the IPL group would recommend this treatment to others.

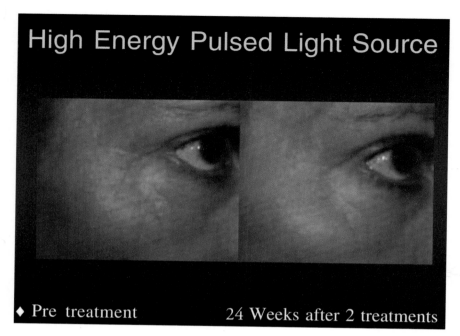

FIGURE 11.3

Before and 12 weeks after 2 treatments with intense pulsed light device.

The only adverse effect reported from the patient survey was purpura noted in the pulsed dye laser group. This side effect lasted about a week. With IPL treatment, mild redness and swelling occurred, which lasted approximately 2 days.

We attempted to correlate the clinical results with histologic improvement. For both techniques, electron microscopy showed increased collagen production in the superficial portion of the dermis (Fig 11-4). This remodeling process also stimulated the production of proteases, as detected by immunocytochemistry, and these proteases contribute to the dynamic remodeling in the dermis. It appears that this induction is not specific to 1 wavelength of light, and this remodeling process does not correlate with clinical improvement.

Our results showed that both the pulsed dye laser and the IPL system are less traumatic than ablative resurfacing methods. However, the clinical results are mild and variable.

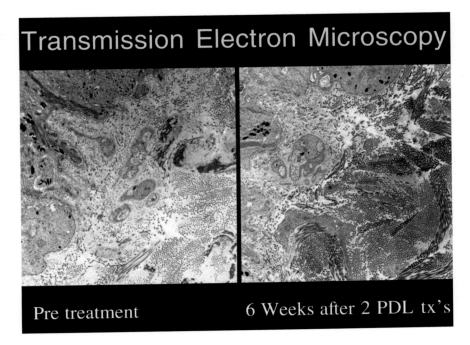

Transmission Electron Microscopy

Pre treatment   6 Weeks after 2 PDL tx's

FIGURE 11.4

Increased collagen production in superficial portion of dermis, evident on electron microscopic image.

VBEAM PULSED DYE LASER

In a preliminary study of the Vbeam pulsed dye laser,[2] we treated 20 subjects with mild to moderate wrinkles using a subpurpuric or purpuric treatment with 2 settings. Ten patients had treatment on 1 side of the face with a 10-mm spot, 595-nm wavelength, cryogen with a Dynamic Cooling Device (DCD) at 30 milliseconds on and 20 milliseconds off, a pulse duration of 20 milliseconds, and a fluence of 4.5 to 6 J/cm². The remaining 10 patients received treatment using the same parameters with the exceptions of a 30-millisecond pulse duration and a fluence of 5 to 7 J/cm². A small amount of purpura washed out within a couple of seconds after treatment. On the other side of the patient's face, we did a control treatment of cooling only.

When we asked the patients which side they thought was more improved in terms of wrinkling, 11 of the 20 patients correctly identified the treatment site; 5 identified the nontreated, or control, side; 3 said neither side was improved;

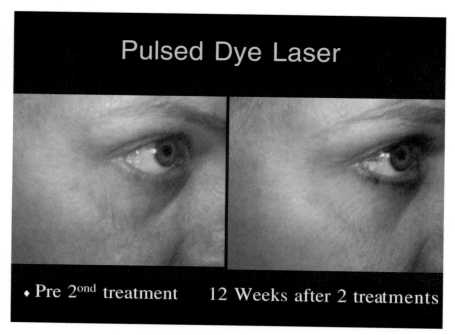

FIGURE 11.5

Patient who noticed mild improvement in wrinkling on herself after pulsed dye laser treatment.

and 1 patient said both sides were equally improved. Patients scored the improvement on a scale of 1 to 4. On average, the 11 patients who chose the correct side noticed an improvement of 3.1, but they also thought the nontreated side had some improvement.

Histologic improvement was noted but did not correlate with clinical results. We performed optical profilometry on a patient who noticed mild improvement on herself (Fig 11-5). The profilometry showed an improvement of approximately 17% on the treated side and 14% on the control side (Fig 11-6). It should be noted, however, that profilometry measurements are difficult to take and to control, because humidity and many other factors can affect the readings. New imaging methods, such as the 3-D in vivo optical skin measuring device, will help quantitate improvements that patients perceive and physicians cannot detect.

In conclusion, I believe that good technology exists for targeting sun-induced telangiectasia and irregular pigmentation. We do not yet have the best technology for nonablative therapy for fine and moderate wrinkles and skin folds. Some of these therapies work, but results are variable and difficult to quantitate.

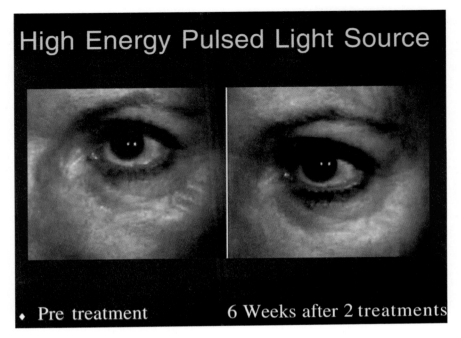

FIGURE 11.6

Same patient as in Figure 11-5 has improvement of approximately 17% on treated side and 14% on control side detected using optical profilometry.

REFERENCE

1. Zelickson B, Kist D. Pulsed dye laser and Photoderm treatment stimulates production of type-I collagen and collagenase transcripts in papillary dermis fibroblasts [abstract]. *Lasers Surg Med.* 2001;(suppl 13):33.
2. Zelickson B, et al. Pulsed dye laser therapy for sun damaged skin. *Lasers in Surgery and Medicine.* 1999;25:229–236.

The study comparing the pulsed dye laser and the IPL was supported in part by research grants from Cynosure Inc, Chelmsford, Mass, and Lumenis, Santa Clara, Calif.

chapter 12

Nonablative Laser Resurfacing

David J. Goldberg, MD

Nonablative technology is at the forefront of skin rejuvenation. Yet photo-rejuvenation and subsurface resurfacing are not an alternative to ablative laser resurfacing. They must be considered as epidermal or dermal remodeling or dermal toning.

The goal of nonablative, subsurface toning or remodeling is to restore damaged collagen without injuring or removing the overlying epidermis. The mechanism of action inherent in all such devices is the selective damage to the dermis (and aged collagen) with light energy, causing an inflammatory response and resultant collagen repair. The collagen and elastic fiber restoration results in decreased wrinkles.[1] Because the epidermis is unharmed, there is no appreciable downtime or recovery period after nonablative laser resurfacing.

Many lasers at different wavelengths as well as light devices are currently being used for nonablative resurfacing. They include the pulsed dye lasers with wavelengths of 585 to 600 nm; the neodymium (Nd):YAG lasers, including the Q-switched with its wavelength of 1064 nm and the 1320-nm Nd:YAG; and the 1450-nm diode laser. In addition, the nonlaser flashlamp device, the intense pulsed light (IPL) device, is used for nonablative resurfacing.

The degree of heat transmission after nonablative resurfacing depends on the laser wavelength, emitted fluence, and depth of absorbing chromophore (eg, dermal water or hemoglobin). Excessive heat production could, in theory, lead to heat-related damage to the epidermis. This would defeat the benefit of nonablative resurfacing, prolong recovery time, and potentially lead to a greater chance of scarring. Some nonablative systems employ epidermal cooling to reduce the risk of this injury. Currently used cooling systems include (1) cryogen spray devices that deliver a burst of cryogen before, during, or after delivery of the laser pulse; (2) contact cooling systems that deliver continuous cooling before, during, or after delivery of the laser pulse; and (3) continuous air cooling systems.

In an attempt to answer the question of whether nonablative laser resurfacing works, my coworkers and I conducted a study using the 1450-nm diode laser.[2]

MATERIALS AND METHODS

The laser used in the study was the 1450-nm diode laser with the Dynamic Cooling Device (Smoothbeam, Candela Corporation, Wayland, Mass). Using a variety of fluences with this laser, we gave 2 to 4 treatments at monthly intervals in 20 patients. We compared efficacy of cryogen laser treatment on 1 side of the face and cryogen alone on the other side. The side that received laser treatment vs cryogen alone was randomized. Three months after the final treatment, we evaluated the results clinically to determine improvement in wrinkles.

RESULTS

On the cryogen laser-treated side, 13 of the 20 patients showed improvement in wrinkles (Fig 12-1), in our evaluation, and the other 7 patients showed no changes at all. However, on the side given cryogen alone, we saw no improvement in any of the subjects (Fig 12-1).

COMMENT

The finding of no improvement in wrinkles on the side given cryogen alone suggests that the cryogen injury itself was not enough to produce an improvement. In most cases, the 1450-nm diode laser did produce an improvement, demonstrating the efficacy of this laser system.

Nonablative resurfacing can improve skin quality, tone, and texture. Because these techniques are all fairly new, long-term data must await several more years of clinical treatment. Ideally, nonablative resurfacing techniques are combined with other adjunctive agents, such as botulinum toxin injections, dermal fillers, and microdermabrasion.

REFERENCES

1. Hruza G. Laser skin resurfacing. *Arch Dermatol.* 1996;132:451–455.
2. Goldberg DJ, Rogachefsky AS, Silapunt S. Non-ablative laser treatment of facial rhytids: evaluation of a 1450-nm diode laser with Dynamic Cooling Device. *Lasers Surg Med.* 2001;21(suppl 13):31.

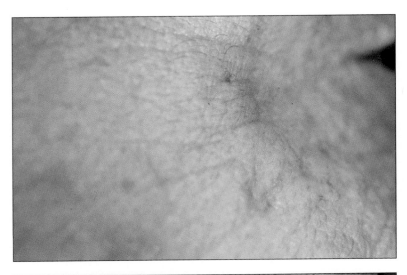

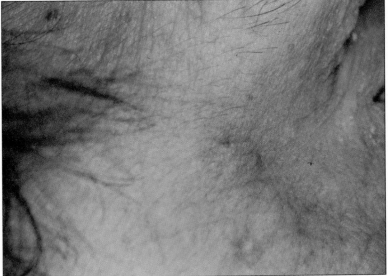

FIGURE 12.1

Three months before (top) and after (bottom) cryogen plus laser treatment on patient's right side or cryogen treatment alone on patient's left side. Improvement is seen on laser-treated side but not on side treated with cryogen alone.

Photorejuvenation and Subsurface Resurfacing

Robert A. Weiss, MD

My perspective is very similar to that of the other speakers. My interest in photorejuvenation began when patients asked me, "What can you do for me except that horrible burning laser?", meaning ablative resurfacing. All of us here know that if laser resurfacing is done correctly, problems such as severe burning can be avoided, but because many patients have a negative impression of ablative resurfacing, I instead offer to perform photorejuvenation. In my office, we use a variety of nonablative techniques, including intense pulsed light (IPL) photorejuvenation and the 1320-nm neodymium (Nd):YAG laser (CoolTouch II, CoolTouch Corporation, Roseville, Calif).[1-4] For patients who want milder treatment, we use the pulsed dye laser with air cooling (Photo-Genica V-Star, Cynosure Inc, Chelmsford, Mass) and a pulse duration of 2 to 20 milliseconds.

In patients who want a very mild treatment, we may not necessarily need to use a laser or light source. We regularly use microdermabrasion alone or in conjunction with any of these other tools. Occasionally we still perform chemical peels, usually in patients who have had the procedure done for years.

TREATMENT ALGORITHM

To determine which technique to employ, we use the following problem-oriented treatment algorithm:

- Telangiectasia: IPL
- Mottled pigmentation: IPL, microdermabrasion, or possibly the long-pulse dye laser
- Mild wrinkles: IPL or the 1320-nm Nd:YAG laser
- Moderate wrinkles: 1320-nm Nd:YAG laser
- Erythematous acne scars: IPL or the pulsed dye laser
- Nonerythematous acne scars: 1320-nm Nd:YAG laser

- Skin atrophy: IPL

This is what we do and, obviously, is not the only way to make a treatment decision. We give patients treatments every 3 to 5 weeks, for a total of 2 to 5 treatments. The number of treatments depends on the spot size, maximum surface temperature (Tmax), condition needing treatment, and the patient's response. Moderate improvement of rhytids typically requires 1 to 4 treatment sessions. Treatment of scarring may take 3 to 6 sessions. After the final treatment, we wait 3 months and then reassess whether more treatment is needed.

RESULTS

Many of our patients are extremely pleased with the results of nonablative resurfacing. One patient objectively had only slight improvement in skin texture but raved about the results of IPL (Fig 13-1). Another patient treated with IPL experienced improvement of telangiectases and elimination of some keratoses (Fig 13-2). He is no longer embarrassed in social situations and feels his rejuvenated appearance is important in his business.

Results of IPL-induced collagen remodeling are shown in Figure 13-3. A patient who had a traumatic scar for 1 or 2 years underwent 5 IPL treatments over 1 year and had remarkable improvement in the scar.

The 1320-nm Nd:YAG laser is effective in treating fine or deeper lines (Fig 13-4), especially around the eyes, and acne scars. This laser is useful in patients of all skin types and colors. Good results also can be achieved when combined with microdermabrasion.

MAXIMIZING RESULTS OF INFRARED LASERS

A number of conditions are necessary to achieve improvement with the 1320-nm Nd:YAG laser. A subclinical injury must be generated. To obtain damage and spongiosis along the dermal-epidermal junction, the laser surgeon must achieve skin temperatures at the skin surface of 45° to 48°C, as measured by the photometer.[4] Three days after laser treatment, there were still points of attachment of the epidermis, as seen with histologic analysis, but to the eye, only erythema was evident, and that lasted only 30 minutes (Fig 13-5). We observed much less damage in many of the other histologic specimens (data not shown). Multiple laser passes are required to achieve acute histologic changes.

What we did in this patient was sort of partial ablative resurfacing, thus bridging the gap between ablative and nonablative resurfacing. It is probably possible to perform this type of treatment with not only the 1320-nm Nd:YAG laser but also other lasers.

Photorejuvenation and subsurface resurfacing really work. However, clinicians do not yet agree on the best treatment sequence. I think that in the next few years, there will be more answers.

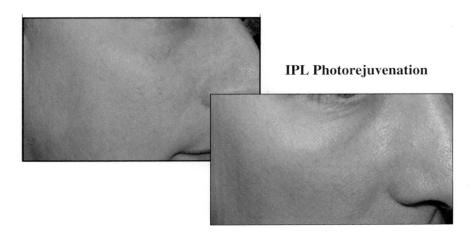

FIGURE 13.1

Moderate improvement in skin texture after one IPL treatment.

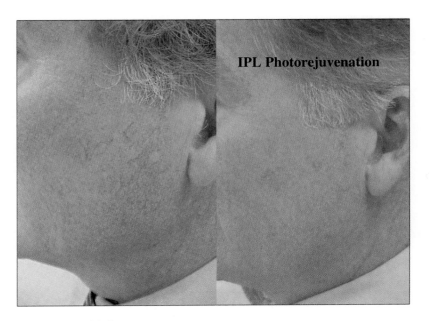

FIGURE 13.2

Improvement in telangiectasias and keratoses after 3 IPL treatments at 4 months posttreatment.

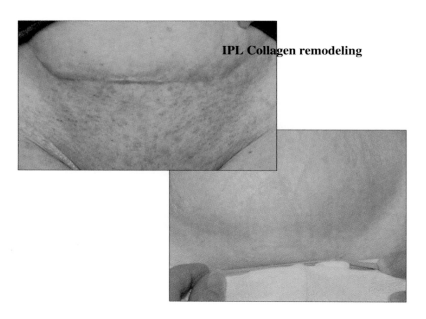

IPL Collagen remodeling

FIGURE 13.3

Scar improvement after 5 IPL treatments. Scar originates from abdominal surgery 2 years before final treatment; patient undergoing hair removal by IPL.

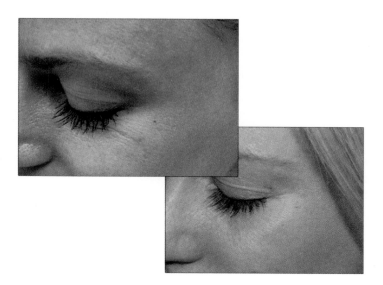

FIGURE 13.4

Improvement in rhytids following 3 1320-nm CoolTouch treatments delivered 1 month apart.

3 Days After Treatment With CoolTouch- Histologic Changes

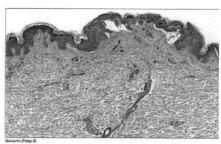

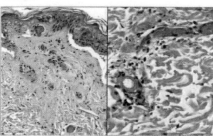

- micro-thrombosis
- widened vessels
- sclerosis of the vessel-walls
- infiltration of neurophilic granulocytes

FIGURE 13.5

Histologic changes seen at 3 days post 1320-nm laser treatment. *Source:* Fatemi A, Weiss MA, Weiss RA. Short-term histologic effects of nonablative resurfacing: results with a dynamically cooled millisecond-domain 1320 nm Nd:YAG laser. *Dermatol Surg.* 2002:28:172–176. Used with permission from Blackwell Science Ltd.

REFERENCES

1. Goldman MP, Weiss RA. Treatment of poikiloderma of Civatte on the neck with an intense pulsed light source. *Plast Reconstr Surg.* 2001;107:1376–1381.
2. Weiss RA, Goldman MP, Weiss MA. Treatment of poikiloderma of Civatte with an intense pulsed light source. *Dermatol Surg.* 2000;26:823–827.
3. Bitter PH. Noninvasive rejuvenation of photodamaged skin using serial, full-face intense pulsed light treatments. *Dermatol Surg.* 2000;26:835–842.
4. Fatemi A, Weiss MA, Weiss RA. Short-term histologic effects of nonablative resurfacing: results with a dynamically cooled millisecond domain 1320nm Nd:YAG laser. *Dermatol Surg.* 2002;28:172–176.

PART THREE DISCUSSION

Jeffrey S. Dover, MD, FRCPC, *Moderator*

Dr Dover: Those of you who were at this meeting in 2000 will notice a paradigm shift from what was presented last year to the conclusions reached this year. The consensus last year was that we did not know for sure whether nonablative resurfacing works. Five excellent presentations this year gave actual data showing the efficacy of nonablative techniques, which I think is impressive. The late plastic surgeon Joel Noe once said, "In God we trust, but from everyone else we want data." Now we actually have some data.

Mitchel P. Goldman, MD: I have 2 comments. First, I thought it was interesting that Dr Zelickson's patients improved with use of cryogen spray cooling and Dr Goldberg's patients did not. I am wondering whether the difference is related to a geographic phenomenon. Second, Dr Bjerring compared efficacy, using fluences of 2 to 3 J/cm^2 with the pulsed dye laser and 7 J/cm^2 with intense pulsed light (IPL), which are 400% less than what we use clinically. I believe that his study is fundamentally flawed in design.

David J. Goldberg, MD: I would like to address the cryogen issue first. I do not know what parameters Dr Zelickson used, but I suspect we probably used different cryogen parameters. There is nothing hocus-pocus about laser or light causing an injury in the dermis. There are many ways to do that. I would not be surprised if he used a greater cryogen spray than we did, and that may have made the difference in our results.

Brian D. Zelickson, MD: Our data were actually patients' subjective data, rather than clinical, objective data, which we do not yet have. We used a cryogen spray of 30 milliseconds with a delay of 20 milliseconds.

Dr Goldberg: We used different cryogen parameters.

Peter Bjerring, MD: In answer to the second question, we used quite different laser parameters. We used wavelengths of 520 to 750 nm, and our energy settings went up to the pain limit that the patients could tolerate. The energy levels used were adjusted to fit visible light and not infrared.

Dr Dover: Is there anything else that could explain the difference between these 2 types of pulsed dye laser? There is a dramatic difference in your data—traditional pulsed dye laser vs this fast uptake or fast-emission pulsed dye laser (NLite, ICN Pharmaceuticals, Costa Mesa, Calif). Could there be variations in the devices that would explain the difference in results, at least in the outcomes of the suction blisters in your study?

Dr Bjerring: I don't know whether there might be other differences except for light spectrum, energy levels, pulse durations, and pulse shapes. In our opinion, it seems to be important that the pulse duration is short and the energy is adjusted to be just below the limit for purpura. What we are aiming at is the biological end point, which is a transient purpura. In bright light, you can see purpura beginning just after the laser pulse and then disappearing again within a second.

Kenneth A. Arndt, MD: I have a question about the components of the pulsed dye laser. I wonder if we are comparing apples and oranges. We are discussing pulse duration of varying lengths, but within that pulse, there are subpulses. I think the pulse characteristics are different for each of these 3 instruments.

Emil A. Tanghetti, MD: I have a lot of experience with the PhotoGenica V-Star (Cynosure Inc, Chelmsford, Mass). Pulses longer than 0.5 milliseconds consist of 3 subpulses, and typically pulse forms are made up of three 200-microsecond pulses. For instance, there are 3 pulses within 40 milliseconds of treatment, so one is able to target small vessels by the subpulses; the large vessels see the 40 milliseconds. Likewise, as I understand it, with the Vbeam (Candela Corporation, Wayland, Mass), you have four 120-microsecond pulses buried within the 40-, 30-, and 20-millisecond pulse durations. Again, the pulses are made up of smaller pulses, so small vessels may see the smaller pulses, and I think the larger vessels may see the combination.

Dr Arndt: Is there a subset of the pulses within the NLite pulsed dye laser, and how is it different from the other 2 pulsed dye lasers? Are we talking about the micropulse or the macropulse?

R. Rox Anderson, MD: I agree that with short pulses, meaning less than 1 millisecond, the laser surgeon will be within the thermal relaxation time for many small vessels that are present throughout the tissue. I think it is probably not so much capillaries, but the postcapillary venules, where most of the cellular action is, where mediators are released, where the mast cells live, where T cells climb in and macrophages climb in and out of. Anatomically, the skin has its postcapillary venular plexus near the surface, in the lower portion of the papillary dermis. I think if you were going to guess at a vascular target that would be most involved in pulsed dye laser responses, it would probably be postcapillary venular plexus, and the vessels are fairly small. There are very good optical and thermal models that have been used to study all the various pulse durations and pulses within pulses, in an attempt to determine which combinations of these pulses will heat which vessels. However, I have not yet seen these studies correlated to either histologic or clinical results.

Dr Arndt: Dr Bjerring, are there pulses within your pulse, or is it a single pulse with the NLite?

Dr Bjerring: It emits a single pulse of 0.2 milliseconds.

Melanie C. Grossman, MD: I want to share a couple of observations I made using the Q-switched neodymium (Nd):YAG laser. I noticed early on that people who had collagen injections about 1 to 3 months before laser treatment seemed to get redness in the area of the injections; this outcome has now become almost predictive, in my experience. Redness develops in the nasolabial folds or under the mouth. Additionally, 1 of these patients reported to me that the results of her collagen injections now last longer, up to 12 months. The doctor who injected the collagen in this patient also noted the same result.

The other observation is that I have found old scars in patients undergoing treatment of wrinkles with the Q-switched Nd:YAG laser, and the scars became red after a few passes and then improved substantially. I have no explanation for this effect but wondered whether anybody else had seen it and if it has been seen with other wavelengths.

Roy Geronemus, MD: One of the things I showed with the 3-dimensional (3-D) optical skin imaging device (Primos, G. F. Messtechnik, Teltow, Germany) is that the scars do improve. I believe that the Q-switched Nd:YAG laser is one of the few laser devices available for the treatment of pitted scars. My experience with ablative resurfacing is that some of the pitted scars have actually worsened, although we are seeing substantial improvement with this nonablative technique. Any of the nonablative technologies I have used—and particularly the CoolTouch II (CoolTouch Corporation, Roseville, Calif), which has a larger spot size and the ability to deliver energy more consistently—work very well on scars. I have actually greatly reduced the amount of resurfacing I do for scar treatment and have switched over to the nonablative technologies for the treatment of scars.

Another thing I have noticed, which is also interesting, is that patients who undergo laser resurfacing first seem to have better results of nonablative procedures than do patients who had no prior resurfacing. This is an anecdotal report; we have not yet analyzed whether there is a benefit from resurfacing before nonablative rejuvenation.

Robert M. Adrian, MD: I am concerned that the benefits of nonablative resurfacing are being overstated. For example, beauty salons in my state now treat patrons using various nonablative machines, including the NLite, and tell their customers that with 1 or 2 treatments their wrinkles will go away within 4 to 6 months. We need to be very careful to confirm our data in independent studies, comparing 1 pulse duration with another. I commend Dr Geronemus on his objective data, because I think that photography is worthless in quantifying the results of any of these procedures. No matter how hard the photographer tries to have the parameters the same before and after the procedure, 1 slight difference in placement of the patient's face toward the camera, the time of day, lighting in the room, and so on, can make the patient look better or worse. It is important that we study the data and decide whether good results are based on luck or skill. We need to ask, is the rapid temporal rise 350-microsecond pulse the only way to go, or is 200, 250, or 450 microseconds a better approach? We should not overstate the benefits.

Dr Geronemus: I'm glad you brought up the topic. This has been a major problem. I think a fault in all of our presentations on nonablative techniques is that no one talked about side effects. Side effects can occur with each and every one of these devices, whether short-term purpura, long-term atrophic scars, or prolonged postinflammatory hyperpigmentation. These devices must be used properly, to minimize side effects. More complications of these devices are occurring in the hands of nonphysicians or untrained operators without supervision. The American Society for Dermatologic Surgery has a registry of reported complications, many of which are disfiguring and certainly distressing. My concern is that in the wrong hands, these wonderful devices may develop a bad reputation that ultimately could hurt all laser surgeons. I think it is important we ensure that people who are using these devices are appropriately trained and carefully monitored and that they understand how to use the device and, just as importantly, understand what they are treating.

Brian S. Biesman, MD: I also have been struggling with how to quantify these results in an objective way. I do not have the Primos 3-D system. One thing that we have not talked much about is, for those patients who do not seem to respond as well to treatment, why not? What do we need to do differently? Do we need to use a different wavelength or to change the fluence? My coworkers and I, like Dr Geronemus, studied changes in skin stiffness after laser treatment. Using a fluence-dependent model with the 810-nm diode laser, we found that in a certain range of fluences, skin stiffness increased, and then, somewhat inexplicably, above that level skin stiffness decreased. Dr Geronemus, did your skin stiffness data correlate with your 3-D photography findings in a direct fashion?

Dr Geronemus: We did not find a complete correlation. One of the concerns we have is the difference in results between men and women, and we are wondering if skin stiffness and compliance are the appropriate parameters. Perhaps we should be looking at it a bit differently. There were significant baseline differences between men and women, in which the men had much less skin stiffness and then showed dramatic changes over time, or where the difference in stiffness was less dramatic in women over multiple treatment sessions. Therefore, skin stiffness and compliance may not be the right parameters for them. Or perhaps we are dealing with other chromophores in men where you will see more of a change, particularly with the increased number of follicular apparati.

Roland Kaufmann, MD: Patients may complain about wrinkles that are invisible or hardly visible. It is, of course, very difficult to prove any visible improvement of this invisible disease. I am fascinated about Dr Geronemus' highly sophisticated techniques to make this visible, but the most fascinating thing is that the patients are so happy with skin photorejuvenation.

Lisa Kellett, MD: We have been using photorejuvenation for about 3 years now, and patients are very happy.

Dr Dover: What technique and device are you using?

Dr Kellett: We use IPL. We also offer a package, a combination of IPL, Q-switched Nd:YAG laser treatment, and microdermabrasion. In patients with postresurfacing erythema, we have routinely been using IPL, 550 and 570 nm filters, with very good results. Has anyone else recently been using photorejuvenation after resurfacing?

Robert A. Weiss, MD: Over the last 4 years we have seen approximately 25 patients for evaluation of prolonged, streaky erythema after carbon dioxide (CO_2) resurfacing, and IPL has worked very well in treating the erythema. In fact, we are preparing a manuscript to describe our findings.

Mark S. Nestor, MD, PhD: I have a comment related to the one made about collagen injections. I'm not too worried because the skin redness will go away. I am more concerned about patients who have had liquid injectable silicone before treatment with either IPL or the 1320-nm Nd:YAG (CoolTouch) laser and there has been some inflammatory change around the silicone. The immune effects may be causing some reaction pattern. We should thoroughly consider whether rejuvenation is indicated for patients who have had prior silicone injections.

I also want to mention combination procedures, which have not been talked about a lot here. With all the skin rejuvenation procedures, the CO_2 and erbium:YAG lasers, for instance, we are finding that combination procedures have better results than do either procedure alone for some patients. In my practice, I often use combinations of techniques, such as IPL and the CoolTouch Nd:YAG laser. We get wonderful results with both skin type I and II changes of photorejuvenation.

Richard E. Fitzpatrick, MD: I just wanted to make a comment regarding the pulse width of photorejuvenation using a pulsed dye laser. I do not think that the short pulse width could have any bearing on effects. In an ongoing study, my coworkers and I are comparing the long-pulse dye laser on half the face vs cryogen on the other side. At approximately 6 and 40 milliseconds, 3 laser treatments are given at 1-month intervals. Both the 6-millisecond and 40-millisecond pulse widths have produced significantly better results than cryotherapy at 3-month follow-up.

Christian Raulin, MD: Dr Bjerring, you had a great result in the patient with a full-face treatment. What were the exact parameters used in this patient? I have another question for the panel. After 1 year of treatment, what is the percentage of patients who recommend the treatment to others, and what is the percentage of who have complaints?

Dr Bjerring: I cannot answer your second question specifically, because we do not have enough data yet after 1 year. The special pulsed dye laser treatment is new. Some of our patients are choosing to return to us after about 9 months to have another treatment, so they must be happy. We have not had any long-term side effects or any complaints yet.

Whitney D. Tope, MPhil, MD: For those of you on the panel who have actually measured collagen production after these techniques, what is the longest date after treatment that you have tested collagen production? In other words, what is the duration of the effect that you can measure in collagen production? There is at least 1 study that has demonstrated recidivism of clinical improvement 6 months after treatment.

Dr Bjerring: We only measured the maximum rate of collagen production about 72 hours after treatment, so that is our end point so far.

Dr Tope: So the question remains: How long does this effect last?

Dr Bjerring: That is still to be answered.

A physician: Others have published a description of results 6 months after a fourth treatment, that is, roughly 10 months after the first treatment. Therefore, at least histologically, one can see evidence of the laser-induced injury long term.

Dr Tope: That is correct, but as mentioned earlier, we must continue to follow up these patients so we know better what the real duration of treatment is.

I have questions for Dr Geronemus. The Primos 3-D imaging and the biomechanical assessment of the skin are very impressive, but I think people were equally impressed with optical profilometry 4 or 5 years ago, and I see no one using that technique now. What do you think these 2 techniques are capable of? Are they difficult to perform and do they get reproducible results? Also, in the color infrared image (Fig 9-1) that showed depth of scarring in the skin, the blue areas, which were the deep areas if I am interpreting correctly, still look blue in the postoperative image. Were the scars still as deep as they were before treatment? Agreed, there was more yellow or superficial involvement of the scars, but the blue areas were still blue, and it is the deep scars about which my patients complain.

Dr Geronemus: That is an important observation. We do not remove all of the scars, nor do we promise that to our patients. However, if you look at that image again, there is less blue, and the blue areas are not as blue. There are more yellow and orange areas, which indicate more superficial involvement of the scars, as well as more uniformity. In terms of reliability of the device, particularly with the Primos 3-D system, we work with the Canfield photographic device with head mount to make sure the head is stabilized. I think we have been able to keep some standardization. Optical profilometry had problems with application of the topical substance and transferral of the substance so it is read somewhere else, and the molding would often crack and break. The 3-D imaging system appears much more reliable. We can actually ensure that we are imaging the exact spot as in the initial pretreatment photograph or image.

Dr Tope: I think it is important, however, to recognize that the data are only as good as what you put in. The 3-D imaging system is complicated to use; if the operator does not identically line up the images before and after treatment, you won't get anything out. On the other hand, if photography is really good, it can show some improvement. I disagree that photography is useless; it just depends on how well it is done. I think that if a professional photographer took the before and after photographs and the photographs were in a grid and the face wasn't positioned any differently, one would be able to see the improvement. I think there is a role for photography, and there is also a role for these other mechanical measurements.

Dr Geronemus: In terms of the long-term benefit of nonablative skin rejuvenation, I tell patients that we have turned back the clock but we are not turning off the clock. I tell them that they had better plan on some maintenance therapy and advise them to come back periodically for additional treatments.

Henry H. Chan, MD: I'm going to put some cold water on this topic and voice my concern regarding long-term complications of photorejuvenation. Although we protect the epidermis during photorejuvenation, we are actually delivering a large amount of energy to the dermis. The question I want to ask the panel is, Could that eventually lead to dermal aging or premature fibroblastic apoptosis? Are we inducing a sunbath phenomenon to our patients? The dangers of ultraviolet A (UV-A) radiation were not really detected until much later on. I'm not saying that we should *not* do nonablative skin rejuvenation, just that perhaps we should have a guideline limiting the number of treatments we should perform. What is the opinion of the panel?

Dr Goldberg: I think that is a question that ought to be raised. However, it reminds me a little of when people expressed concerns about whether laser treatment of congenital nevi could lead to melanoma and whether it is appropriate to treat children's port-wine stains for years and years. Physicians have performed laser removal of tattoos since approximately 1980, and concerns were raised about the safety of that treatment. They are fair questions, but the light source used for photorejuvenation is not UV-A. It's not x-rays and not UV-A. These systems are visible light or of the near infrared type.

Cyrus Chess, MD: I would like the panel to address 2 issues. The first is that it appears to me and from the photographs shown during the presentations that periocular rhytids are more effectively treated nonablatively than rhytids elsewhere on the face. I am curious whether that is everybody's opinion and, if so, why that would be.

Second, Dr Bjerring stated that when one compares the clinical results using the pulsed dye laser (NLite) with data in the literature about effectiveness of the CO_2 laser in reduction of wrinkles, the NLite allows 80% the effectiveness of CO_2 resurfacing. If I heard that correctly, I would like the panel or the people who spoke earlier who have great expertise in CO_2 resurfacing to say whether that is a valid and reliable conclusion.

Dr Bjerring: This analysis was comparing data from a 1996 study (Fitzpatrick RE, Goldman MP, Satur NM, Tope WD. Pulsed carbon dioxide laser resurfacing of photo-aged facial skin. *Arch Dermatol.* 1996;132:395–402) with the new data, using exactly the same scale of wrinkles. Of course, it was done by 2 independent research groups, but the data should be comparable.

Dr Weiss: Never say never, but for now, I think to use the data of ablative resurfacing to compare it with nonablative resurfacing is absurd. With all due respect, I think it hinders what we are trying to do with nonablative resurfacing.

Jean Carruthers, MD: I agree with all the comments being made about photography. I find that the best camera to photograph pigment or redness is the instant-picture camera (Polaroid). I have 2 different digital cameras, and the flash in each of them bleaches out pigment, wrinkles, and redness. The 35-mm photography also actually produces lovely photographs of wrinkles. The Canfield system, so the photographs are taken in the same room, with the same illumination, in which the patients have no makeup and are positioned exactly the same way every time, is time-consuming but really what we need to do for high-quality studies. I would like to make a plea for everybody to change the technique of photographing crow's feet. Rather than a before picture of just the crow's feet, I believe the corner of the mouth also should be shown. I would love to see photographs of crow's feet be a bit larger on the face.

Some interesting comments have been made about combined therapy. Canadian physicians enjoy the use of a couple more dermal fillers than are available in the United States. An excellent filler for type V acne-scarred skin is Artecoll, a microimplant composed of tiny acrylic beads suspended in a collagen vehicle that is injected subdermally. After injecting this filler, I use the 1320-nm Nd:YAG (CoolTouch) laser. That combination therapy has produced wonderful results. In addition, I have used IPL to reduce erythema after CO_2 resurfacing and have some photographs showing the beautiful results.

Dr Arndt: How does the laser surgeon choose what techniques to do? In patients undergoing partial-face resurfacing, many physicians may choose to perform one of a variety of photorejuvenation techniques after botulinum toxin (BOTOX) injections. There are now so many combination therapies, it is getting a little confusing as to what is rational and particularly what is the place of botulinum toxin in this spectrum of adjunctive procedures.

Dr Carruthers: I think that they are additive. Certainly, when we use the 1320-nm Nd:YAG laser (CoolTouch) around the eyes, we always inject botulinum toxin as well.

Dr Arndt: Then how do you evaluate the effects of the laser?

Dr Carruthers: One can use the laser first and then inject Botox to smooth out the residual wrinkles. But here is an interesting finding. I can do 6 treatments of the 1320-nm Nd:YAG laser in the periocular region, and she has exactly the same very thick, sausage-like rhytids while smiling that patients have after CO_2 resurfacing who have not received botulinum toxin injections. So I believe that with any resurfacing modality, if you do not do something to the expressive musculature under the skin, it is going to ruin the result, no matter how aggressive the treatment is and whether it is ablative or nonablative. I think that botulinum toxin injections with all types of resurfacing are a natural treatment combination.

ADDENDUM

Jo S. Bohannon, MD: One laser company claims that the success of its cosmetic results depends on where the collagen is deposited in the dermis—that deposition of collagen higher up is better. Comments, please?

R. Rox Anderson, MD: Dr. Bohannan just asked if there is any science behind this business about the anatomical depth of the thermal injury in the dermis and the final clinical result. Dr. Ross has studied that in some detail.

E. Victor Ross, Jr, MD: One critical consideration is where the peak temperature should be—in the papillary dermis, the deep reticular dermis, or the deep, deep reticular dermis, down to the fat? Nobody really knows. Another argument is whether one should use discrete chromophores or bulk heating with a water-based chromophore. Certainly the cosmetic results of nonablative rejuvenation have not been comparable to those obtained with traditional laser skin resurfacing using an erbium:YAG or carbon dioxide laser. My rationale for using a 1450-nm or 1320-nm laser is that if the parameters are manipulated correctly, one can heat probably about 300 µm deep in the dermis. That is where the solar elastosis is on dermatopathologic slides stained with hematoxylin-eosin, so that is what one should heat. What has not been shown is that if that layer is heated, with very high temperatures or gentle heating, whether the patient obtains the same type of cosmetic improvement possible with more traditional, top-to-bottom laser skin resurfacing. So far, I would have to say no. However, I do not think it makes sense to heat really deep in the dermis, such as 1 mm down. We know from pigskin experiments that we conducted using the erbium:YAG laser, in which we overcooled the skin and heated very deep, that we produced only pitted scars or no change. Therefore, I don't think it is advisable to heat that deep. I also do not think one should heat too close to the dermal-epidermal junction, because it basically challenges the cooling device too much. The area of 200 to 500 µm is somewhat safe, and it might be somewhat effective.

Roy Geronemus, MD: I do not think we know the answer to the question about the deposition of collagen or changing collagen in different levels of the dermis. These claims being made by the laser companies are strictly conjecture. My coworkers and I have tried to affect different levels of the dermis using a combination of 2 lasers. With the use of the 1320-nm neodymium:YAG laser, we cool before treatment and a second pass after treatment, so there is no cooling until after the second pass with the cooling device, after the laser has been admitted. Then we follow through with a different technique with a different laser, theorizing that we are reaching different levels of the dermis with collagen deposition. We are seeing a large degree of patient satisfaction.

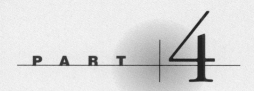

Novel Approaches to Skin Rejuvenation (Excluding Photorejuvenation)

chapter 14

A Novel Radiofrequency Technology

Michael S. Kaminer, MD

An investigational new radiofrequency device (ThermaCool, Thermage, Hayward, Calif) has been cleared by the Food and Drug Administration (FDA) for nonablative skin rejuvenation. Radiofrequency is the delivery of electrical energy. This device is not a laser. Animal and in vitro studies have been completed and clinical trials are in progress, but the device is not yet commercially available. I have used the device and will describe it.

The concept of using electrical energy on the skin is not new. Other radiofrequency devices have been used over the years. A Bovie, for example, is a radiofrequency device used for electrocautery. The Visage ablative electrosurgical device (ArthroCare Corp, Sunnyvale, Calif) is an ablative use of this similar concept, of using electrical energy for destruction. The ThermaCool device is a different approach, however—a nonablative approach.

VOLUMETRIC TISSUE HEATING

Radiofrequency works very differently from lasers (Table 14-1). The biggest difference is the concept of volumetric tissue heating. Whereas a laser selectively heats a target, this radiofrequency technology heats an entire environment. Like some lasers, simultaneous contact cooling is an important part of this device.

TABLE 14.1

Comparison of Laser and Radiofrequency (ThermaCool) Devices

Parameter	Laser	ThermaCool
Energy source	Light	Electricity
Mechanism of action	Heat	Heat
Efficacy	Target driven	Volumetric
Easy-to-understand physics	No	No

When electricity is delivered to tissue, the tissue will generate heat based on the resistance of tissue to electron movement (Ohm's law) instead of photon absorption, as with lasers. Ohm's law involves the concept of impedance. Impedance (R = ohms, or Ω) to the movement of charged particles creates heat relative to the amount of current (I = amperes) and time (t). The formula derived is as follows: Energy (in joules) = $I^2 \times R \times t$.

One can create heat with a laser, by heating a target and using thermal relaxation times, or one can create heat by moving electrons through it, and the resistance to tissue then creates heat in a given location. The advantage of the radiofrequency concept is that the operator can control how much energy to deliver. The operator can control depth and intensity of energy delivery.

In theory, with modification of some of the technology, the operator can deliver energy in smaller or bigger areas, higher or deeper in the dermis.

POTENTIAL CLINICAL TARGETS

Numerous clinical targets are possible, including skin (epidermis, papillary dermis, and reticular dermis), fat, perhaps cellulite, and wrinkles.

It is possible that this radiofrequency device can be used to target structures that lasers cannot reach. It has the potential to distribute joules in deeper dermis. The operator does not necessarily need to target a particular structure; he or she can target its environment as well.

A comparison of laser and this radiofrequency technology is given in Table 14-1. The physics of both technologies are not easy to understand. It will take some time for clinicians to get used to how this radiofrequency device works and to completely understand what the science is, as well as for the technology to evolve and improve. Currently, the ThermaCool device is a promising non-ablative treatment option, potentially with efficacy beyond rejuvenation. More clinical work is needed to confirm efficacy and safety for numerous clinical targets and to establish a definitive mechanism of action.

Dr Kaminer is a member of the Thermage Scientific Advisory Board, Hayward, Calif.

chapter 15

A New Nonablative Radiofrequency Device: Preliminary Results

Suzanne L. Kilmer, MD

The ThermaCool radiofrequency (RF) device (Thermage, Hayward, Calif) is the only nonablative device I am aware of that does not use photons. It is a volumetric way to heat up tissue. The operator will be able to put heat into the dermis, or hopefully any other area, and still have sparing of the epidermis. The technology is still in the rudimentary stages but has progressed since the original ThermaCool device was made (Fig 15-1). It is 510(k) approved by the Food and Drug Administration (FDA), but it is not yet commercially available, because the company continues to refine it.

COOLING

Parallel contact cooling makes this device very different from the previous RF devices. The cooling comes from within this device. A cryogen spray goes onto the plate, which is then placed on the skin to cool the epidermis (Fig 15-2). There is precooling, cooling during the treatment, and postcooling. The device provides gradations of cooling, with the skin coolest at the surface and not as cool as the heat is deposited deeper. By varying the cooling times, the heating times, the electrodes, and all the different settings, the operator can change the schematic tremendously (Fig 15-3). There is great potential for changing the settings and figuring out what to target. A thermographic photograph shows the cooling at the surface, and the heating below in the dermis (Fig 15-4).

ANIMAL STUDIES

Ross and coworkers conducted the initial animal studies of this RF device in guinea pigs, and they found some initial contraction that was probably muscle contraction. Measurements of the treated area obtained 2 to 4 weeks after application of the RF device showed a residual 5% to 10% contraction of tissue.

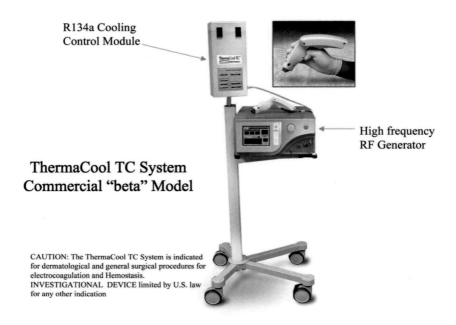

R134a Cooling
Control Module

High frequency
RF Generator

ThermaCool TC System
Commercial "beta" Model

CAUTION: The ThermaCool TC System is indicated
for dermatological and general surgical procedures for
electrocoagulation and Hemostasis.
INVESTIGATIONAL DEVICE limited by U.S. law
for any other indication

FIGURE 15.1

Photograph of original ThermaCool radiofrequency device. (Note: The American Medical Association does not endorse or recommend any particular type or brand of high frequency radiofrequency device.)

Histologic analysis demonstrated thermal damage, activated fibroblasts, and some collagen remodeling. Fat lysis was present, but there were some cases of epidermal loss.

CLINICAL TRIALS

To test the safety of the RF device in humans, I used it to treat an area of skin that was scheduled for excision in patients undergoing abdominoplasty (unpublished data, 2000 to 2001). I tested different conservative doses and performed follow-up for up to 2 months after treatment. We did not see skin contraction,

ThermaCool heating/cooling schematic

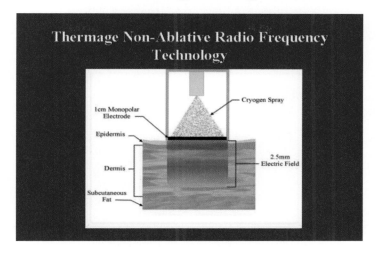

FIGURE 15.2
Schematic of ThermaCool's cryogen spray cooling.

Reverse Thermal Gradient Depiction

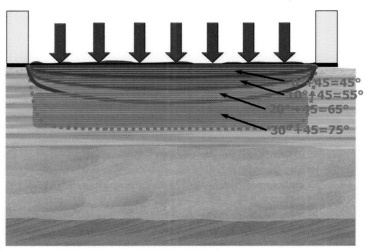

FIGURE 15.3
Depiction of reverse thermal gradient.

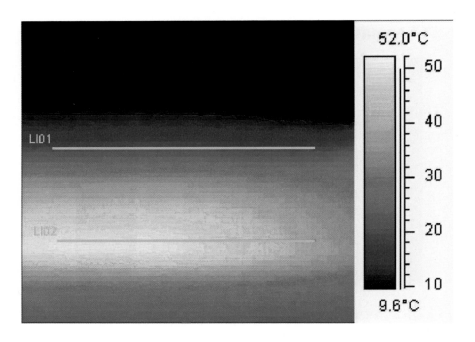

FIGURE 15.4

Thermographic photograph shows cooling at top layer of skin (blue areas) and heating below (red and orange areas) with ThermaCool device.

probably because we used lower doses. There were some collagen changes, and there was inconsistent fibroblast activity, again probably related to the dose. We had a very low burn rate, but we did have some "edge effects," or small burns at the edges of the electrode. Radiofrequency is a little unusual in that it does have an edge effect, but the researchers are working on improving that. Erythema was present immediately after treatment and to some extent 24 hours later (Fig 15-5). However, 7 days after treatment, the skin had healed, and at 3 weeks after treatment, there was no residual erythema left (Fig 15-5), and histologic analysis

Immediate post TX   **24 hours post TX**

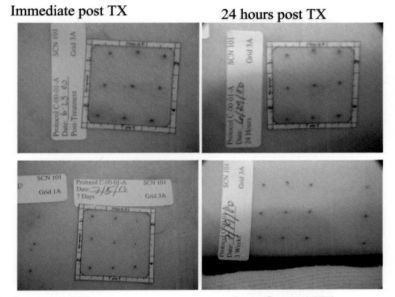

7 days post TX   **3 weeks post TX**

FIGURE   15.5

Radio frequency treatment sites viewed at four post-treatment times.

revealed increased epidermal thickness, increased fibroblasts, and probably some thickening and changes in the collagen.

Another subject was treated in the submental area and had skin tightening (Fig 15-6).

A multicenter clinical trial is ongoing to study the efficacy of the RF device for tightening of periorbital skin. Clinical trials also are planned for evaluation of efficacy in skin tightening in other areas, submental reduction, wrinkle reduction, and treatment of acne scarring. I think this new technology holds possibilities for being able to remove fat and cellulite, remodel scars, and treat striae. More research is needed before the potential of the ThermaCool device is fully known.

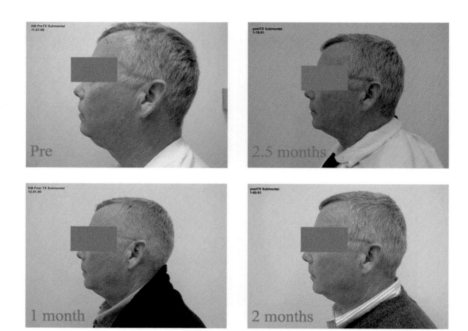

FIGURE 15.6

Skin tightening at the submantal area after radio frequency device treatments.

Dr Kilmer is a member of the Thermage Scientific Advisory Board, Hayward, Calif, and received research grant support from the company.

Volumetric Heating of Skin Using Radiofrequency: Preliminary Findings

Javier Ruiz-Esparza, MD

I am one of the coprincipal investigators of a new radiofrequency technology, which I refer to as radiodermoplasty. My coworker is Julio Manuel Barba Gomez, MD, in Guadalajara, Mexico. I will present the preliminary clinical findings in a few selected patients.

There are 2 probable mechanisms of action that are hypothesized for radiodermoplasty: (1) dermal tightening, which we can use as a lifting force for eyebrows, the submental region, face, and breasts; or (2) dermal remodeling, to improve the surface of the skin, such as in wrinkles, stretch marks, or acne scars.

SUBJECTS AND METHODS

We initiated a clinical study of a novel radiofrequency device, which uses volumetric tissue heating (ThermaCool, Thermage, Hayward, Calif). A total of 96 subjects were entered in the study at monthly intervals in groups of approximately 15 to 20, so that we could vary the parameters depending on what our findings were. All skin types and both sexes were represented in the study population, and the age of subjects ranged from the second to the seventh decade. A formal protocol with approval from 2 separate ethics committees was followed. Appropriate informed consent was obtained from all study subjects.

The procedure was performed in most subjects using topical anesthesia. In the first group (n =17), the treatment goal was to establish safe doses with some evidence of efficacy. Targeted treatment areas were those considered the safest in the face and neck for the intended degree of tissue heating. Treatment areas included preauricular skin, the temporal area along the hairline, the submental region, and, in a very limited fashion, the outer canthal areas. The energies used were in the lower end of the energy delivery capabilities of the device. In other words, higher energies are possible with this technology. Precooling times were long, in an attempt to minimize the risk of epidermal burns. Monopolar and bipolar electroplates with different depths of heat delivery were tried (deep dermis, subcutaneous fat, and superficial dermis).

The technique of electroplate application to the targeted skin was refined over time. In the first group, a freehand delivery approach was used. In the second group, we used a more precise pattern of delivery to a target treatment area—a grid marking system. Squares were drawn on the intended treatment areas and numbered, and the energy and cooling times were recorded for all treatment squares, in an attempt to identify the variables that could explain any positive or negative results of efficacy and safety. A 16-week follow-up is available for the first and second groups.

RESULTS

A woman in the first treatment group, who received an eyebrow lift, was treated with radiodermoplasty in the temporal area along the hairline. By treating the temporal regions, we modified the arch of the eyebrow. A month after treatment, the tarsal crease appeared less deep, and the rhytids in the outer canthi were softened (Fig 16-1).

Results of lifting of loose skin in the submental region showed only a modest improvement in skin tone (Fig 16-2). Contour improvement was not as impressive as that seen with submental liposuction.

We performed full-face treatments, to see whether we could do a similar procedure to a face-lift but without incisions. Tissue tightening was observed in 2 of 5 subjects. One subject is shown 16 weeks after 3 procedures in Figure 16-3.

We treated the upper side of the breast along with the pectoral area, to determine whether contraction of that skin would bring some lifting of the breast. In the first person we treated, we treated only the right breast and kept the left as a control. There was a slight modification of the shape of the breast (Fig 16-4).

For treatment of wrinkles, we have had mixed results using radiodermoplasty. When we used very high energies, we shrunk the skin, and the wrinkles appeared more prominent in the short term. Then there was a late phase during which we saw some improvement. Therefore, we are not sure how useful the technique is for this indication. We are working on new treatment algorithms using less energy and more treatment sessions. We are also treating only the skin above the lateral canthus.

While treating a subject for facial lines, we noticed that his acne scars improved, so we selectively treated the acne scars in another subject. We have had very good early results both with ice-pick scars (Fig 16-5) and "rolling hill" scars (Fig 16-6).

Then we tried the technology on striae distensae. The subjective improvement of all treated subjects has been favorable. Photographic documentation of improvements has been difficult, but objective improvement can be seen when contrasted with untreated areas (Fig 16-7).

In the nearly 100 individuals treated with the radiofrequency device, there has been no downtime and a low incidence of complications. An edge effect was ob-

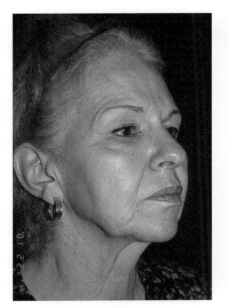 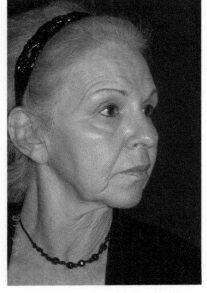

Rt side Pre-op   One month after one session

FIGURE 16.1

Before (left) and 1 month after (right) eyebrow lift using non-ablative radiofrequency on temporal and frontal skin along hairline.

served after radiodermoplasty, but it went away within 3 weeks, and the burns were small and manageable (Fig 16-8). Patient acceptance was extremely high.

COMMENT

Although patient satisfaction with this radiofrequency device was very high, there was a small amount of bias, because subjects participated in clinical trials and were not charged for the procedure. The improvement was modest and best noticed when preoperative and postoperative photographs were compared.

This technology is still evolving, and much remains to be defined regarding the optimal combination of parameters, tissue response, technique, frequency, and number of treatments. We believe we initially used a suboptimal radiofrequency energy. The effect of radiodermoplasty awaits further evaluation with good therapeutic doses and longer (6-month) follow-up. Additionally, we plan to perform a blinded evaluation. With the process of administering repeated treatments to many of these subjects, we expect results to improve, as they do with laser. More data are needed to establish the reproducibility of clinical results.

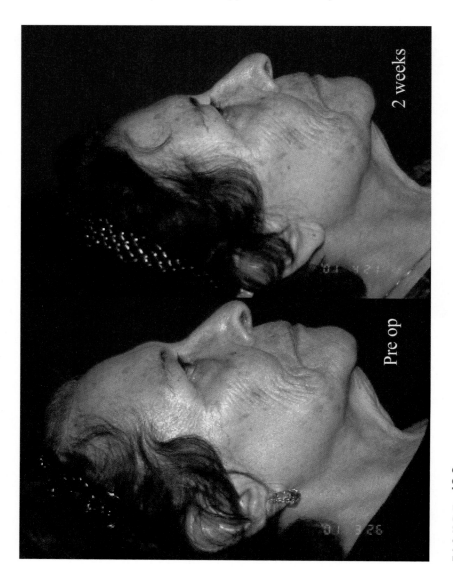

FIGURE 16.2

Before (left) and 2 weeks after (right) after non-ablative radiofrequency on the submental area.

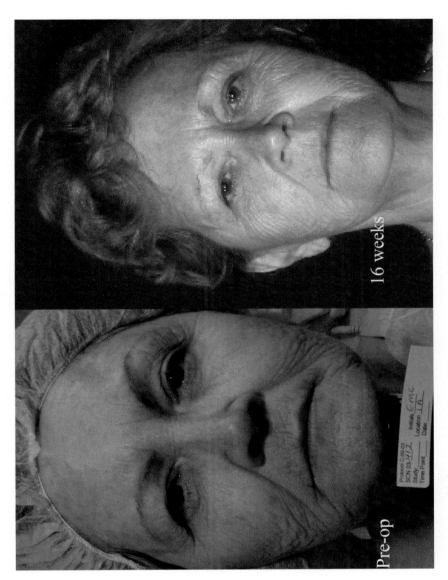

FIGURE 16.3

Before (left) and 16 weeks after (right) full-face radiodermoplasty in 3 stages.

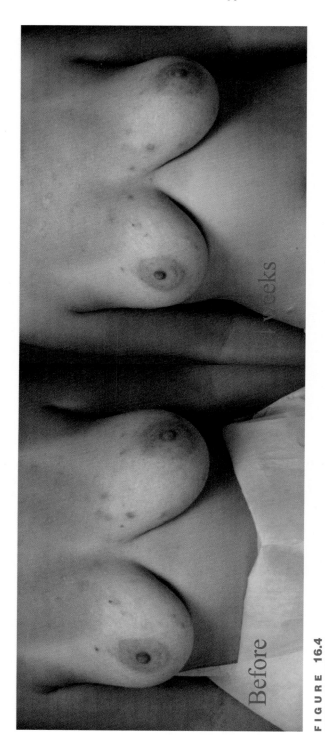

FIGURE 16.4

Radiofrequency for breast lift and contouring. right breast was treated. Left breast: control.

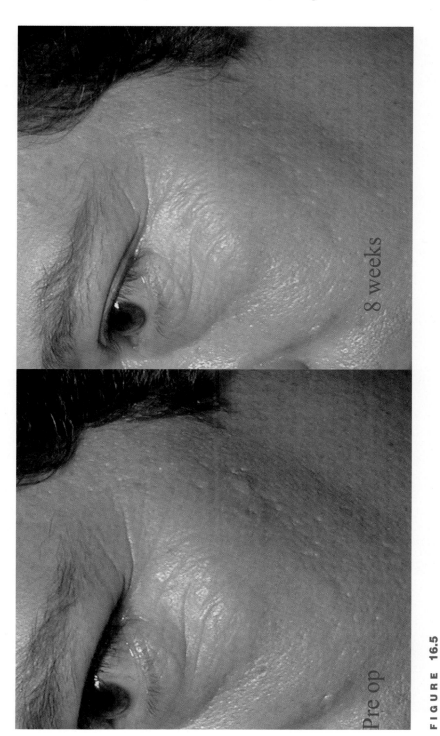

FIGURE 16.5

Ice-pick scars before (left) and 8 weeks after treatment (right) with non-ablative radiofrequency.

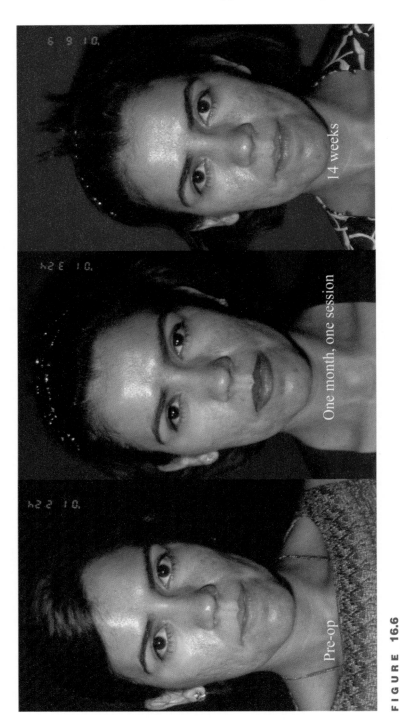

FIGURE 16.6

Acne scars on cheeks after 1 month and 14 weeks after radiodermoplasty (1 treatment session on right cheek and 2 treatment sessions on left).

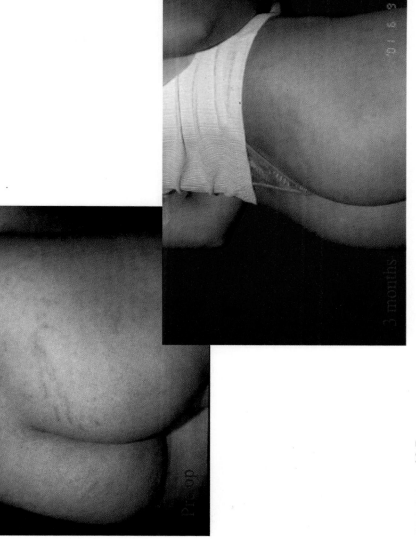

FIGURE 16.7

Red striae distensae pre-operatively and 3 months after treatment using radiodermoplasty.

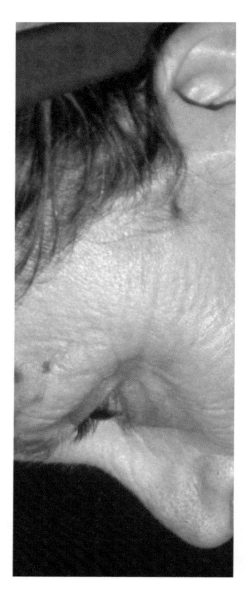

FIGURE 16.8

Only minor complications: Superficial focal burn on tail of eyebrow.

chapter 17

Nonlaser Methods for Dermal Therapy

Jerome M. Garden, MD

The use of radiofrequency to heat tissue for medical applications is not new. I have not used the ThermaCool radiofrequency device (Thermage, Hayward, Calif), which is under investigation. However, from my review of the company's product literature, it appears that the manufacturer is trying to control the flow of electrons per unit time (current).

RADIOFREQUENCY VS MICROWAVE

This technology differs from microwave, which involves an introduction of electromagnetic radiation, with the ability to select out different structures within the skin due to dielectric property differences. Hair shafts seemed to absorb microwaves much better than the surrounding connective tissue area, so there was some science behind it. It is the only system I have ever used that treated white hairs (unpublished observations, 1999). Unfortunately, a microwave system is very difficult to control.

Advances in radiofrequency technologies have been made. Years ago, I would never have thought that the Bovie cautery one day would be able to be used in a nonablative type of process, but, indeed, it seems that researchers have been trying to control this energy.

The images of the ThermaCool device shown in Chapter 15 show sufficient cooling of the top layers, and yet there is still volumetric tissue heating; the whole area is being heated. There may be some differences with the flow of electrons between some structures and others. The science still is not totally understood.

A WORD OF CAUTION

My hope is that the new device will be introduced in a safe and slow way. I am concerned that if the development of this technology is pushed forward too quickly, safety cannot be ensured and we will run into the same issues as encountered with other systems, such as the microwave systems. Whether or not the developers of this radiofrequency device will be able to surmount these problems that the microwave systems had remains to be seen. I hope that it works, because if the developers are able to control this device, the ThermaCool device will be another system for us to use for skin rejuvenation, which may be even better than what we have today.

PART FOUR DISCUSSION

Kenneth A. Arndt, MD, *Moderator*

Dr Arndt: Last year we talked about photorejuvenation, and we had no data. This year was exciting because we have data about many systems.

Roland Kaufmann, MD: Could you provide some information about the fluences, energy densities, and depth of energy delivery using the radiofrequency device?

Javier Ruiz-Esparza, MD: The fluences have been in the range of 75 J up to 250 J for a single session. We can vary the depth, to the papillary dermis, for example, for treatment of superficial processes such as the *striae distensae* and to middermis for treatment of wrinkle lines, acne scars, and fat. We have treated a few cases of cellulite and have not seen any clinical changes, so I am not convinced yet that we have the right parameters for cellulite. The beauty of this technology, however, is that one can choose the level of the skin to be treated.

Dr Kaufmann: With deeper delivery of energy did you, by chance, observe loss of blond hair as a side effect?

Dr Ruiz-Esparza: We have not seen that. The hair continues to grow, but follow-up has been only 4 or 5 months.

Michael S. Kaminer, MD: At this meeting, laser technology is discussed by a group of several hundred experts who still have not quite got everything figured out. Yet everybody here would agree that lasers hold great promise, and how one harnesses the technology is as important as the technology itself. Likewise, I think it is important to acknowledge that this radiofrequency technology is perhaps only a year old, and there is a lot that is yet to be figured out, but it is very promising. What is interesting about this new technology is that the operator can deliver heat and move it up, down, and sideways; can change its shape; can deliver as much energy as desired; and can cool deep or cool less. All that can be done. We can state that unequivocally. The only question that now remains is how does one harness that technology? Where does one decide to put the energy, and when one puts it there, what is it going to do? The first variable must be safety. The second variable is efficacy, and that is not yet fully known. What we do know is that we can make this technology move around the way that we want it to in 3 dimensions. That is an amazing feat, given all the troubles that have arisen with some other technologies over the years.

Harvey H. Jay, MD: If the basic heat generation is from resistance and one is dealing with different structures, different composition, completely different conductivity, why are you saying that you are dealing with just a volume area? There really should be completely different heat generation in different structures.

Suzanne L. Kilmer, MD: You bring up a good point, in that the device is not as easy for us to control as we like, because we are still learning about this technology. When we performed the first clinical trials, just the amount of anesthesia in the area mattered, hydration vs no hydration, whether we used a eutectic mixture of lidocaine and prilocaine (EMLA), and whether there were sebaceous glands and hair follicles. There are lots of parameters that we are still refining. One of my patients had a burn on her forehead, and that was partly because of the way the device was controlled; it was a feedback mechanism, an impedance-controlled mechanism.

There may be ways that we can manipulate this device so that we can target sebaceous glands or other appendages. Right now, however, this technology is sort of a black box, if you will, an unknown in that we are trying to figure out how to make it work better.

Dr Jay: That makes a lot of sense, but I think the concept of volumetric heating as a uniform temperature does not seem to hold.

Dr Kaminer: It is important to distinguish between volumetric and uniform. Volumetric heating simply means that an area can be heated. There may or may not be differences between the temperatures relative to the hair follicle or around blood vessels. We don't know. But the term *volumetric* does not mean that everything is heated uniformly and one gets the same exact energy delivery with the same exact microheating. Those are the variables that we do not know yet. Volumetric heating means one can heat a given area of tissue. Volumetric heating is not determined specifically by how an area absorbs energy using a chromophore, as do lasers. We are bulk heating something, and how tissue absorbs heat and what happens in that area are what we are trying to learn.

Dr Jay: I still do not follow that concept, because the term *volumetric* sounds as if one is heating a specific volume. Even when using a laser or light, a physician is treating a certain volume. I think the term *volumetric* probably needs to change.

R. Rox Anderson, MD: I used to be an electrical engineer. I think there are some simple ways to think about this concept that might be helpful. The energy is deposited at sites where the product of the square of the current (I^2) multiplied by the impedance is the highest. In the skin, this current passes around and always tries to take the path of least resistance. The thing that dominantly controls the impedance of the tissue is the freedom with which charges can move. So the easier that charges can move, the lower the resistance, or impedance, is. That is pretty much where water and electrolytes are. That is what is carrying the current, these little sodium and chloride ions that were made in an aqueous environment. Thus, the major sites where there is high impedance are where lipid is located. The skin is pretty much wet everywhere with the exception of where there is lipid. Lipid is in the sebaceous glands, which are middermal structures, and also in the subcutaneous fat.

My point is that there is a big difference in where this energy gets deposited whether things are in series or in parallel. This is unproven, but I believe the sebaceous glands are high-impedance structures that are in parallel with the rest of the dermis between them, and the current will flow around them. Therefore, I would not expect to see selective injury of sebaceous glands with this device. This is just a guess from a former electrical engineer. It is exactly the opposite in the subcutaneous fat. If one forces the current to go through an entire layer that is made out of mostly lipid, that entire layer has high impedance compared with the dermis, and so I would expect to see more heating where the impedance is high. What will come out of study of this new technology, I hope, is a lot of knowledge about how to control the current paths to force them to go through lipid-rich structures when those are the targets, or through some aqueous area of the tissue. I would expect to see large differences between lipid-rich and lipid-poor structures, and that, in the long run, will be one of the things that will differentiate radiofrequency from other technologies. It is very exciting, because no other tools are available now that act this way in clinical practice.

Richard E. Fitzpatrick, MD: In a parallel circuit, particularly if one envisions these little lipid-rich structures as being small resistors in a parallel circuit, I^2 will always favor the high-current area as far as the heat generation. Therefore, those areas will subsequently be relatively spared. Animal studies of radiofrequency were performed in guinea pigs, which have a broad band of fat at the base of the dermis. With the electrodes, we forced a series circuit because of the geometry involved, and we saw that fat was considerably more damaged than the upper part of the dermis and even the tissue below that. Clearly in that situation, the fat was acting in a series-type circuit and getting very high heat. However, as we have seen in humans so far, I think—I do not have all the evidence that the panelists do—there is relative sparing. So it depends largely on how you envision that circuitry. Just go back to Kirchoff laws when you were in college and high school and how you envision how the circuitry is going to go.

I think that *volumetric heating* is a good term. For most purposes, it is mostly water through the dermis. If you argue that radiofrequency is not volumetric heating, one could make the same argument for the 1320-nm neodymium:YAG laser (CoolTouch II, CoolTouch Corporation, Roseville, Calif) or the diode 1450-nm laser (Smoothbeam, Candela Corporation, Wayland, Mass). I would say those lasers use volumetric heating, too. We are certainly sparing small areas where there is no water, but the dermis is still 80% or 90% water. Yes, there are small foci where there is not going to be heating, but I think overall heating is fairly volumetric and fairly even.

PART 5

How Have Millisecond-Domain Lasers Changed the Approach to Treatment of Vascular Anomalies and Ectasias?

Improved Results in the Treatment of Facial Vascular Lesions Using Millisecond-Duration Lasers

Arielle N. B. Kauvar, MD

The introduction of millisecond-duration laser pulses has greatly improved the way we treat cutaneous vascular lesions. The 450-microsecond pulsed dye laser set the standard for the industry, with dramatic improvement in capillary vascular malformations as well as other cutaneous vascular lesions. However, the laser produced a dramatic, intense, blue-black purpura from hemorrhage and delayed vasculitis that would last 10 to 14 days. In addition, the 450-microsecond laser was relatively ineffective for treatment of larger diameter vessels. Based on a report by Dierickx et al[1] several years ago, it appeared that pulse durations in the 1- to 10-millisecond range were more ideally suited to the treatment of port-wine stains, and pulse durations of 10 milliseconds or greater were better suited to the treatment of telangiectasia. In more recent years, a wide variety of laser technologies has been developed for the treatment of vascular lesions. This new technology includes not only longer pulse durations but also the addition of longer wavelengths, higher fluences, and skin cooling.

PURPURA

It is difficult to separate out the effect of lengthening of the pulse durations alone, since many other laser parameters have changed as well. Longer pulse durations are necessary for the uniform heating of larger vessels and for decreased purpura. Compared with the intense blue-black purpura observed after treatment with a 0.45-millisecond pulsed dye laser, the purpura observed with a 1.5-millisecond pulsed dye laser is less intense and shorter-lived With the addition of cryogen spray cooling, there is a further reduction in purpura (Fig 18-1). In a study by Kauvar et al[2], side-by-side comparison of a 1.5-millisecond pulsed dye laser using a 7-mm spot and a fluence of 7 J/cm^2 with cryogen spray cooling demonstrated a reduction in purpura and other side effects. Complete healing took place in 5 days, compared with 9 days without the cryogen cooling.

PORT-WINE STAIN AND HEMANGIOMA TREATMENT

Using 1.5-millisecond, 595-nm pulsed dye laser in combination with higher fluences and cryogen spray cooling, Kauvar et al[3] have been able to achieve improved clearance of port-wine stains. We performed a prospective study comparing fluences greater than 10 J/cm^2, in which one half of the lesion was treated at 12 to 14 J/cm^2 and the other half at 10 J/cm^2. Better clearance with eradication of hypertrophic vascular blebs was achieved compared with cryogen cooling after

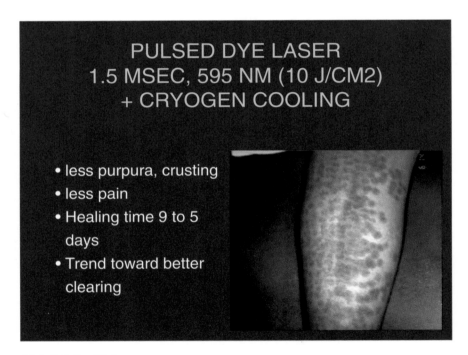

PULSED DYE LASER
1.5 MSEC, 595 NM (10 J/CM2)
+ CRYOGEN COOLING

- less purpura, crusting
- less pain
- Healing time 9 to 5 days
- Trend toward better clearing

FIGURE   18.1

Side-by-side treatment with 1.5-millisecond pulsed dye laser with and without cryogen cooling shows decreased purpura and edema on cryogen-treated side. *Source:* Kauver ANB et al. The effect of cryogen spray cooling on pulsed dye laser treatment of vascular lesions. *Lasers Surg Med.* 1998 (suppl 10):211. Coypright John Wiley & Sons. Reprinted with permission of Wiley-Liss, Inc., a subsidiary of John Wiley & Sons, Inc.

just 3 treatment sessions. The 1.5-millisecond, 595-nm laser at high fluences can also be used to achieve improved clearance, compared with historical controls, in superficial and mixed-type hemangiomas after 3 treatment sessions.

In another study, published in the *Archives of Dermatology* last year, we used the 1.5-millisecond pulsed dye laser at high fluence, with a wavelength of 595 nm, in conjunction with cryogen spray cooling.[4] Compared with historical controls, there was greater clearance of port-wine stains in an infant population using these parameters. On average, we achieved greater than 75% clearance of lesions after 3 to 4 treatment sessions.

A dose-response study performed by Geronemus and Lou[5] used exposures of 1.5 to 40 milliseconds on a new variable-pulse-duration dye laser that is available with a fixed wavelength of 595 nm. This study demonstrated that purpura was necessary to achieve clearance of port-wine stains. The combination of a 10-millisecond pulse duration and a fluence of 10 J/cm^2 produced moderate purpura and good clearance of lesions. With the use of longer pulse durations that precluded the development of purpura, clearance of lesions was poor. Some presence of purpura also appears to be necessary for the clearance of discrete linear or arborizing facial telangiectasia.

PULSE DURATION

In collaboration with Kist and Zelickson,[6] we have been using confocal microscopy. Earlier this year the preliminary results were presented of a study to investigate the effect of pulse duration on pulsed dye laser treatment of port-wine stains. We have data only from several histologic samples and 1 patient with a hypertrophic port-wine stain. It appeared that we achieved better clearance of port-wine stain vessels at 10 milliseconds than at shorter pulse durations of 0.45 and 1.5 milliseconds. Histologic analysis demonstrated that after treatment with the high-fluence, short-pulse duration parameters, we produced what we termed cluster reangiogenesis, the replacement of large ectatic vessels with numerous small-diameter blood vessels. This reangiogenesis may contribute to the appearance of persistent erythema in these patients. We also showed that there was decreased perivascular innervation in unheated port-wine stains compared with normal skin, and that there was increased perivascular innervation after treatment, particularly with the longer pulse durations. Further studies are required to corroborate these findings.

FACIAL TELANGIECTASIA AND POIKILODERMA OF CIVATTE

There are multiple systems with millisecond pulse durations that can be used to treat without purpura. The 532 potassium-titanyl-phosphate (KTP) laser, using millisecond pulse durations, is an excellent modality for the treatment of linear or arborizing telangiectasia. The intense pulsed light (IPL) source can treat poikiloderma and facial erythema.[7] We use a pulsed dye laser with nonpurpuric pulse durations of 6 to 10 milliseconds to treat facial erythema associated with rosacea or poikiloderma of Civatte. We are investigating a long-pulse neodymium (Nd):YAG laser at 1064 nm for the treatment of facial telangiectasia. Using pulse durations of 10 to 30 milliseconds, we can achieve purpura-free treatment of facial telangiectasia (Fig 18-2).

Multiple wavelengths can now be used with millisecond pulse durations to provide purpura-free treatment with the laser. A 14-year-old patient with a history of an extensive mixed capillary/cavernous hemangioma had multiple venulectasias and telangiectasia remaining following regression. She was treated at 1064 nm for the blue veins, 532 nm for the red telangiectases, and a pulsed dye laser at 6 milliseconds for the background erythematous scars. There was no purpura after treatment, and after 3 treatment sessions, she had excellent clearance of the lesions.

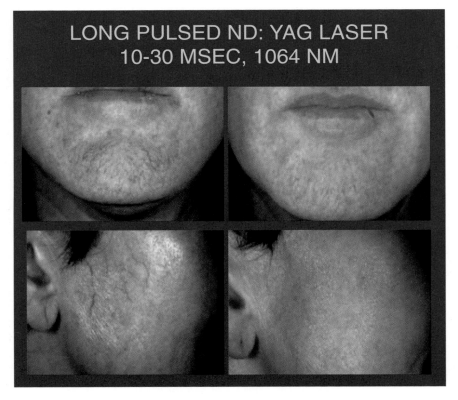

FIGURE 18.2

Small, fine, red, discrete telangiectasia before (left) and 1 month after (right) 1 treatment with 1064-nm long-pulse neodymium:YAG laser using pulse durations of 10 to 30 milliseconds.

In summary, the advantages of millisecond pulse durations are decreased or no purpura; faster recovery; and improved clearance of papillary vascular malformations, telangiectasia, and venulectasia.

REFERENCES

1. Dierickx CC, Casparian JM, Venugopalan V, Farinelli WA, Anderson RR. Thermal relaxation of port-wine stain vessels probed in vivo: the need for 1-10-millisecond laser pulse treatment. *J Invest Dermatol.* 1995;105:709–714.
2. Kauvar ANB, Grossman MC, Bernstein LJ, Kovacs SO, Quintana AT, Geronemus RG. The effect of cryogen spray cooling on pulsed dye laser treatment of vascular lesions [abstract]. *Lasers Surg Med.* 1998(suppl 10):211.
3. Kauvar ANB, Lou WW, Zelickson B. Effect of cryogen cooling on 595 nm, 1.5 msec pulsed dye laser treatment of port-wine stains [abstract]. *Lasers Surg Med.* 2000(suppl 12):24.
4. Geronemus RG, Quintana AT, Lou WW, Kauvar AN. High-fluence modified pulsed dye laser photocoagulation with dynamic cooling of port-wine stains in infancy. *Arch Dermatol.* 2000;136:942–943.
5. Geronemus RG, Lou WW. Treatment of port-wine stains by variable pulse width pulsed dye laser with cryogen spray: a preliminary study. *Dermatol Surg.* 2001;27:903–905.
6. Kauvar ANB, Kist D, Friedman P, Geronemus RG, Zelickson B. Confocal microscopic study examining the effect of wavelength pulse duration and fluence in laser treatment of port-wine stains [abstract]. *Lasers Surg Med.* 2001(suppl 13):26.
7. Goldman MP, Weiss RA. Treatment of poikiloderma of Civatte on the neck with an intense pulsed light source. *Plast Reconstr Surg.* 2001;107:1376–1381.

Treatment With Millisecond-Domain Lasers of Port-wine Stains and Facial Telangiectasia

Pablo Boixeda, MD, PhD

In the last 12 years, we have treated more than 2000 patients with port-wine stains. Computer analysis shows that vascular depth is one of the most important prognostic factors in laser treatment.[1] Superficial lesions, no matter what color, respond very well to laser treatment (Fig 19-1), but deep-saturated lesions, pink or dark colors, have a less complete response (Fig 19-2). Treatment with the high-energy long-pulse dye laser can improve results in patients with port-wine stains that are resistant to treatment with the standard pulsed dye laser. With the long-pulse dye laser (Vbeam, Candela Corporation, Wayland, Mass), we have performed more than 1000 treatments in the past year. Higher fluences with sufficient epidermal cooling have improved the outcome in many patients. In addition, we can use longer pulses, multiple pulsing, or other lasers or light sources. For equal test results and for shorter-lasting purpura, we should use the longest pulse with the lowest energy (Fig 19-3).

Very bulky and exophytic lesions are probably best treated with continuous-wave lasers, such as the carbon dioxide (CO_2) laser. Even with millisecond lasers, it is difficult to eradicate port-wine stains in many patients (Fig 19-4).

FACIAL TELANGIECTASIA

Many laser systems can be used for the treatment of facial telangiectasia, generally with excellent outcomes (Fig 19-5). The 450-microsecond pulsed dye laser can treat many vessels (especially small-diameter telangiectases) in each session and is more effective in patients with diffuse background facial redness. The problem with the pulsed dye laser, however, is purpura. Many people have misused the term *purpura* to describe the resulting damage of the ectatic blood

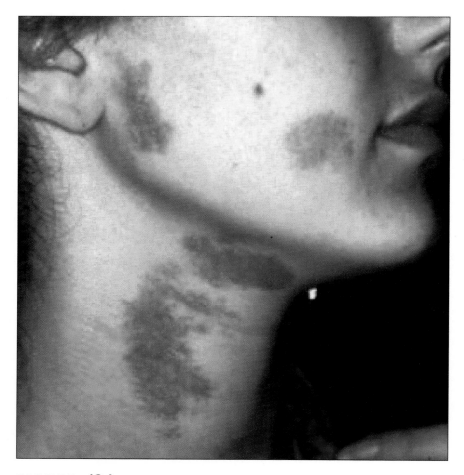

FIGURE 19.1a

Superficial port-wine stains (pink or dark colors) before laser treatment.

vessels. Purpura is correctly defined as the extravasation of blood. With very short pulse length, extravasation occurs as a result of the mechanical disruption of the vessel wall. At longer pulse lengths, no vessel rupture and no extravasated blood occur, although clinically the same blue-gray color is still observed. This color may be caused by platelet aggregates and agglutination of erythrocytes or thrombosis within the vessel lumen. Zachary[2] proposed that the appearance of purpura is related to loss of oxygen-carrying capability of the intravascular erythrocytes. Purpura can be minimized using a larger spot size (10 mm), lower fluences, or longer pulses. Long-millisecond-domain lasers allow treatment of larger vessels without purpura (Fig 19-6). Yet with purpura, results occur more quickly. The patient thus has the choice between faster results with purpura and

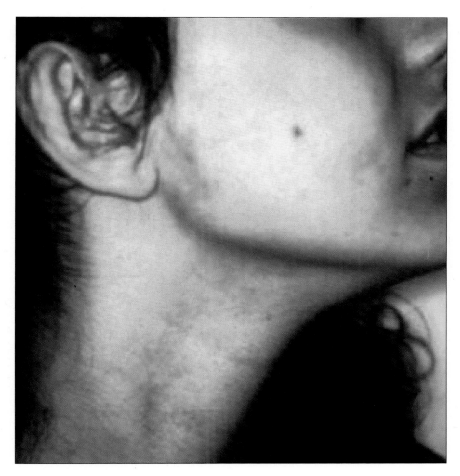

FIGURE   19.1b
Superficial port-wine stains after laser treatment.

no downtime with more treatments. A patient treated with the long-pulse dye laser is shown in Fig 19-7.

OVERLAPPING PULSES

We were able to treat large vessels with the short-pulse dye laser with multiple passes. Multiple passes produce an accumulative increase in temperature in blood vessels, leading to thermal coagulation. Histochemical analysis with ni-troblue tetrazolium chloride has been shown to be specific for the exact defini-tion of tissue thermal damage induced by the argon laser (Fig 19-8) and selective photothermolysis with the pulsed dye laser (Fig 19-9).

FIGURE 19.2a

Deep lesions are less responsive to laser treatment.

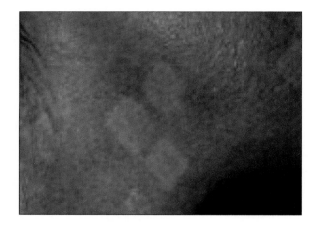

FIGURE 19.2b

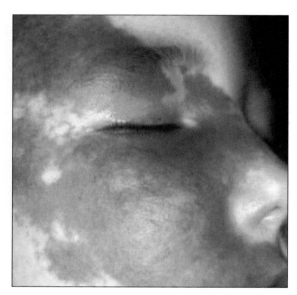

Overlapping pulses produce an increase in temperature in laser-irradiated blood vessels by 2 mechanisms: direct light absorption by blood and direct bilateral thermal heat conduction from adjacent blood vessels. Treatment with a multiple number of passes or overlapping spots (several "stacking" laser pulses) has been tried. Multiple passes below or equal to subpurpuric threshold seem to be safe and effective and have been extensively used with long pulses for treatment of facial telangiectasia. However, concentrations of superficial large and dense vessels need more time to cool off after laser treatment, so excessive stacking pulses are less safe. Even with epidermal cooling systems, excessive overlapping with higher purpuric fluences can induce perivascular coagulation with epider-

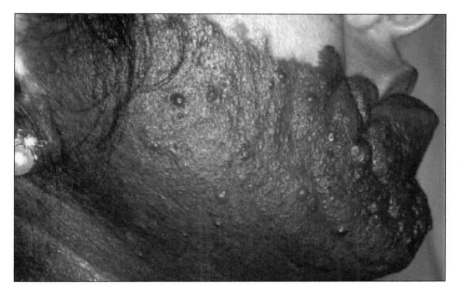

FIGURE 19.2c

FIGURE 19.2d

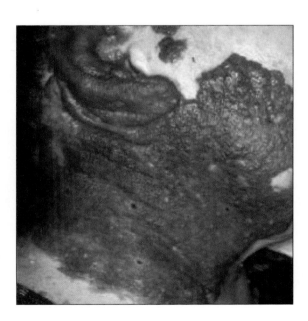

mal and dermal injury (vacuolization and necrosis). In some cases, there is an increased risk of ulceration and atrophic or hypertrophic scars.

In a patient who received 2 stacking pulses, using the same parameters, the second pulse induced more coagulation than the first but was still safe (Fig 19-10). In

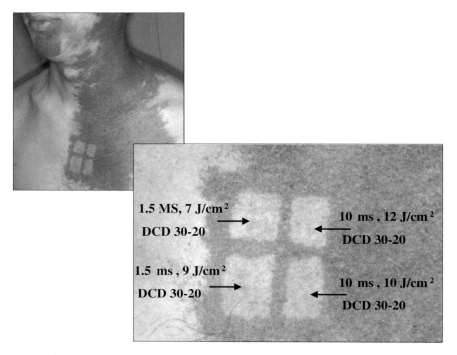

FIGURE   19.3

For equal test results, longest pulse should be used with lowest energy to get shorter-lasting purpura. DCD indicates Dynamic Cooling Device.

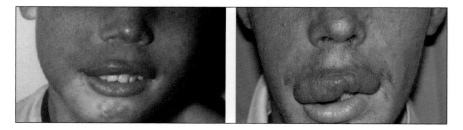

FIGURE   19.4

Port-wine stain (left) resistant to laser therapy (right).

another patient, there was good coagulation with 1 pulse, but with 2 stacking pulses at the same parameters there was nonselective thermal damage, with rings of radial heat diffusion evident (Fig 19-11). Superficial large and dense vessel concentrations need more time to cool off, so stacking pulses are less safe. In a third patient, 1 long pulse (10 milliseconds) was safe (Fig 19-12, upper left), but 3 stacking pulses led to nonselective thermal damage in the dermis and epidermis,

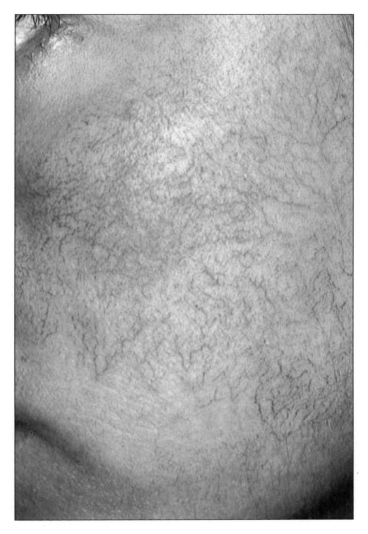

FIGURE 19.5a

Facial telangiectases before treatment with pulsed dye laser.

especially in the center of the spot (Fig 19-12, upper right). These 3 pulses, delivered at 1-minute intervals, produced more and deeper coagulation than with 1 pulse and were still safe, because separated passes allow enough time for vessels to cool (Fig 19-13, bottom). There was also vasodilatation.

Dierickx et al[3] showed that the fluence required to produce purpura increased as the pulse interval between 2 pulses increased. Thus, the time between passes should always be mentioned. In terms of spot size, the 10-mm spot size is probably the safest for using multiple pulses.

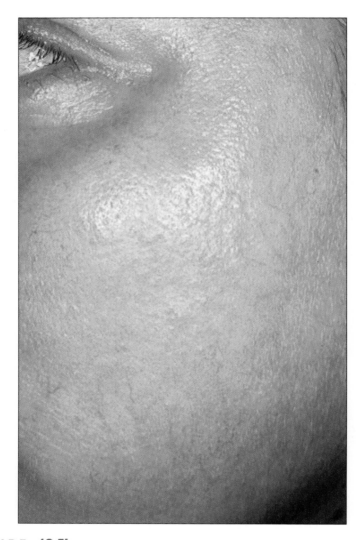

FIGURE 19.5b

Facial telangiectasia after treatment with pulsed dye laser.

In conclusion, for facial telangiectasia, longer pulse duration and wavelength improve our ability to treat larger vessels with less purpura and less pain. For port-wine stains, treatment with the long-pulse dye laser can obtain greater clearing, but the combination of parameters should be optimized in each patient.

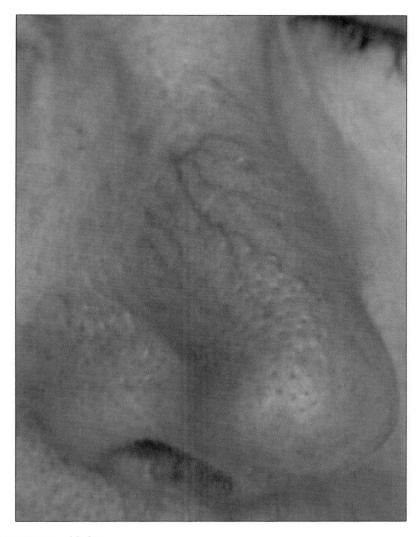

FIGURE 19.6a

Larger vessels on nose before treatment with long-pulse dye laser.

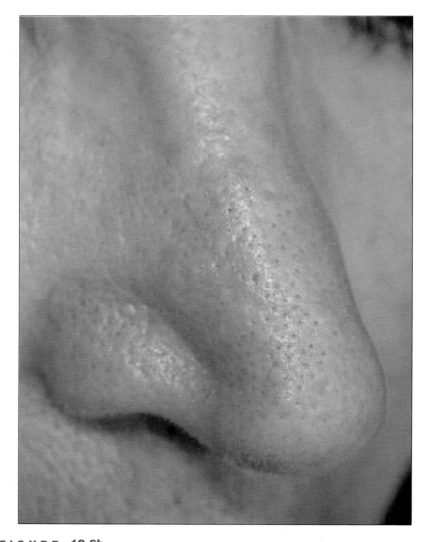

FIGURE 19.6b

Larger vessels after treatment with long-pulsed dye laser.

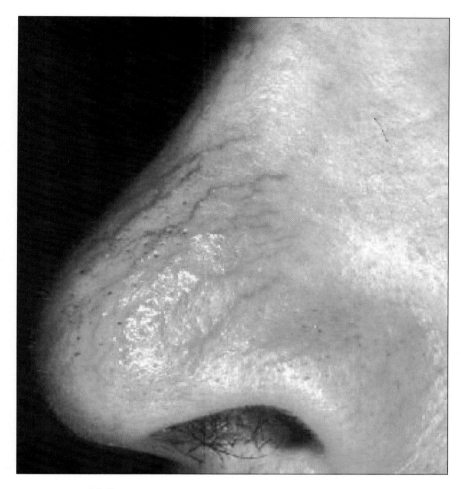

FIGURE 19.6c

Larger vessels before treatment.

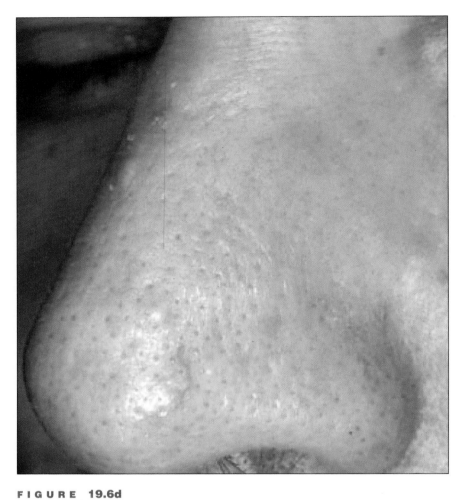

FIGURE 19.6d
Larger vessels after treatment with long-pulse dye laser treatment.

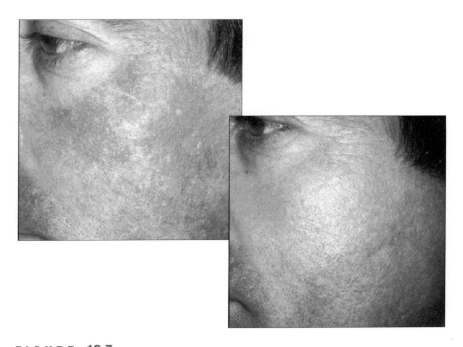

FIGURE 19.7

Facial telangiectases before (left) and after (right) treatment with long-pulse dye laser.

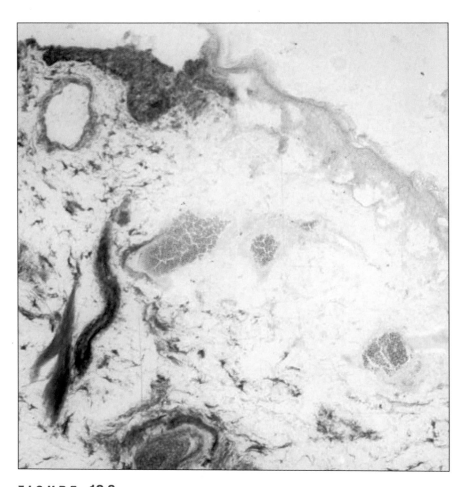

FIGURE 19.8

Argon laser damage (nitroblue tetrazolium chloride stain).

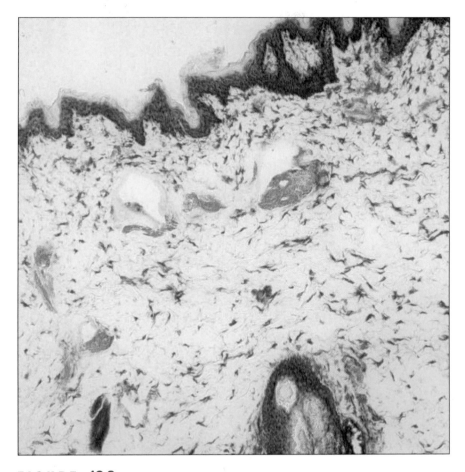

FIGURE 19.9

Selective photothermolysis with pulsed dye laser (nitroblue tetrazolium chloride stain). DCD indicates Dynamic Cooling Device.

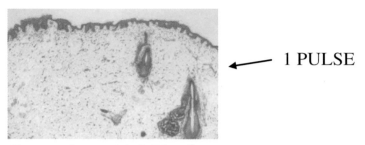

← 1 PULSE

7 mm, **6 ms, 11.5 J/cm²**
DCD: 30-20

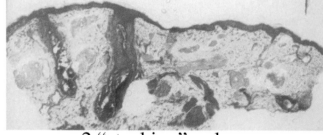

2 "stacking" pulses

FIGURE 19.10

Poor coagulation with 1 pulse (top) and selective coagulation with 2 stacking pulses (bottom). DCD indicates Dynamic Cooling Device.

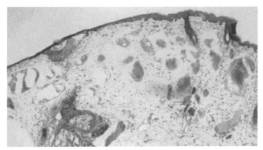

7 mm, **6 ms, 12 J/cm²**
DCD: 30-20

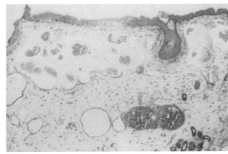

2 "stacking" pulses

FIGURE 19.11

Radial waves of dermal damage by heat propagated from concentric rings of heated blood vessels. Also apparent is epidermal damage, which can lead to scarring and pigmentary changes. When targets are closely spaced and with use of high fluences and long pulses, more skin cooling is needed. DCD indicates Dynamic Cooling Device.

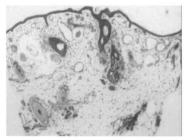   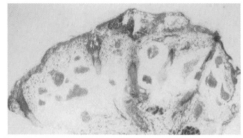

7 mm, **10 ms , 10 J/cm²**   3 "stacking" pulses
DCD: 30-20

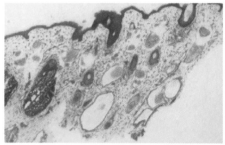

3 "passes" (1 min)

FIGURE 19.12

With 10-millisecond long pulse, 1 pulse is safe (upper left), but 3 stacking pulses with same parameters in same patient (upper right) lead to nonselective thermal damage (by direct radial thermal diffusion from vessels) of epidermis (especially in center of beam) and dermis. With these 3 pulses with 1-minute interval between them, there is exponential decay in temperature and more coagulation and vasodilatation as physical consequence, but epidermis and perivascular dermis are not damaged (bottom). DCD indicates Dynamic Cooling Device.

REFERENCES

1. Fiskerstrand EJ, Svaasand LO, Kopstad G, Dalaker M, Norvang LT, Volden G. Laser treatment of port wine stains: therapeutic outcome in relation to morphological parameters. *Br J Dermatol.* 1996;134:1039–1043.
2. Zachary CB. Purpura after use of the 585-nm pulsed dye laser. *Dermatol Surg.* 1996;22:191.
3. Dierickx CC, Farinelli WA, Anderson RR. Multiple-pulse photocoagulation of portwine stain blood vessels (PWS) with a 585 nm pulsed dye laser [abstract]. *Lasers Surg Med.* 1995(suppl 7):56.

chapter 20

Influence of Varying Pulse Durations, Different Types of Lasers, and Intense Pulsed Light on Vascular Anomalies and Ectasias

Christian Raulin, MD

The historical development of pulsed phototherapy is as follows. Initially, the short-pulse dye laser was used. Then came the development of the intense pulsed light (IPL) technology, the potassium-titanyl-phosphate (KTP) laser, and the medium-pulse dye laser (wavelength range, 585 to 600 nm). Afterward, the long-pulse neodymium (Nd):YAG (532 to 1064 nm), long-pulse alexandrite (755 nm), and long-pulse dye lasers (595 nm) were invented. The current devices are much smaller than the original ones.

My experiences with the treatment of port-wine stains, hemangiomas, telangiectases, venous malformations, and leg veins are reported herein.

PORT-WINE STAINS

In an ongoing study of 15 patients with port-wine stains, my coworkers and I compared the 0.5-millisecond, 585-nm pulsed dye laser with the 595-nm pulsed dye laser at pulse durations of 0.5 and 20 milliseconds. We have evaluated data from 5 patients. Thus far, the conventional, short-pulse, 585-nm dye laser appears to give better results than the short-pulse, 595-nm dye laser (Fig 20-1), and there are no advantages with longer pulse durations.

On the other hand, port-wine stains that were treated several times with a conventional pulsed dye laser also improved with treatment with the long-pulse dye laser. We also obtained improvement with the IPL technology. A patient who

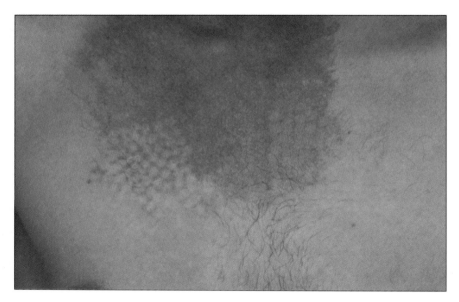

FIGURE 20.1

Clearance of port-wine stain 4 weeks after treatment with short- and long-pulse dye lasers. Treatment parameters, using spot size of 7 mm, were as follows: patient's right side: 585 nm, 0.5 milliseconds, and 5.5 J/cm²; middle: 595 nm, 0.5 milliseconds, and 5.5 J/cm²; and left side: 595 nm, 20 milliseconds, and 13 J/cm².

was treated with 6.5 J/cm² with a conventional pulsed dye laser and had no improvement was then given 4 IPL treatments, and he had nearly full clearance of his port-wine stain (Fig 20-1). So, I think it makes sense to combine several lasers and IPL technology to improve the treatment of port-wine stains.

HEMANGIOMAS

A study we conducted compared the pulsed dye laser, with a pulse duration of 0.5 milliseconds, with the KTP laser, at 50 milliseconds, in the treatment of hemangiomas. The pulsed dye laser achieved better results but clearly produced more side effects.[1]

TELANGIECTASES

When treating rubeosis and small vessels less than 0.1 mm in patients with telangiectases, I prefer using the short-pulse dye laser over the long-pulse dye laser. For treatment of thicker vessels, I think that IPL, the KTP laser, or the long-pulse dye laser (2 to 40 milliseconds) yields better results than does the short-pulse dye laser. When longer pulse durations are used with the pulsed dye laser, I think that some purpura is needed. In my experience, treatment without purpura does not have a good effect.

VENOUS MALFORMATIONS

For treatment of venous malformations, I think IPL technology has the best results. I prefer a pulse duration of 8 milliseconds and triple pulses with IPL. We are beginning studies with the long-pulse dye laser and the long-pulse Nd:YAG laser (1064 nm). The long-pulse Nd:YAG laser seems to be effective for venous malformations as well.

LEG VEINS

Treatment of leg veins is a challenge in the field of laser therapy. In my opinion, sclerotherapy is the best and least expensive treatment of leg veins. Most patients' expectations of laser therapy are too high. They want clearance without side effects, and this is, I think, not possible. Laser is only an option if sclerotherapy fails, especially for small vessels. However, when we used the KTP or the long-pulse dye laser, there was a short-lived clearance, and then the vessels reappeared and were worse than before treatment. The same results occurred with IPL. I cannot speak about the effects of the long-pulse Nd:YAG lasers at 1064 nm, as we have no results yet.

In conclusion, I think that longer pulse durations widen the spectrum of the indications for laser treatment and reduce the spectrum of side effects.

REFERENCE

1. Raulin C, Greve B. Retrospective clinical comparison of hemangioma treatment by flashlamp-pumped (585 nm) and frequency-doubled Nd:YAG (532 nm) lasers. *Lasers Surg Med.* 2001;28:40–43.

I would like to thank Stefan Hammes, MD, who provided substantial research assistance with the study mentioned herein.

Role of Millisecond-Domain Lasers and Intense Pulsed Light in the Treatment of Vascular Anomalies and Ectasias

Mark S. Nestor, MD, PhD

The concept of selective photothermolysis consists of 3 factors working together: (1) wavelength, (2) pulse duration, and (3) fluence. Wavelength influences absorption by the target and the depth of penetration. Pulse duration affects the rate of energy, transmission, and thereby the size of the affected vessel, and the degree and type of damage. The fluence represents the amount of energy delivered and affects the degree and type of damage.

The types of vascular anomalies (targets) treated include port-wine stains, hemangiomas, venous lakes, poikiloderma of Civatte, telangiectases, small facial veins, and leg veins. Patient concerns include effectiveness of treatment, the number of treatments, downtime, pain, and complications.

The lasers I use include the potassium-titanyl-phosphate (KTP; 532 nm), 1 to 100 milliseconds; long-pulse dye (585 to 600 nm), 1.5 to 40 milliseconds; alexandrite (755 nm), 20 milliseconds; and neodymium (Nd):YAG (1064 nm), up to 50 milliseconds or more. I also use intense pulsed light (IPL) devices (505 to 1300 nm) up to 500 milliseconds. The pulsed dye and Nd:YAG lasers and IPL have cooling devices.

IMPROVED EFFECTIVENESS

There have been a number of changes in millisecond-domain lasers and IPL. The effectiveness of these devices has improved. We can treat larger vessels because of the longer pulse durations. There is certainly decreased downtime (purpura), which is favorable for the patients. Overall, there is decreased pain, although pain can be increased with longer pulse durations depending upon fluence.

Overall, complications may be decreased. However, the gold standard, the short-pulse dye laser, is very safe, and we certainly have room for improvement with the millisecond-domain lasers.

CHOICES OF DEVICE

For the laser treatment of port-wine stains, I still use the pulsed dye laser. In certain instances, the shorter pulse durations (up to 1.5 milliseconds) work very well. I also use IPL in many of my patients with port-wine stains, and I use combinations of both laser and IPL in certain patients.

For treatment of hemangiomas and venous lakes, I also use the pulsed dye laser. Again, sometimes with short pulse durations, one gets some purpura, but their effectiveness is unmatched. Certainly, the longer pulses can be used if necessary. I have also experienced excellent results with the longer pulse, 1064-nm Nd:YAG laser (Varia, CoolTouch Corporation, Roseville, Calif) at 25- and 50-millisecond pulse durations. With this laser, there is no purpura and quick clearance of the vessels.

When I treat patients with poikiloderma of Civatte, I have switched almost entirely to IPL, because I do not get the purpura, although in certain cases, I also use the pulsed dye laser. Again, the question is short vs long pulse: which works better? Although there is less purpura after treatment with the longer pulses, I think short pulse is more effective.

In cases of telangiectasia due to rosacea and other causes, my mainstay of treatment is IPL. I have both the older IPL device (Photoderm VL 550 nm, Lumenis, Santa Clara, Calif) and the newer system (Quantum SR, Lumenis). The Quantum has a 560-nm filter. Using the same parameters, I find greater improvement in telangiectases with the older Photoderm system, than with the Quantum. However, pigmentation is improved more with the Quantum IPL device. I also use the KTP or the pulsed dye laser for treating telangiectases.

For treatment of small facial veins, I have switched almost entirely to the Nd:YAG (Varia), which has a cooling device. I can even treat the tiny veins around the nose with a 25-millisecond pulse duration in 1 treatment. I still use the KTP laser on occasion. The pulsed dye laser produces purpura, but it is effective. The 1064-nm Nd:YAG (Varia) has great promise for the treatment of leg veins.

ROLE OF SHORT-PULSE LASERS

With the advent of millisecond-domain lasers, are the short-pulse lasers still useful? I believe they are. They are the original gold standard. Short-pulse lasers may be less painful than long-pulse lasers. I have done treatment side by side in keloidal scars, and the short-pulse laser seems to be a little better. For dermal remodeling, short-pulse lasers may be—and, again, this is speculative—a little better. The number of treatments certainly varies. The downtime (purpura) is acceptable for some patients, although obviously not most patients.

For the future, we need better treatment protocols. We need to improve outcomes and maximize safety. I think that combination therapies are also important. We need enhanced visualization of the vessels and more effective cooling devices. Research will ultimately reveal which wavelengths and pulse durations will be most effective for a given vascular anomaly.

Effect of Pulse Duration on Laser Therapy for Cutaneous Vascular Lesions

Jerome M. Garden, MD

It seems that there has been a tremendous shift in laser treatment from port-wine stains toward other vascular lesions, most prominently leg veins. This change is understandable, because many more people have problems with leg veins than with port-wine stains. However, the study of port-wine stains remains important for understanding laser-tissue interaction and, of course, patient care.

The following laser parameters are crucial to the therapeutic outcome of vascular lesions: (1) wavelength emission, (2) pulse duration, (3) energy or power having an impact on the tissue, (4) spot size and shape, and (5) beam quality—whether the light presentation is homogeneous or there are any hot spots.

Pulse duration is the length of time the laser irradiates the tissue. Since there are many available pulse durations, one should choose a time that limits the damage only to the intended target. In vascular lesions, the target is the blood vessel. The desired pulse duration is related to the thermal relaxation time, where the estimated value is approximately the square of the diameter of the vessel. The goal is to target the blood vessels and leave everything else alone. One needs a laser system that treats different types of vessels and has different pulse durations.

Recent study has focused on longer-pulse-duration lasers. The longer pulse durations enhance selective damage of larger-caliber vessels and do spare the epidermis, because the epidermis has a very short thermal relaxation time. However, the small vessels also are spared, and many patients have small-vessel disease. A laser system is not yet available that can effectively spare the epidermis while treating both small and large vessels.

Although longer pulse duration does have some relative epidermal sparing, in order to injure vessels, longer pulses necessitate greater fluences, which may injure the epidermis and surrounding structures. Additionally, certain laser systems at higher fluences, or energies, may be more prone to producing purpura.

PORT-WINE STAINS

Pulse durations for laser treatment of port-wine stains should be less than 10 milliseconds, as several studies have shown.[1-5] Small-vessel lesions may need a pulse duration less than 1 millisecond. A child with a port-wine stain was treated with the 450-millisecond pulsed dye laser, and results were excellent. A coolant can be used with the laser. Unfortunately, in most of my patients, I do not achieve results this good, despite many years of experience. In the patient with a hypertrophic port-wine stain, the pulsed dye laser, even at 1.5 milliseconds, usually is not very effective. It will make the lesion only mildly lighter. A different laser is needed. For a patient like this, I would recommend the longer-pulse, 1064-nm neodymium (Nd):YAG laser. The intense pulsed light (IPL) systems also are wonderful in treating these types of port-wine stains.

FACIAL ECTASIA

Treatment of facial ectasia involving larger vessels also requires longer thermal relaxation time. The 532-nm Nd:YAG lasers have available longer pulse durations and therefore work well in treating telangiectases. The pulsed dye laser also can be beneficial in the treatment of these facial lesions. One can even use the 450-millisecond laser; just set it at 10-mm, low energy, and purpura will not result. Other lasers that can be used, because they have longer pulse durations, include krypton and copper-vapor, as well as the nonlaser IPL.

VENULAR MALFORMATIONS

Venular malformations, or very ectatic capillary malformations, may have vessel sizes in excess of 0.2 mm. We often see patients who have venular capillary malformations or combinations of capillary and venular malformations. Because we have had a hard time eliminating the venular component with the shorter-pulse-duration laser systems, we are now trying the 1064-nm Nd:YAG laser. This laser has a longer wavelength and pulse duration as well as the capability for a large amount of energy. In a typical venular vascular malformation, we were able to get rid of a lot of the larger vessel components and even the deeper lesions that failed to respond to treatment with the pulsed dye laser. I have used the 1064-nm Nd:YAG laser to treat some venular malformations that did not respond to irradiation with the 532-nm lasers, and I obtained partial lightening of the lesions.

We have to look at the total picture when treating vascular anomalies and ectasias, not just at a single parameter. I am hopeful that the laser industry will continue to develop more systems with broader parameters that will enable an approach to treating many of these different types of vascular lesions.

REFERENCES

1. Anderson RR, Parrish JA. Microvasculature can be selectively damaged using dye lasers. *Lasers Surg Med.* 1981;1:263–276.
2. Van Gemert MJC, Welch AJ, Amin AP. Is there an optimal laser treatment for portwine stains? *Lasers Surg Med.* 1986;6:76–83.
3. Garden JM, Tan OT, Kerschmann R, et al. Effect of dye laser pulse duration on selective cutaneous vascular injury. *J Invest Dermatol.* 1986;87:653–657.
4. Dierickx CC, Casparian JM, Venugopalan V, Farinelli WA, Anderson RR. Thermal relaxation of port-wine stain vessels probed in vivo: the need for 1- 10-millisecond laser pulse treatment. *J Invest Dermatol.* 1995;105:709–714.
5. Fiskerstrand EJ, Svaasand LO, Kopstad G, Ryggen K, Aase S. Photothermally induced vessel-wall necrosis after pulsed dye laser treatment: lack of response in port-wine stains with small sized or deeply located vessels. *J Invest Dermatol.* 1996;107:671–675.
5. Raulin C, Schroeter CA, Weiss RA, Keiner M, Werner S. Treatment of port-wine stains with a noncoherent pulsed light source: a retrospective study. *Arch Dermatol.* 1999;135:679–683.

Dr Garden received research assistance from Laserscope, San Jose, Calif, for this work.

PART FIVE DISCUSSION

Kenneth A. Arndt, MD, *Moderator*

Dr Arndt: There is some controversy regarding the treatment of vascular anomalies and ectasias. Dr Raulin, as I understand it, you said that treatment of telangiectasia without purpura was ineffective. Is that correct?

Christian Raulin, MD: Yes, when I used the long-pulse dye laser at 10 or 20 milliseconds, I think we needed a little purpura.

Emil A. Tanghetti, MD: We recently presented data at a meeting; when I treated vessels between 0.2 and 1.2 mm, I could not get clearance reliably in 1 to 2 treatments without getting purpura. That was an absolute. If I tried to achieve sub-purpuric thresholds, I did not get the clearance. I also successfully used multiple passes on these lesions. With multiple passes of 3 seconds apart on buttocks, I lowered the purpuric threshold by only about 1 J. So I did multiple passes and got purpura and reliable clearance.

Dr Arndt: My coworkers and I conducted a study about this issue. We first found out what the purpuric threshold was, then on 1 side of the patient's face treated 1 J above the purpura threshold and on the other side of the face, 1 J below. Both sides improved, but the side with purpura clearly improved better and more rapidly. Patients often will choose to be treated on more than 1 occasion so they do not have purpura, but in our study there was some improvement with subpurpuric levels.

Richard E. Fitzpatrick, MD: The purpura with the long-pulse laser is very different from the purpura with the 450-microsecond laser. With the use of the long-pulse laser, especially in patients with telangiectasia, intravascular purpura almost always results. The laser surgeon does not produce purpura throughout the dermis because the vessel has not been ruptured. Intravascular purpura clears much faster. Usually it lasts only for 3 or 4 days, and patients find that acceptable. When I give patients the choice of treatment with purpura or having multiple treatments without purpura, they invariably choose treatment with purpura, if I explain that the purpura will not last long. However, if one pushes the parameters of the long-pulse laser or tries to clear a lesion in a single treatment, dramatic purpura can result, which patients find unacceptable. However, for dramatic purpura to happen, one has to use the 450-microsecond pulse duration.

Roland Kaufmann, MD: Dr Raulin mentioned the history of pulsed lasers in the treatment of vascular disorders, but before the pulsed lasers, we had the continuous-wave lasers, such as the argon laser. We used the argon laser with good results in many telangiectatic processes and angiomas. We used it at 0.1- and 0.2-second pulse duration, and that was a continuous-wave pulse. Now we have several of these so-called pulsed lasers as long-pulse lasers up to 250 milliseconds, such as the neodymium (Nd):YAG or the diode laser. As far as I can calculate, 200 milliseconds of long pulse is the same as 0.2 seconds of continuous-wave laser light. And as far as I understand from the absorption characteristics, the Nd:YAG laser is even further away from the absorption of hemoglobin than is the argon laser. So after 20 years, do we return to using the argon laser?

Arielle N. B. Kauvar, MD: When we talk about using millisecond pulse durations with new laser systems, we generally use pulse durations of 1 to 50 milliseconds, not 250 milliseconds, as was used with continuous-wave lasers. In addition, the argon laser also had strong absorption by melanin, whereas there is little absorption by melanin at 1064 nm. One of the problems we saw with the argon laser is that the pigment absorption would lead to scarring and depigmentation in patients. By being far removed from the absorption maxima for melanin with these other wavelengths, we can more safely treat at higher fluences and millisecond pulse durations.

Jeffrey S. Dover, MD, FRCPC: We have experience treating patients with diffuse redness of the face using the pulsed dye laser (Vbeam, Candela Corporation, Wayland, Mass), 10 milliseconds, as high a fluence as one can attain, 7.5 J/cm², with a 10-mm spot. We get very good results. If I can see vessels, which I may have to use magnifying loupes to see, the vessels do not clear. Some physicians have told us that if we double pass or triple pass, we can destroy visible vessels. Having tried that in split-face comparisons, we have not found that successful. From what Dr Boixeda said, however, it matters whether the passes are done immediately, one after the other.

Thomas E. Rohrer, MD: When we first started using the longer-pulse dye lasers, we tried a single pass, as we used our short-pulse dye lasers. We found that we were getting not the same results as with the short-pulse laser. What we found worked well was stacking the pulses. Typically, I will stack them immediately, so if it's a pulse that is not going to cause purpura, or if it causes just intravascular purpura, I will stack the pulses on top of each other, 1, 2, 3 pulses in a row. We find that we get great clearing with that.

Dr Dover: Are these just tiny vessels or even modest-sized vessels that you are treating?

Dr Rohrer: We are getting good clearance of moderately sized vessels that are on the ala nasi, even up to half a millimeter, as well as of diffuse erythema on the cheeks and the tiny vessels.

Dr Dover: Have you seen any epidermal necrosis? Histologic findings would suggest that some epidermal necrosis occurs.

Dr Rohrer: I was surprised to see the nonselective damage in Dr Boixeda's histologic images. We have not seen any epidermal necrosis with this technique. The only adverse effect I have seen with this technique that differs from our other techniques is an increase in the number of patients with postoperative edema. To prevent this complication, when we are treating full cheeks with 2 or 3 passes, we typically start patients on a course of steroids.

Dr Arndt: Are these patients left with purpura?

Dr Rohrer: No, they have no purpura, even with the 3 stacked pulses.

Pablo Boixeda, MD, PhD: Multiple passes will depend on several points. With regard to the patient, the following should be taken into consideration. First, the vessel size and density are important, because larger vessels need more time for cooling by heat conduction (directly proportional to the square of the target size). Therefore, multiple pulses are safer with smaller vessels and with less vessel density. Second, the quantity of red blood cells inside the vessels (target chromophore) should be considered. Third, the vessel depth is important, as multiple passes favor the increase in temperature in vessels that are optically shielded, and perhaps it is possible to go deeper. Fourth, the epidermal pigmentation is also important. Fifth, we must consider that with multiple pulses there is vasodilatation.

Regarding the laser, we have to consider, first, the fluence. There is greater risk with higher energies. Multiple passes at a subpurpuric or just purpuric threshold are probably safe. Second, time intervals between pulses are important, as I showed. Short intervals produce a more rapid increase in temperature. Third, the spot size is probably safer with a 10-mm spot. Fourth, pulse width is important, as longer pulses need more time to cool off. Finally, the cooling parameters are important. All these parameters must be considered for multiple pulses with the pulsed dye laser to be safe.

A physician: When we have done triple passing, or stacking as Dr Boixeda called it, if we looked with a magnifying loupe, we could see purpura within just the vessels (not in the full circle), which lasted much longer with each successive pulse. It looks as if this is similar to augmenting the thermal injury, as long as one does repeat the pulse before the thermal effect of the first pass goes away or is washed out.

Dr Rohrer: Right; that is why I try to get the pulses in very quickly. If one waits too long, often what happens is the vessel will collapse and the target is lost. That obviously will not increase efficacy.

A physician: Are you performing this technique with a cooling device?

Dr Rohrer: Yes, we are.

R. Rox Anderson, MD: That is a very important point. One can keep putting energy in, but as soon as the bulk temperature of the dermis rises over about 60°C, a third-degree burn will result. It is quite possible to do that. What goes on with multiple pulses is multiple thermal cycles, which are fairly complicated. At a basic level, the protein coagulation that occurs due to heating is cumulative. So during a thermal cycle, proteins are damaged irreversibly. The laser surgeon "cooks" part of the protein and cooks more and more, and each cycle adds up. In dermatologic and ophthalmologic laser surgery and in some other specialties, there is a rule of thumb that applies to multiple pulses: the amount of injury is such that the threshold fluence for a given amount of injury is equivalent to the fourth root of the number of pulses. Two to the fourth power is 16. Therefore, as we have shown, the laser surgeon must put in 16 pulses to get the equivalent of doubling the fluence from a single pulse. In other words, with 16 pulses, the laser surgeon can use half the fluence per pulse and produce the same type of thermal injury that is possible with a single pulse. Pulse stacking is helpful, but it is not simply linearly additive, and it has some quick limits to it.

The other point I want to make is that these vessels are alive. The vessel collapse phenomenon, in which the chromophore is lost, has also been studied in detail. There is a fluence at which an intravascular coagulum is produced, which is seen as an immediate graying; it's a form of purpura. As the fluence is increased with these long pulses, the laser surgeon will reach a fluence that is about 1.5 times the coagulation threshold at which the vessel is devoid of blood. However, if the first pulse or a subsequent pulse truly clears the chromophore from being in the vessel, I do not think there will be any effect. Absorption of the light energy must occur to have an effect.

I think multiple pulses are clinically useful. In studies, we cleared port-wine stains remarkably well using pulse stacking. Difficult-to-remove lesions were essentially cleared in a single treatment that took hours to complete because we applied hundreds of pulses.

Clinicians keep trying to figure out the best parameters by evaluating the immediate skin response. We need a laser device with a feedback system to help determine what the best parameters should be.

Dr Dover: We have been talking about pulsed dye lasers, but for years we have been essentially doing double and triple pulses with the IPL.

Christopher B. Zachary, MBBS, FRCP: At least 10% to 20% of port-wine stains are so thick that they cannot be improved much with laser treatment. I think that laser surgeons who treat many patients with port-wine stains need at least 2 lasers now, particularly a long-pulse, 1064-nm Nd:YAG. In my own practice, I like to use the long-pulse 1064-nm Nd:YAG. I tend to use a 3-mm spot, and I use a pulse duration of about 45 to 50 milliseconds and very high fluences of 250, 280, or 300 J/cm^3. These patients get a result that is almost immediate. The patients can hear the laser snapping or popping, and they know something is happening. It takes a lot longer for the resultant skin response to clear up; it is not like a 5-day bruise. Then I will immediately—within a couple of minutes—treat over the port-wine stain with a standard pulsed dye laser or the Vbeam pulsed dye laser, to treat the superficial component, which, of course, would not be affected.

Christine C. Dierickx, MD: I would like to encourage physicians who have the GentleLASE long-pulse alexandrite laser (Candela Corporation, Wayland, Mass) to start using it for treatment of certain vascular lesions. With the GentleLASE, I routinely treat all my patients with deep-purple lesions and port-wine stains, nodular lesions such as nodular port-wine stains, blue rubber bleb nevus syndrome, and hemangiomas. I use a very high fluence, between 60 and 80 J/cm^2. My end point is purpura, but the results are so remarkable that I get clearing of the nodules in a single treatment. One hemangioma cleared completely in 2 treatments.

Milton Waner, MD: Dr Dover, the intravascular purpura that you saw is just a coagulum. When we used the old argon, dye, and copper-vapor lasers with small spot sizes and loupes, the first thing we would see is the coagulum, and then we would see the vasospasm. There was a time sequence.

What are the best parameters for port-wine stains? I know that's a difficult question. Is a pulse duration of 20 or 30 milliseconds the only way to go? Speakers at last year's meeting reported that 1.5 milliseconds, with a wavelength of 595 nm, seemed to give the best results.

Jerome M. Garden, MD: The smaller vessels do better with shorter pulse durations, and the wider vessels fare better with longer pulse durations. So I think the best laser system out there is one that gives our patients multiple choices—a system, perhaps, such as a diode laser, with which one can tune in different wavelengths, different pulse durations, and different energies. What the laser surgeon needs to do is put test sites down on each patient, in different areas of the lesion because every area is different, and determine which settings seem to be most responsive.

About 10 years ago at another meeting, I presented the results of a study in which we compared different wavelengths: 577, 585, 590, and 595 nm. Some patients with port-wine stains had extremely good results at 585 nm; other patients did better at 577 nm. The difference was in the type of port-wine stain and the anatomical area. Sometimes there was a substantial difference within the same patient.

Dr Fitzpatrick: I'm trying to understand the multiple pulsing technique. If 16 consecutive pulses are required to double the fluence, and more coagulum develops with each pulse, it seems to me that multiple pulsing may be far safer than high fluence. High fluences clearly are more effective at eliminating vessels, but they have a much higher risk. During multiple pulsing and cryogen with each pulse, aren't there multiple coolings? And what happens when there is both multiple cooling and multiple pulsing? Is this a good technique? Should we be triple pulsing, that is, triple stacking, or quadruple stacking every spot on a port-wine stain?

Dr Anderson: Cumulative thermal damage with thermal cycles assumes that each cycle is identical. That's when this fourth root of the number of pulses applies. If you're going to pulse stack rather rapidly, you have to care deeply about the residual thermal footprint from the previous treatment pulse. I guarantee that pulse stacking with no cooling at all will lead to third-degree burns and bad results. Early in my experience with pulse stacking, I learned that it is possible to create a scar with a pulsed dye laser if pulses are stacked on the same area. Two pulses are safe. In most fair-skinned individuals, the bulk temperature jump, with no cooling whatsoever in the dermis, for most of the lesions that we treat is approximately 15°C. The vessels become a lot hotter than that, then cool off (thermal relaxation), and then if the interval before the next pulse is not long, the bulk temperature rises 30°C, and that is barely tolerable. If this occurs a third time, the story's over and a burn results.

Many of the new pulsed dye lasers are coupled with dynamic cooling. Other lasers have more aggressive bulk cooling devices. With a cold sapphire window cooling device or using cold air, the laser surgeon actually extracts a total number of calories greater than what one extracts with a Dynamic Cooling Device (DCD). The DCD is cooling the skin exactly where and when it needs to for most of these vascular lesions, so it is a brilliant invention. The question, with pulse stacking, is, Does each pulse cool the skin a little more or heat the skin a little more? The answer varies with the patient, the lesion, the pigmentation, the setup of the DCD, and the selected fluence. In an experimental setting, we avoided this issue by making the pulse "stacking" tens of seconds apart so that the skin returned to an ambient skin temperature. The way we did that, which is actually clinically practical if one is treating a large lesion, is by not stacking the pulse immediately one after the other. We treated the whole lesion, went back and then treated the whole lesion again, and then treated the whole lesion a third time. This was done with a computer-driven scanning system, a laboratory system that would not be suitable for the clinic, but under those conditions, we got fantastic results. Some of the best clearing of port-wine stains by a pulsed dye laser that I have seen was with this repetitive pulsing experiment.

I think pulse stacking or repetitive pulsing is a good thing to try, as long as it is done cautiously. Be very careful if you have no cooling system.

Dr Boixeda: As predicted in a theoretical model (Verkruysse W, van Gemert MJ, Smithies DJ, Nelson JS. Modelling multiple laser pulses for port wine stain treatment. *Phys Med Biol.* 2000;45:N197–203), multiple-pulse laser irradiation improves the outcome of port-wine stains by an accumulative increase in vessel temperature, which leads to higher temperatures in optically shielded vessels. With multiple pulses, the smaller structures such as the epidermal cells and melanocytes can cool (especially with epidermal cooling systems), whereas the larger structures such as the blood vessels will retain the heat and thermocoagulate. We can get better results, but we must consider all the points I mentioned earlier to optimize the parameters in each patient.

The figure I showed (Fig 19-12) was the result of 3 stacking or repetitive pulses and 3 passes with a 1-minute interval between pulses. We used a cooling device (30 milliseconds on and 20 milliseconds off), and there was epidermal or dermal damage with stacking. Perhaps with more cooling, the treatment would have been safer. Further studies with cooling are needed.

PART 6

Advances in the Use of Lasers and Light Sources in the Treatment of Leg Veins

Role of Lasers in the Treatment of Leg Veins

Arielle N. B. Kauvar, MD

Treatment of leg veins with lasers remains challenging. Most of the cutaneous vascular lesions that we treat are composed of relatively monomorphous, small-diameter vessels. However, leg veins are heterogeneous, in terms of diameter, depth, and degree of oxygenation, and that has made it very challenging to treat these vessels effectively. Early on, the application of existing vascular technology to the treatment of leg veins was relatively disappointing because of limitations in the technology. The limitations of these lasers included insufficient depth of penetration; insufficient fluence, resulting in incomplete intravascular coagulation; and a risk of epidermal damage when high fluences were attempted. More recently, the technology has moved to longer wavelengths for increased depth of penetration, longer pulse durations for more ease in heating larger diameter vessels, and higher fluences in conjunction with epidermal protection and skin cooling. A wide variety of devices are now used for the treatment of leg veins (Table 23-1).

Epidermal cooling methods have increased the ability to effectively treat leg veins because of the ability to safely use high fluences. Almost all the lasers used to treat leg veins now have some form of cooling device, such as cryogen spray cooling, the sapphire cooling tip, or the cooling chamber. We tested the ScleroLase flashlamp-pumped pulsed dye laser (pulse duration,

TABLE 23.1

Lasers and Light Sources Used in Treatment of Leg Veins

Device	Wavelength, nm	Pulse Width, ms
Pulsed potassium-titanyl-phosphate	532	1–100
Tunable pulsed dye	585–600	1.5–40
Long-pulse alexandrite	755	3–20
Diode	800, 930	1–250
Long-pulse neodymium:YAG	1064	1–500
Flashlamp (intense pulsed light)	500–1100	2–20

1.5 milliseconds; wavelength, 595 nm; Candela Corporation, Wayland, Mass) with cryogen spray cooling.[1] We found that by using higher fluences, up to 23 J/cm², we were able to get more effective clearance of vessels, compared with results of studies by other investigators.[2,3] With 1 treatment, we had greater than 75% clearance at 3 months in 80% of patients with veins up to 1 mm in diameter.

The trend now is to use longer wavelengths in conjunction with higher fluences, allowing us to treat deeper veins and larger diameter veins. A variety of wavelengths have been tested, including the alexandrite, diode, and neodymium (Nd):YAG lasers.

ALEXANDRITE LASER

The alexandrite laser was first studied by McDaniel and associates.[4] They used a long-pulse alexandrite laser at fluences of 20 J/cm² tested on vessels up to 1.2 mm in diameter and had moderate success.

Kauvar and Lou[5] evaluated the 3-millisecond, 755-nm laser at much higher fluences, up to 80 J/cm², in the treatment of veins up to 3 mm in diameter, and we achieved excellent clearance (Fig 23-1). Thirty-three (65%) of 51 patients had greater than 75% clearance 12 weeks after just 1 treatment session.

DIODE LASER

A variety of 800-nm diode lasers as well as a 930-nm diode laser have also been explored for the treatment of leg veins. These lasers have been successfully used to treat vessels measuring 0.5 to 2 mm in diameter.

NEODYMIUM:YAG LASER

The first report using Nd:YAG lasers to treat leg veins came from Weiss and Weiss,[6] who showed excellent clearance of veins up to 3 mm in diameter using the Vasculite system (Lumenis, Santa Clara, Calif). A wide variety of long-pulse Nd:YAG lasers are now available. They all have various methods of cooling and can achieve high fluences, up to 250 or 300 J/cm?. These lasers are being tested for treatment of both large and small leg veins. I explored the use of the 1064-nm long-pulse Nd:YAG laser (CoolGlide, Altus Medical, Burlingame, Calif) as treatment of reticular veins and large telangiectases, and found good clearance after 1 treatment session.[7] Although treatment of these larger vessels is effective, it is very painful. Proper laser cooling and a topical anesthetic are necessary to make the treatment tolerable for the patient. Thrombus formation is possible with treatment of the larger vessels (2 mm and larger), and compression hose may therefore be useful in treating larger veins with the long-pulse Nd:YAG lasers (Fig 23-2, top).

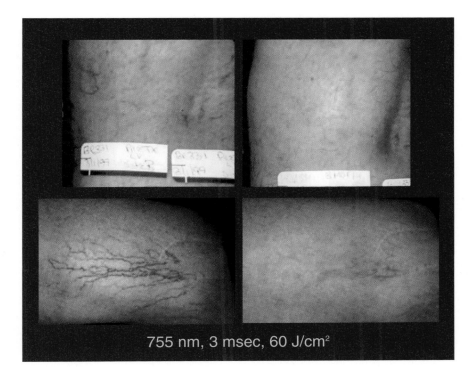

755 nm, 3 msec, 60 J/cm²

FIGURE 23.1

Vessels in popliteal fossa 3 months after 1 treatment session with long-pulse alexandrite laser.

I also explored the treatment of smaller-diameter vessels with the CoolGlide system and was able to achieve vessel clearance in early studies.[8] We are presently fine-tuning the parameters. Initially we used a 7-mm spot with fluences of 100 to 120 J/cm². We are now using a 3-mm spot with fluences of 130 to 150 J/cm², with good results.

We performed a similar study using another 1064-nm long-pulse Nd:YAG laser (Lyra, Laserscope, San Jose, Calif) for treatment of reticular leg veins and telangiectasia.[9] Good to excellent clearance was obtained for both veins (Fig 23-3, bottom) and telangiectases after 1 treatment session.

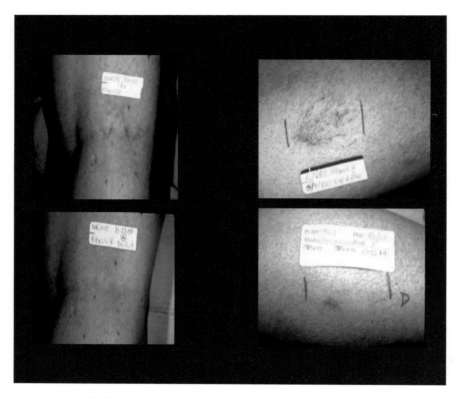

FIGURE 23.2

Evidence of thrombus formation approximately 1 month after treatment with 1064-nm long-pulse neodymium:YAG laser (top), 50 milliseconds, 100 J/cm^2, 10-mm spot size. Complete clearance was obtained 3 months after treatment (bottom).

INDICATIONS

The pulsed dye and pulsed KTP lasers are generally good for treating leg vessels up to 1 mm in diameter. The alexandrite and diode lasers appear to be most effective for the treatment of vessels measuring 0.5 to 2 mm in diameter. The Nd:YAG lasers are now being explored for their effectiveness in treating both small and large vessels.

Laser technology for the treatment of leg veins has greatly improved over the last few years but is still evolving. Laser parameters are still being fine-tuned. There is a need for improved predictability of outcomes compared with sclerotherapy, which in most cases gives more consistent results. However, there are specific instances when laser treatment is the preferred approach. Laser treatment should be considered first in patients who are fearful of needles or have responded poorly to superficial sclerotherapy. Presently, laser therapy also is preferred for isolated, nonarborizing, superficial telangiectases of the legs measuring less than 0.3 mm in diameter and for postsclerotherapy telangiectatic matting.

SIDE EFFECTS

There are side effects associated with laser treatment. Treatment of larger vessels is painful. There also is a potential for matting or erythema, blistering or crusting, and thrombus formation. As with sclerotherapy, transient hyperpigmentation after laser therapy of leg veins is a common occurrence, but the combination of longer wavelengths and improved skin cooling methods should help decrease the incidence of pigmentation.

REFERENCES

1. Kauvar ANB, Lou WW, Quintana AT. Effect of cryogen spray cooling on treatment of leg telangiectasia with 595 nm, 1.5 msec and 755 nm, 3 msec lasers [abstract]. *Lasers Surg Med.* 1999 (suppl 11):19.
2. Hsia J, Lowery JA, Zelickson B. Treatment of leg telangiectasia using a long-pulse dye laser at 595 nm. *Lasers Surg Med.* 1999;20:1–5.
3. Bernstein EF, Lee J, Lowery J, et al. Treatment of spider veins with the 595 nm pulsed dye laser. *J Am Acad Dermatol.* 1998;39:746–750.
4. McDaniel DH, Ash K, Lord J, Newman J, Adrian RM, Zukowski M. Laser therapy of spider leg veins: clinical evaluation of a new long pulsed alexandrite laser. *Dermatol Surg.* 1999;25:52-58.
5. Kauvar ANB, Lou WW. Pulsed alexandrite laser for the treatment of leg telangiectasia and reticular veins. *Arch Dermatol.* 2000;136:1371–1375.
6. Weiss RA, Weiss MA. Early clinical results with a multiple synchronized pulse 1064 nm laser for leg telangiectasias and reticular veins. *Dermatol Surg.* 1999;25:399–402.
7. Kauvar ANB. Treatment of reticular leg veins with a 1064 nm long pulsed ND:YAG laser [abstract]. *Lasers Surg Med.* 2001(suppl 13):24.
8. Kauvar ANB. Optimizing treatment of small (0.1–1.0 mm) and large (1.0–2.0 mm) leg telangiectasia with a long pulsed Nd:YAG laser [abstract]. *Lasers Surg Med.* 2001(suppl 13):24.
9. Kauvar ANB, Friedman P. Long pulsed Nd:YAG laser treatment of leg veins [abstract]. *Lasers Surg Med.* 2001(suppl 13):48.

chapter 24

Photothermal Treatment of Leg Telangiectasia

Mitchel P. Goldman, MD

The key factor determining the success of laser treatment of leg veins is the long-term effect. Any reticular vein can be treated and stay clear for a short time, but physicians want long-term effects. Without long-term effects, there is no reason to use a $60,000 or $70,000 laser when we basically can treat leg veins with a $2 syringe and needle.

A leg vein is much different from a tattoo particle, port-wine stain, or nevus of Ota, for which there is a simple target. A leg vein is a very broad type of system. The physician treating leg veins must know something about phlebology, the treatment of venous disease. The physician must know how to cut off the reflux from the saphenofemoral or saphenopopliteal junction, and there now are intraluminal lasers that can do that. The physician needs to know how to do ambulatory phlebectomy for larger veins (greater than 4 mm). Even though it is possible to treat larger veins with lasers, it is much too painful, and it is my hypothesis that they are all going to recur for reasons I will explain later. After acquiring the necessary knowledge to treat leg veins, the physician should start performing sclerotherapy. Only after you do all these things is it appropriate to use a laser or intense pulsed light.

COMPLETE THERMOCOAGULATION

If a patient has small telangiectases, the physician must understand that the telangiectases are connected to a very broad venous network. It is not appropriate to treat a section without fully realizing what is going on with the rest of the venous system. The endothelial cells will migrate centimeters from a point of injury to reconstitute the blood vessel. It can take approximately 1 year for the endothelial cells to migrate back and establish their vascular channel. Therefore, a 3-month follow-up is insufficient in evaluating the effectiveness of treatment of leg veins.

A number of studies show that every single telangiectasis is fed by a reticular vein.[1,2] So, if the physician just closes off the telangiectasis and does not take care of the feeding reticular vein, there will be problems. Even though the

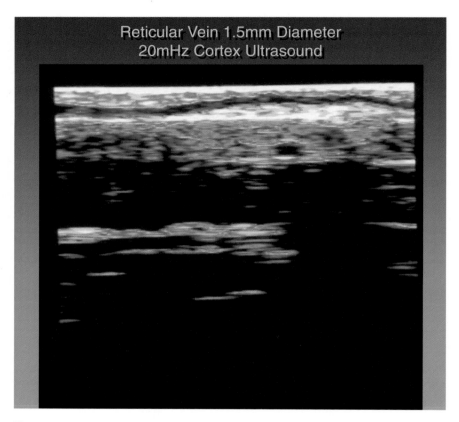

FIGURE 24.1

Cortex ultrasound image of reticular vein measuring 1.5 mm in diameter.

1064-nm neodymium (Nd):YAG lasers cannot penetrate 3 or 4 mm into the skin, a 1.5-mm reticular vein (Fig 24-1) is sometimes located right next to the dermoepidermal junction. The laser surgeon can definitely spot-"weld" the vein but is not going to treat the deeper portion, which is under the skin and not visible. The endothelial cells are going to migrate and reconstitute the telangiectasis. It therefore makes no sense to try to laser-treat reticular veins that are 3 to 4 mm in diameter.

CRITICAL LASER PARAMETERS

The following are the most important parameters for laser treatment of leg veins: (1) wavelength that allows selective absorption by the red blood cells and penetrates to the vessel depth; (2) pulse duration of 5 to 20 milliseconds for veins 0.1 to 0.2 mm in diameter; (3) fluence related to the optimal absorption, for example, 7 J/cm^2 for a 585-nm wavelength and 100 J/cm^2 or more for 1064 nm; and (4) spot size greater than 5 mm in diameter.

AVOIDANCE OF EPIDERMAL DAMAGE

Avoidance of epidermal damage during laser treatment is critical, to protect the skin, minimize pain, and achieve a deeper effect. There are many different ways to accomplish cutaneous cooling. Ice cooling has been known for decades to be effective.[3] Air cooling is extremely effective as well.[4] There are many other ways to cool the epidermis, including gels, contact cooling, or dynamic cooling. A comparison of contact and dynamic cooling is shown in Table 24-1. The advantage of dynamic cooling over all other cooling methods is that one knows exactly what one is getting each time. Then there are the cryogen techniques with the long-wavelength lasers, such as the 1064-nm Nd:YAG (Varia, CoolTouch Corporation, Roseville, Calif), which uses thermal quenching. This technique gives not only dynamic cooling but also then another cooling spurt to cool the epidermis when the heat from the vessel returns to the epidermis.

To determine whether cooling is really necessary for effectiveness, I conducted an experiment on myself. My normal skin temperature is 33°C. After I used a 15-millisecond pulse of 70 J/cm^2 with the 1064-nm Nd:YAG laser, the skin temperature increased to 43° to 45°C. It decreased with contact cooling to 15°C and with dynamic cooling to 12°C. The skin can be heated to no more than 45°C before thermal damage occurs.

The 1064-nm Nd:YAG laser can cause complications such as ulcerations. An ulceration described by Albert Ramelet, MD (written communication, 2001) was not caused by overheating the skin; it most likely resulted from closing off an arterial feeding vessel.

TABLE 24.1

Contact vs Dynamic Cooling

Cooling Method	Temperature Timing	Reduction (°C)	Visualization
Contact	Must maintain contact for effect	10–19	Slightly more difficult
Dynamic	Occurs synchronized with laser pulse	17	Easy

THE FUTURE

An optimal laser is already available, with all the wavelengths and pulse durations and optimal fluences. However, we must take the art out of the technique and have a more scientific way of determining parameters. As has already been suggested, laser surgeons need some kind of retrofeedback cooling protection for the skin so that we can match the pulse duration to the vessel diameter. We need to match the combinations of wavelengths to the depths of the blood vessels and also retrofeedback to ensure that the vessel is destroyed.

For laser treatment of leg veins to improve, we need to prevent inadequate treatment by completely thermocoagulating the vessel, and we need to prevent excessive treatment that leads to epidermal damage.

REFERENCES

1.   Weiss RA, Weiss MA. Doppler ultrasound findings in reticular views of the thigh subdermic lateral venous system and implications for sclerotherapy. *J Dermatol Surg Oncol.* 1993;19:947–951.
2.   Mariani F, Trapassi S, St Manchini S, Muncini S. Telangiectases in venous insufficiency: investigations of refluxes and sclerotherapy. *Acta Phlebol.* 2000;1:33–38.
3.   Hohenleutner U, Walther T, Wenig M, Baumler W, Landthaler M. Leg telangiectasia treatment with a 1.5 ms pulsed dye laser, ice cube cooling of the skin and 595 vs 600 nm: preliminary results. *Lasers Surg Med.* 1998;23:72–78.
4.   Raulin C, Greve B, Hammes S. Cold air in laser therapy: first experiences with a new cooling system. *Lasers Surg Med.* 2000;27:404–410.

Dr Goldman served as a paid consultant or received discounted equipment, honoraria, or research grants from Lumenis, Santa Clara, Calif; Coherent Medical, Palo Alto, Calif; CoolTouch Corporation, Roseville, Calif; Altus Medical, Burlingame, Calif; Cynosure Inc, Chelmsford, Mass; Sciton Inc, Palo Alto, Calif; and Candela Corporation, Wayland, Mass.

chapter 25

Treatment of Leg Veins With Lasers and Intense Pulsed Light

Robert A. Weiss, MD

Laser treatment of leg veins has several problems compared with treatment of facial veins. There are extensive interconnections between groups of telangiectases, so spot treatment on the leg can lead to many problems with laser treatment. Hence, sclerotherapy is still the gold standard in treatment of leg veins. In addition, bright-red telangiectases on the leg are often mixed with the more mature, violaceous venulectases, and problems also exist with hydrostatic pressure. Other problems in the laser treatment of leg veins, compared with that of facial veins, include thicker vein walls, larger veins, and a much larger surface area. These are all problems that need to be addressed to make this treatment better.

ALGORITHMIC TREATMENT APPROACH

The algorithmic approach to laser treatment of leg veins initially involves elimination of high-pressure reflux. Fortunately, endovenous techniques are available to accomplish this using lasers or radiofrequency. The next step is to treat the primary branches off the greater saphenous vein and then the reticular veins. Often the reticular veins are treated at the same time as the associated telangiectatic webs. From my experience, most patients are much more gratified when I treat their larger veins, and I would encourage laser surgeons to add treatment of large veins to their practice. Larger veins actually are much easier to treat than small telangiectases because they respond with the fewest treatments.

Ways to overcome problems of laser-treating leg veins include the following: longer wavelengths (810 to 1064 nm), deeper penetration, epidermal cooling, larger spot sizes, higher fluence, and longer pulse durations. I expect a feedback mechanism to be implemented in lasers in the next year.

INTENSE PULSED LIGHT

Good results of treatment of smaller leg veins can be obtained with intense pulsed light (IPL) or the long-pulse dye laser. The output of IPL is shown in Fig 25-1, and the relative intensity peaks at a wavelength of approximately 600 nm.[1] When a leg has smaller vessels that are telangiectatic and is sun-damaged, IPL can achieve very good results (Fig 25-2). IPL is also useful for treating individual telangiectases not associated with any hydrostatic pressure.[2]

PULSED DYE LASER

My coworkers and I are conducting a study with the long-pulse dye laser (PhotoGenica V-Star, Cynosure Inc, Chelmsford, Mass), employing a 20-millisecond pulse duration with fluences of 7 to 9 J/cm^2. We used, rather than a triple pass, 3 stacked pulses (pulses delivered one immediately after the other), and increased safety with use of continuous air cooling. Preliminary data

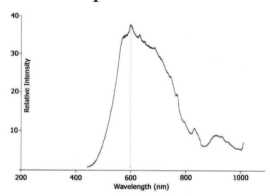

Output of IPL

FIGURE 25.1

Output of intense pulsed light. Reprinted with permission of the *Archives of Dermatology* (1999;135:679–683). Copyright 1999, American Medical Association.

(R. A. Weiss, MD, M. A. Weiss, MD, K. L. Beasley, MD, unpublished, 2001) demonstrated the results in patients who failed to respond to either sclerotherapy alone or sclerotherapy combined with 1064-nm neodymium (Nd):YAG laser treatment.

INDICATIONS FOR 1064-NM NEODYMIUM: YAG LASER

Larger violaceous vessels are better treated with the 1064-nm Nd:YAG than with the long-pulse dye laser.[3] It is possible to penetrate to at least depths of 2 to 3 mm with a 1064-nm Nd:YAG. I find it very helpful for treating veins around the ankles; I perform 1 treatment. Another good indication for using a 1064-nm Nd:YAG laser is when telangiectases come from arteriovenous (AV) malformations. Results are comparable to those of sclerotherapy in similar regions using the same parameters, but laser treatment causes more pain. Other indications for treatment with the 1064-nm Nd:YAG laser include patients who do not want treatment with needles or who are allergic to sclerosing solution as well as patients with reticular veins.

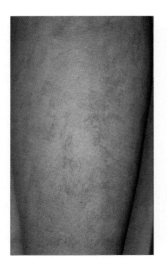 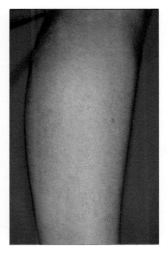

FIGURE 25.2

IPL treatment of superficial telangiectases of the leg.

Value of Endovenous Techniques

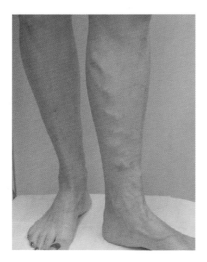 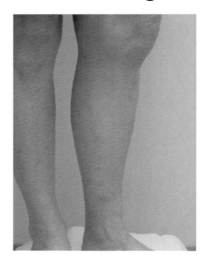

FIGURE 25.3

Before treatment (left); after treatment 95% improvement in varicose veins treated with endovenous fiberoptic radiofrequency (right).

ENDOVENOUS TECHNIQUES

A new fiberoptic design using a conical fiber achieves good narrowing of the vessels and uniform constriction. We did the procedure through a single puncture and actually closed off the patient's greater saphenous vein, without doing anything else except reduction of the pressure. The patient had 95% improvement in her leg veins (Fig 25-3), and sclerotherapy can eliminate the rest of them.

In conclusion, I offer these tips for treatment of leg veins: know the principles of hydrostatic pressure;[4] do not depend entirely on the laser; learn how to perform sclerotherapy; use a combination of sclerotherapy and laser, especially in patients who ask for laser therapy; know how to treat the common side effects of treatment of leg telangiectasia; and know how to treat larger veins also.

REFERENCES

1. Raulin C, Schroeter CA, Weiss RA, Keiner M, Werner S. Treatment of port-wine stains with a noncoherent pulsed light source: a retrospective study. *Arch Dermatol.* 1999;135:679–683.
2. Weiss RA, Sadlick NS. Epidermal cooling crystal collar device for improved results and reduced side effects on leg telangiectases using intense pulsed light. *Dermatol Surg.* 2000;26:1015–1018.
3. Weiss RA, Weiss MA. Early clinical results with a multiple synchronized pulse 1064 nm laser for leg telangiectasias and reticular veins. *Dermatol Surg.* 1999;25:399–402.
4. Weiss RA. Endovenous techniques for elimination of saphenous reflux: a valuable treatment modality. *Dermatol Surg.* 2001;27:902–905.

Cynosure Inc, Chelmsford, Mass, provided a research grant for the study using the long-pulse dye laser.

Clinical and Histologic Findings of Leg Veins Treated With Laser

Robert M. Adrian, MD

Before any physician attempts to use lasers for the treatment of leg veins, that person should thoroughly study and understand the anatomy, physiology, and pathophysiology of the venous circulation of the lower extremity. I have performed sclerotherapy for approximately 20 years and was not successful with this technique until I enrolled in a course in venous anatomy. At this point, after having a firm understanding of venous anatomy, I realize the importance of first performing a thorough physical examination of the lower extremities to make sure that there is no reflux in large veins, tributaries, and other small veins off the saphenous and popliteal system. One must also understand the role of both centric and eccentric perforators in the pathogenesis of venous disease of the lower extremities. After ruling out large-vessel disease, it is quite easy to move on to cutaneous laser treatment or sclerotherapy, with which most dermatologists are familiar.

One of the most important concepts to understand in the use of lasers for lower-extremity vessels is that not all lasers will treat all veins. Small vessels that are less than 1 mm tend to respond well to pulsed green and yellow light lasers, with larger vessels often showing better response to alexandrite, diode, and neodymium (Nd):YAG lasers. Many different types of lasers can provide good results in the treatment of leg veins as long as one selects a laser based on size and color of the vessel to be treated. Over the past 8 years, I have had experience with numerous pulsed and continuous-wave lasers in the treatment of leg veins and would like to share with you some of my experience.

In the treatment of small red and pink vessels, 532-nm potassium-titanyl-phosphate (KTP) and 585- and 595-nm pulsed dye lasers provide the best results. The 755-nm alexandrite, 800-nm diode, and 1064-nm Nd:YAG lasers have proved to be quite effective in the treatment of blue telangiectases and small reticular veins of the lower extremities. One must pay attention to end points in the treatment of leg veins, with the end point for small vessels being vessel disappearance and for large vessels the establishment of a persistent

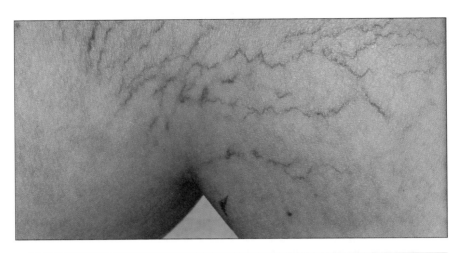

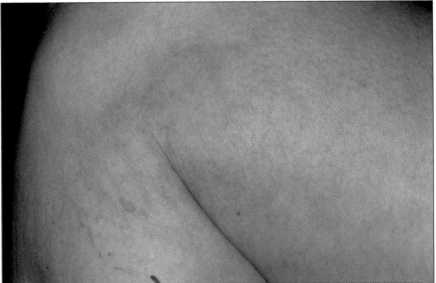

FIGURE 26.1

Telangiectasia of lower extremity before (top) and 3 months after (bottom) treatment with neodymium Nd:YAG laser (VersaPulse, Lumenis, Santa Clara, Calif) at 532 nm, 50 milliseconds, and 20 J/cm².

intravascular clot. In published studies, the long-pulse green 532-nm Nd:YAG laser (VersaPulse, Lumenis, Santa Clara, Calif) has proved effective in the treatment of small red and blue telangiectases of the lower extremities (Fig 26-1). Comparative studies using the alexandrite (Fig 26-2), diode, and Nd:YAG lasers (Figs 26-3 and 26-4) have shown all of them to be effective in the treatment of small blue telangiectases and reticular veins of the lower extremities.

HISTOLOGIC FINDINGS

Of interest is the fact that, regardless of the laser used, histologic analysis after treatment shows similar clinical effects. Over the years, we have obtained biopsy specimens from a number of vessels after treatment with all of the above-mentioned lasers (Fig 26-5) and have found rather typical histologic findings of intravascular coagulation, disruption of the endothelial lining, and thermal coagulation of the vessel and the perivascular tissue (Figs 26-6 and 26-7). Despite differences in the laser used, histologic findings are similar, which would indicate that a similar mechanism of action that is thermal in nature plays a role in the destruction of these vessels.

COMPLICATIONS

Complications from laser treatment of leg veins are reduced by operator education and experience and are most often limited to hypopigmentation and hyperpigmentation at the site of treatment.

Hyperpigmentation can be a major problem with the use of the alexandrite, diode, and Nd:YAG lasers to treat large vessels; however, it can be reduced by the use of compression hose after the laser procedure in a similar fashion as is used after sclerotherapy. Telangiectatic matting and blushing have been seen as a result of laser treatment and may be unavoidable in certain instances. Finally, it is very important to provide the patient with realistic expectations as to one's degree of success in using lasers to treat leg veins. It is important to not exaggerate the benefits of this technology, so that patients will not be disappointed when all vessels do not respond or adverse effects are noted.

In summary, sclerotherapy remains the treatment of choice for most lower-extremity leg veins. The use of lasers as an ancillary procedure has provided patients another treatment option for this troublesome clinical problem.

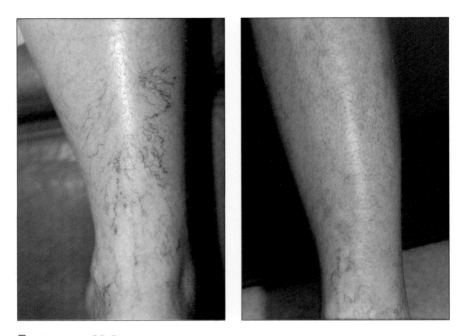

FIGURE 26.2

Lower-extremity telangiectasia before (left) and after (right) 755-nm alexandrite laser treatment.

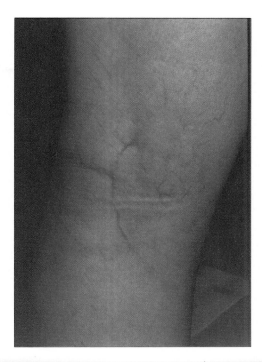

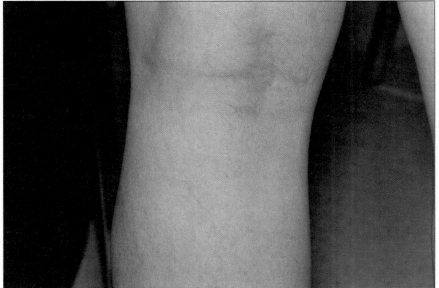

FIGURE 26.3

Small reticular vein of lower extremity before (top) and after (bottom) 1064-nm Nd:YAG laser treatment (Varia, CoolTouch Corporation, Roseville, Calif).

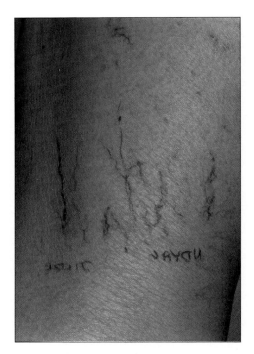

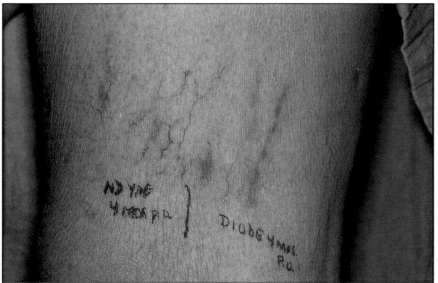

FIGURE 26.4

Comparison of Nd:YAG and diode lasers (left and right side of leg, respectively) in treatment of leg veins before (top) and 4 months after treatment (bottom). Note hyperpigmentation at both sites.

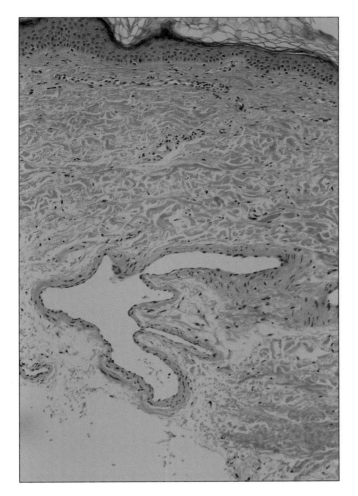

FIGURE 26.5

Typical lower extremity telangiectasia approximately 700 µm deep on histologic analysis.

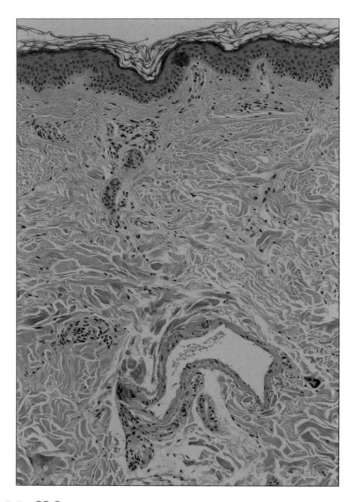

F I G U R E 26.6

Histologic analysis of leg telangiectasia immediately after treatment with 532-nm Nd:YAG laser (VersaPulse). Note endothelial damage and coagulative changes in vessel wall and perivascular area.

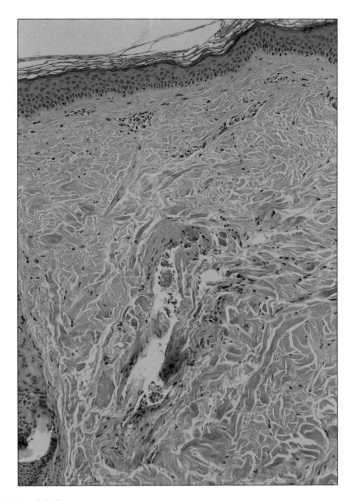

FIGURE 26.7

Histologic analysis of leg telangiectasia 5 days after treatment shows extensive vessel necrosis and infiltration with inflammatory cells.

PART SIX DISCUSSION

Jeffrey S. Dover, MD, FRCPC, Moderator

Dr Dover: All 4 speakers made similar points. First, sclerotherapy is the treatment of choice for most leg veins. Second, only when one is a master of sclerotherapy should one consider using lasers to treat leg veins. Are there any comments or questions?

Milton Waner, MD: Dr Weiss, the complications of venous radiofrequency techniques have been quite severe. I understand there has been 1 death and 1 pulmonary embolism. Would you like to tell us about the complication rate and some of the complications?

Robert A. Weiss, MD: The complications have been distorted out of proportion. A feasibility study was done in the United States in 1997 for endovascular radiofrequency shrinkage of varicose veins. The Food and Drug Administration was getting very particular about inclusion and exclusion criteria through the cardiovascular committee, and the manufacturer of this equipment, VNUS Medical Technologies Inc in San Jose, Calif, decided to go directly to Europe to study this device. Radiofrequency ablation was not considered a new procedure. VNUS went to a number of vascular surgeons in Europe, who do not have the understanding of the skin that dermatologists do, and they did things like putting the patient under general anesthesia and placing the catheter into the vein without any local anesthesia, without any protection of the skin. In young, thin men, particularly when the surgeon tried to close off the greater saphenous vein from the knee down, there were about 3 or 4 patients who had skin burns because the saphenous vein was extremely superficial and directly under the skin. In the technique that we use, which uses tumescent anesthesia, skin burns have not occurred.

The case of the pulmonary embolus occurred in a woman who was treated and discharged, and then injured her ankle and was prescribed bed rest for 3 days. It is not known whether the pulmonary embolus that developed was related to the procedure itself or to the bed rest.

Mitchel P. Goldman, MD: Dr Weiss and I have performed more than 300 of these cases, and we have never had a complication. Pulmonary emboli are rare, actually much rarer with the venous techniques than with just a ligation and stripping procedure. We leave intact the collateral venous system going into the saphenofemoral junction, which prevents the development of pulmonary emboli, unless there are other circumstances, such as a patient's extended inactivity. We hope that these unusual complications will not scare people away from what is an outstanding and safe surgical procedure.

Dr Weiss: A vein drains the lower abdomen, the superficial epigastric vein that drains into the saphenofemoral junction, and that is a little more superior than the terminal valve, so you actually leave that intact. I think we are going to actually have less recurrence in surgery because when we look at the surgical recurrences, what happens is that lower abdominal drainage has to go somewhere, and then you start getting these larger varicosities on the central part of the anterior thigh. We are not seeing that, and this is even at 2 years' follow-up. Unfortunately, they are saddled with those reports of side effects, but it is really a safe procedure.

Dr Waner: In your hands, the procedure may be safe, but less experienced physicians will be performing this procedure, so complications may well happen again.

Dr Weiss: There is a higher incidence of pulmonary emboli with ligation and stripping of the veins.

Dr Waner: There have been many more surgical procedures done than venous closure procedures, so, clearly, we do not know the true incidence.

Dr Weiss: Physicians who perform the procedure should do it with tumescent anesthesia.

Whitney D. Tope, MPhil, MD: Is there any way to avoid the ulcerations that have been seen with neodymium (Nd):YAG laser treatment? Is there a handheld Doppler device that one might use to check areas suspected of containing an arterial feeding vessel?

Dr Goldman: That is a great question. Even in sclerotherapy, ulceration infrequently develops. Usually, the ulcerations are small. Causes of such ulcerations include closing off an arterial feeding vessel and pulse stacking.

A physician: From my review of the original patient's chart, there appeared to have been many overlapping pulses because the laser surgeon saw no visible response, so I think it was due to pulse stacking.

Dr Goldman: In answer to the original question about avoiding this complication, I think that if one runs a Doppler device over the area and hears strong arterial sounds, that means there must be an arteriovenous (AV) anastomosis. From histologic findings, it is known that approximately 1 in every 26 telangiectases that are biopsied have an AV anastomosis feeding into them as well.

Dr Dover: Another possible cause of ulceration is inadequate skin cooling. Full-thickness necrosis of the skin can occur with use of any of the long-pulse Nd:YAG lasers if there is insufficient cooling. I have seen that happen twice, unfortunately. I am sure other laser surgeons have experienced this problem as well, whether the procedure is on leg veins or facial veins.

Dr Goldman: I think laser surgeons often inadvertently hit arteries. One cannot always see them. One would think that an artery would be far harder to hurt thermally than it is, but I think laser surgeons do occasionally hurt them. One of the feedback systems that perhaps laser manufacturers should provide, if possible, is a way to read bulk temperature. With pulse stacking, the bulk temperature of the skin rises to a point at which the skin "cooks." That is my hypothesis. It would be very interesting to further study that.

A physician: In the mid-1980s, there was evidence that laser treatment of coronary arteriosclerosis, depending on the type of laser and parameters used, induces either vasospasm or vasorelaxation. Has the interaction between the laser parameters used and the effect of vasospasm or vasorelaxation been studied in the leg veins?

Dr Goldman: The experiments you allude to used intravascular lasers, and there was an intravascular argon laser in the 1980s. The laser we use now is the diode, and we are using it at such high fluences that, literally, we are almost blowing holes in the veins. So I cannot imagine that the vein is just going to go into spasm and do nothing else. We have 3 or 4 months of follow-up using the diode laser intravascularly, and the veins are cooked; they are not growing back. If they were in spasm, we would see them coming back within a week.

Arielle N. B. Kauvar, MD: I have a comment regarding the use of 1064-nm Nd:YAG lasers for the treatment of leg veins. Technique is extremely important. When choosing laser parameters, you cannot necessarily extrapolate data from one device to another. Cooling is important. When using a 1064-nm Nd:YAG laser, the tissue effect of the laser and necessary cooling depends not only on the fluence but also on the spot size. From the standpoint of pain alone, there is much more pain with larger spot sizes than with smaller ones. When using larger spot sizes and higher energy, the laser surgeon requires a lot more cooling. For instance, I am using now a 3-mm spot on leg veins with the CoolGlide Nd:YAG system (Altus Medical, Burlingame, Calif) with post-treatment cooling alone. If the laser surgeon cools small telangiectases with a contact cooling system before laser treatment, he or she will compress the veins and will remove the hemoglobin target, preventing effective treatment. On the other hand, when treating larger vessels with higher fluences and a bigger spot size, both precooling and postcooling may be necessary, and one cannot stack laser pulses at all. Sometimes the laser surgeon needs to leave a couple of millimeters between individual pulses to avoid skin damage and ulceration. These lasers are extremely technique-dependent. I think it behooves laser surgeons to have proper experience with any specific system in the treatment of different-sized leg veins.

A physician: That is an important point. It gets back to what Dr Goldman said earlier. It would be nice to take the art out of this, but I don't think we can; what you just described is true art. We have a lot of trouble with treating leg veins. We have tried reproducing good experimental results in the clinical setting, and it was very difficult to do. I think that is because laser treatment is more than just point and shoot.

Robert M. Adrian, MD: I do mostly clinical practice, and we treat 150 to 200 patients with leg veins a month, or some 2000 cases a year. One must be careful when treating leg veins with an Nd:YAG or diode laser. It is possible to induce a severe venulitis using the diode laser. These complications are uncommon, but they can happen.

E. Victor Ross, Jr, MD: I have encountered a couple of patients in whom ulcerations occurred. I was pulse stacking about 2 years ago and inadvertently went with a high repetition rate. Initially I saw some skin lightening and some sort of bumping up of the skin. I stacked pulses, at about 5 or 6 pulses at 2 to 3 Hz. I was getting full-thickness denaturation of the skin, and there was no blood there, so I think there was some water heating, resulting in bulk heating of the skin.

I think one can go to different areas of the skin where there is not a vessel. Certainly, treatment may have taken longer, but it may have reduced the risk of ulcers. With the 1064-nm Nd:YAG laser, the energy goes everywhere, and the laser surgeon does have to worry about the bulk heating effect. I think smaller spot sizes can avoid some of those complications. Cooling is very important too, and water also is a cooling tool. Water has a very small absorption.

Richard E. Fitzpatrick, MD: I would like to ask the panel about facial veins and the potential problems of thrombus on the face.

A physician: I think what you're talking about is blue facial veins, usually periocular veins, treated with the long-pulse Nd:YAG laser, correct?

Dr Weiss: Some of the larger violaceous veins in men, yes, we do, but one must turn the fluence down. On the devices I use, I turn it down to 70 or 80 J/cm^2.

Dr Dover: Which devices?

Dr Weiss: The 1064-nm Nd:YAG laser, the Varia (CoolTouch Corporation, Roseville, Calif) and the Vasculight (Lumenis, Santa Clara, Calif).

Dr Dover: These devices are different.

Dr Weiss: That's right. One laser has a 5.5-mm spot, and the other has a 6-mm spot.

Dr Dover: But basically you use a fluence lower than what you would use to treat leg veins?

Dr Weiss: Yes. Leg veins are treated at a fluence of 120 to 140 J/cm^2, and facial veins are treated at 70 to 90 J/cm^2.

Laser, Scalpel, Diamond Knife, Shaw Scalpel—And the Winner Is . . . ?

chapter 27

Incisional Laser Surgery

Brian S. Biesman, MD

The ideal device for surgical incision and dissection would have at least 3 major components. It should accomplish its objective in a quick and efficient manner; be cost-effective; and provide excellent intraoperative hemostasis, which would then allow superb visualization of anatomical structures. It should also minimize unnecessary tissue injury, which will lead to wound dehiscence and scarring. To date, such a device has not been identified.

Many incisional devices are available. For the purposes of this discussion, I will consider the free-beam carbon dioxide (CO_2) and erbium:YAG lasers as well as the CO_2 laser coupled with a diamond knife. I will also compare incisional laser surgery with the scalpel. Traditional surgery performed with scalpel and scissors requires the use of either monopolar or bipolar cautery, a fact that some people forget when talking about cold-steel surgery. When these techniques are used to perform surgery in a very vascular area, such as the periorbital region, substantial intraoperative bruising and swelling often result. Although this usually does not adversely affect the final result, it delays the patient's return to normal activities and should be avoided if possible. Some people have suggested that laser incisional techniques offer the advantage of less intraoperative bruising and swelling.

There have been many claims over the years that laser decreases postoperative swelling and ecchymosis, but it has been difficult to prove, at least for blepharoplasty surgery, that there is a difference. In a multicenter, double-blind study that I helped organize, we evaluated 35 patients who underwent upper eyelid blepharoplasty, 1 side with laser, 1 side with cold steel (Biesman BS, Buerger DE, Yeatts P, et al, unpublished data, 2000). We were unable to demonstrate a statistically significant difference between laser and cold steel.

COMPARISON OF CO_2 LASER WITH OTHER INCISIONAL METHODS

Use of the CO_2 laser decreases the operative time compared with other incisional methods.[1] It accomplishes this by providing hemostasis when operating in anatomical regions where most blood vessels have an internal diameter less than 1.0 mm, by acting as both a blunt and sharp dissecting tool, and by acting as a cautery. Hence, 1 device essentially acts as 3, decreasing excessive handling of instrumentation.

In the 1980s, the prevailing opinion was that CO_2 lasers produced too much thermal damage to be useful in cutaneous surgical procedures.[2] Today, scarring and wound dehiscence can be minimized with good surgical techniques and modern surgical devices. I think there is no longer much difference between the CO_2 laser and traditional incisional techniques in terms of scarring and wound dehiscence.

In terms of disadvantages, use of the laser has a higher cost as well as a learning curve. The most notable difference between performing incisional surgery with a laser and using standard instruments is the lack of tactile feedback from the laser. The complications of laser incisional surgery that are of greatest concern include postoperative scarring, wound dehiscence, and infection. When appropriate precautions are taken to reduce the risk of these problems, their incidence should be extremely low. Important measures include limiting the zone of lateral thermal injury, not making incisions perpendicular to relaxed skin tension lines, using permanent monofilament sutures to close wounds, and leaving sutures in place 7 to 10 days.

HISTOLOGIC STUDY OF LASER INCISIONS

Histologically, when parallel incisions are made in a piece of eyelid tissue in vivo, there is hemorrhage around the cold-steel incision and no hemorrhage around the laser incision. At a higher magnification, a zone of thermal injury can be seen around the CO_2 incision that measures approximately 150 μm on each side. It seems to be biologically well tolerated. This amount of thermal injury can be decreased to about 75 μm with the erbium:YAG laser. Not surprisingly, hemostasis is not quite as good with the erbium:YAG as with the CO_2 laser.

DIAMOND LASER KNIFE

A recently introduced device combines traditional incisional techniques with laser surgery. The Diamond Laser Knife (Clinicon Corporation, Carlsbad, Calif) is a diamond knife coupled to a CO_2 laser. The device is supposed to have the advantage of very fine cutting plus hemostasis. In vitro studies in human eyelid tissue comparing the Diamond Laser Knife with a CO_2 system and micropoint monopolar cautery demonstrate a smaller zone of lateral thermal injury associated with the Diamond Laser Knife than with the other devices (S. Baker, MD, oral communication, January 3, 2001). Inexperience with the device, however, can lead to problems resulting from zones of lateral thermal injury up to 400 μm. The Diamond Laser Knife is not useful for blunt dissection but does provide good tactile feedback. Because only a few units were made, I have not yet used this device. Additional studies with this device are needed before its proper role in incisional surgery is defined.

INDICATIONS FOR LASER

In my practice, I am selective in my use of laser but believe that in certain situations lasers offer advantages over other techniques. Examples of such situations include many, but not all, cosmetic blepharoplasty procedures; correction of upper eyelid retraction; correction of severe blepharoptosis, including congenital ptosis; and when I operate on patients who are unable to discontinue use of anticoagulants. I generally do not use lasers to make skin incisions in patients with "tight" eyelids, those with prominent epicanthal folds, or in external lower blepharoplasty.

In conclusion, I do not think it is appropriate to be only a laser surgeon or to completely eschew laser techniques in favor of cold steel without at least trying laser surgery. In my opinion, the winner is not any one of the surgical devices we are discussing but rather the surgeon who is able to keep an open mind, be familiar with the technologies, and then decide which technology best fits the needs of the patient.

REFERENCES

1. Glassberg E, Babapour R, Lask G. Current trends in laser blepharoplasty: results of a survey. *Dermatol Surg.* 1995;21:1060–1063.
2. Wesley RE, Bond JB. Carbon dioxide laser in ophthalmic plastic and orbital surgery. *Ophthalmic Surg.* 1985;16:631–633.

chapter 28

Advantages and Disadvantages of the Laser, Scalpel, and Diamond Knife in Cutaneous Surgery

Roland Kaufmann, MD

The laser, scalpel, and diamond knife might all be winners, depending on which features are considered: economical aspects, cutting precision, procedural ease, speed of work, and indications for use. The advantages and disadvantages of the various cutting instruments are compared in Table 28-1 and in the text.

LASER

Thermally interacting devices, whether electrosurgical blades or carbon dioxide (CO_2) lasers, are used in certain anatomical sites, such as the anogenital area and the eyelids. Compared with scalpel incisions, due to the thermal tissue injury,

TABLE 28.1

Comparative Evaluation of Cutting Instruments

Criterion	Scalpel	Laser	Diamond Knife
Precision	Low	Variable	Very high
Cutting depth	Unlimited	Variable	Designed for superficial cuts
Cost	Low	High	High
Versatility	High	Low	Low
Handling	Easy	Demanding	Limited
Hemostasis	No	Yes	No
Other features	Disposable blades	Special equipment required	Thousands of corneal incisions possible

CO_2 laser cuts have less defined borders, heal more slowly, and produce more collateral tissue damage and fibrosis.[1] Moreover, laser cuts will usually require several passes within the same line of incisions to finally reach the desired depth. As with hemostatic electrosurgical devices, "dry" cuts are produced, but in contrast no tissue contact is established during the laser beam cutting process. Therefore, there is no feedback for the surgeon with regard to the size of the incision, and much more experience is required to avoid complications.

Carbon dioxide lasers are widely used as a cutting device in different techniques of lower and upper eyelid blepharoplasty, when hemostasis might be advantageous in deeper incisions and also during vaporization of fat pads.[2] As an alternative to combining scalpel blades for cutting and electrocautery for hemostasis, the CO_2 laser can be used as the exclusive cutting and cauterizing tool and the handpiece also can be used for blunt dissection within the soft tissue.[3] Especially in lower eyelid blepharoplasty, the CO_2 laser transconjunctival approach has gained much attention because of its benefits regarding procedural ease, reduction of operative time and bleeding, and superior intraoperative visibility.[4–6] However, results with the CO_2 laser can be comparable to those with the scalpel (Fig 28-1).

Laser cuts also can be created by erbium (Er):YAG laser incisions, leading to excellent wound healing due to the lack of relevant heat coagulation.[7] In some indications, such as hair grafting in cicatricial alopecia, Er:YAG lasers might offer advantages over conventional metal-blade instruments.[8] Newer Er:YAG lasers also allow thermal application modes with some hemostasis functions if required. However, I personally do not use this laser for performing any longitudinal incisions.

CO₂ Laser   Scalpel

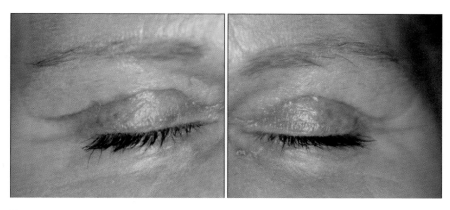

FIGURE 28.1

No difference in result of blepharoplasty is apparent between incisions made with carbon dioxide laser in right eye (left) and those made with scalpel in left eye (right) 5 weeks after surgery. Courtesy of Alina Fratila, MD.

METAL-BLADE KNIVES

Disposable scalpel blades, razor blades, ring knives, and punch knives all have major advantages in cutaneous surgery due to an easy handling and extremely high versatility for all types of routine skin surgery. A surgeon's tactile perception of the cutting surface while applying pressure and dissecting tissue is unaffected with use of metal-blade knives, as is the "feeling" for the depth and extent of the appropriate incisional work.[9] Moreover, the cost of these instruments is low, although they usually are designed for single use only.

DIAMOND KNIFE

For many years, diamond knives have been used clinically exclusively in ophthalmic surgery, such as to make highly controlled incisions in the cornea for refractive surgery.[10,11] They also are used in histopathologic microtomes to create thin or semithin sections.[12] The diamond knife is an extremely fine, precise, and sharp instrument compared with the scalpel blade. These knives usually are designed for fine, superficial incisions, compared with the unlimited cutting depth of the scalpel. A diamond knife has less versatility and ease of handling than does a scalpel. In addition, hemostasis is not possible with the diamond knife.

For nonlaser incisional work in cutaneous surgery or for the excision of superficial tiny skin lesions, a metal-blade scalpel, ring knife, or even fine scissors will be appropriate instruments in most of the indications. However, laser ablation can help to improve the tissue-sparing approach in removing very fine circumscribed lesions with the highest precision. Moreover, in eyelid surgery, healing of the thermally damaged skin incisions is usually fast with a good cosmetic outcome, so that additional tissue-sparing fine cuts would not offer any real advantages over incisions performed with use of the laser or scalpel.

PRACTICAL CONCLUSIONS FOR SKIN SURGERY

If I want to perform a cut that resembles a scalpel cut, I will simply use a scalpel. For routine use in skin surgery (incisions, excisions, and shaving), there is no laser or special cutting material that can replace a steel blade. If I want to avoid bleeding, however, I cannot use a scalpel. In this case, the pulsed CO_2 laser, the coagulative mode of Er:YAG lasers, or electrosurgical devices should be chosen, depending on individual preferences and experience. Definitely, there is no need for diamond knives in cutaneous surgery, since these delicate instruments would offer no advantage in performing skin incisions.

REFERENCES

1. Arashiro DS, Rapley JW, Cobb CM, Killoy WJ. Histologic evaluation of porcine skin incisions produced by CO_2 laser, electrosurgery, and scalpel. *Int J Periodontics Restorative Dent.* 1996;16:479–491.

2. Baker SS, Muenzler WS, Small RG, Leonard JE. Carbon dioxide laser blepharoplasty. *Ophthalmology.* 1984;91:238–244.

3. Biesman BS. Lasers play a useful role in periorbital incisional surgery. *Dermatol Surg.* 2000;26:883–886.

4. David LM, Sanders G. CO_2 laser blepharoplasty: a comparison to cold steel and electrocautery. *J Dermatol Surg Oncol.* 1987;13:110–114.

5. Mittelman H, Apfelberg DB. Carbon dioxide laser blepharoplasty: advantages and disadvantages. *Ann Plast Surg.* 1990;24:1–6.

6. Coleman WP III. Cold steel surgery for blepharoplasty. *Dermatol Surg.* 2000;26:886–887.

7. Kaufmann R, Hartmann A, Hibst H. Skin-ablative and cutting properties of mid-infrared laser surgery. *J Dermatol Surg Oncol.* 1994;20:112–118.

8. Podda M, Spieth K, Kaufmann R. Er:YAG laser assisted hair transplantation in cicatricial alopecia. *Dermatol Surg.* 2000;26:1010–1014.

9. Morrow DM, Morrow LB. CO_2 laser blepharoplasty: a comparison with cold-steel surgery. *J Dermatol Surg Oncol.* 1992;18:307–313.

10. Galbavy EJ. Use of diamond knives in ocular surgery. *Ophthalmic Surg.* 1984;15:203–205.

11. Rowsey JJ, Balyeat HD, Yeisley KP. Diamond knife. *Ophthalmic Surg.* 1982;13:279–282.

12. Reymond OL. The diamond knife 'semi': a substitute for glass or conventional diamond knives in the ultramicrotomy of thin and semi-thin sections. *Basic Appl Histochem.* 1986;30:487–494.

Thermal Scalpel in Incisional Surgery

Milton Waner, MD

I have had a great deal of experience with a thermal scalpel and will limit my discussion to that instrument. The thermal scalpel is simply a knife that cuts and heats, and it allows the surgeon to raise tissue planes. I have used the Shaw scalpel, a thermally activated cutting blade that provides immediate capillary and small-vessel hemostasis. This instrument has temperature-control buttons, enabling the surgeon to work at very reasonable temperatures and to determine the temperature of the tissue flap.

When performing incisional surgery through a vascular malformation, one obviously needs some form of hemostasis. However, when one incises through normal skin to find a hemangioma or some sort of vascular lesion beneath the skin, cold steel is preferable to a thermal scalpel for the initial incisions. The reason is that thermal necrosis occurs with use of a thermal scalpel, and no matter how narrow the zone of thermal necrosis is, I believe it will lead to a worse scar.

The thermal scalpel is useful in the removal of vascular lesions, such as arteriovenous malformations and hemangiomas. It provides a certain amount of tactile sensation and enables the surgeon to cut through tissue planes and locate the exact plane needed without destroying cartilage or facial nerves.

Although I would use cold steel for incisional surgery, very large venous malformations require thermal hemostatic assistance. In this setting, I would not use a laser, because a laser does not provide tactile sensation. In my experience, the surgeon is far more liable to cut through tissue planes with a laser than with a thermal scalpel.

The thermal scalpel, in addition to its ability to preserve tissue planes and provide hemostasis, has the advantage of low cost.

PART SEVEN DISCUSSION

R. Rox Anderson, MD, *Moderator*

Dr Anderson: Do any of the panelists or members of the audience have experience with the harmonic scalpel?

A physician: The manufacturer of this scalpel currently does not make a blade or a tip fine enough to use in the facial area. I guess it is better for abdominal work.

Dr Anderson: Yes, the laparoscopic surgeons apparently like it, for many of the same reasons that we complain about.

Mitchel P. Goldman, MD: It is interesting that hardly any of the panelists have experience with the diamond knife, so let me share ours. In 30 patients, we performed an excision, and one-half of the excision was done with the diamond knife (Diamond Laser Knife, Clinicon Corporation, Carlsbad, Calif) and one-half was made with a scalpel. We found no difference at all in skin appearance between the 2 techniques. There was no thermal damage with the diamond knife. The diamond scalpel blade is expensive, can be used for only maybe 60 surgeries, and is pumped by a small carbon dioxide (CO_2) laser, but at least it offers an alternative. We should have someone with experience say something about it, so that's our experience.

Milton Waner, MD: The reason that there is no experience is that the company made and sold only a small number of units.

A physician: The only diamond knife I could get was from ophthalmologists—the diamond knife without the laser combination, that is, the cold diamond knife. I think in dermatologic surgery, especially in fine areas such as the eyelid, the diamond knife is not needed, because the eyelid skin nearly always heals with almost invisible scars independent from the incisional device used. One can even use a thermal laser, and it makes no difference in healing, so we do not need these very fine devices in cutaneous surgery.

Dr Anderson: Laser surgeons are experts about how to coagulate blood vessels selectively, right? We heard a number of talks about that. Yet I am unaware of any devices in which the hemostasis is being achieved selectively. All the devices we discussed are just cooking the tissue. Obviously, there is the potential to cause thermal damage, but, in fact, we are experts at avoiding that complication. We are experts at coagulating blood without causing unwanted thermal damage. It is interesting that pulsed dye lasers and their ilk have not been used as microvascular hemostasis devices. A colleague who is an otolaryngologist made the interesting discovery that after pulsed dye laser treatment of laryngeal papillomatosis, he incised the tissue in the larynx and it did not bleed. He described the experience as similar to cutting on cadaver tissue, and he liked that he did not have to frequently wipe and mop. I wonder if anybody else has tried using the pulsed dye laser for hemostasis. I have not done so in skin, but we use pulsed dye lasers to treat scars, and they do coagulate blood vessels that bleed, so maybe this idea should be pursued further.

Christine C. Dierickx, MD: I tried it by coincidence. When I started my practice, I had a laser but not an electrocautery machine, and whenever I performed incisional surgery and had pinpoint bleeding, I used either a pulsed dye or a long-pulse alexandrite laser to give 1 pulse. The bleeding stopped, and I could continue my surgery, so the pulsed dye laser is a great tool for stopping bleeding during surgery.

Dr Anderson: Did you use the pulsed dye laser after the bleeding had occurred?

Dr Dierickx: Yes.

Dr Anderson: What's interesting is that if you use it before the incision, I believe there is no bleeding at all.

Javier Ruiz-Esparza, MD: Back when we were working with the argon laser, we used argon laser on small hemangiomas that we wanted to cut without bleeding; then we used a CO_2 laser in incision mode.

Harvey Jay, MD: When using a laser, which does not provide tactile sensation, has anybody tried using automatic sensing, by combining it with Doppler ultrasonography? The exact advantage would be that one would not have to worry about the field. Indeed, if one can somehow evaluate what the tissue is, the laser should be able to automatically be set to penetrate where desired.

Dr Waner: Surgeons who perform surgery at the base of the skull and endoscopic sinus surgery, where the position is very important, have ways they can determine the precise location. They take a computed tomographic (CT) scan and feed all the 3-dimensional information into a computer. The magnet that is at the end of the instrument is a 3-dimensional frame, actually an XYZ frame, that is put on the patient's head during surgery, so that wherever the instrument is placed, the surgeon can see the location on the screen in 2 or 3 dimensions. So these surgeons do not use Doppler; they use CT with a 3-dimensional printout. Doppler is very expensive and is not practical. Tactile sensation is something that a surgeon learns. When lifting up a skin flap, a surgeon needs to be able to feel while cutting, to stay in the right plane. One loses tactile feedback when using an instrument that cuts through tissue like butter, such as a contact neodymium:YAG laser or a CO_2 laser.

Dr Jay: I know that in robotic surgery some people believe it is safer to use a laser, because it can be put in certain positions that would prevent causing unnecessary damage.

Dr Anderson: A couple years ago in my laboratory, we became curious about the question of whether it is possible to make a laser surgical tool with excellent tactile feedback, and there is a way to do that. I don't know whether people have heard of evanescent optical waves. When light bounces off a prism, the light goes outside the prism before coming back in, and there is energy on the outside of a glass prism where the light is reflected. We built some experimental tools that were surgical incisional devices in which laser light crawled over the surface, but there is no beam emitted. These devices give tactile feedback like a scalpel but have all the other interactions of a laser. We never built a practical device or tried to perform surgery with it, but there are several articles published in the physics literature about this. I think if there is a real need for the combination of tactile feedback and selective hemostasis during laser surgery, there is probably a way to do it.

Dr Goldman: That is what this diamond knife does. With the combination of the CO_2 laser, it does exactly what the surgeon is doing. It behaves like a laser plasma around the diamond, and it has outstanding tactile feel. The problem is that the diamond is very sharp and, despite what you said earlier, it can cut deeply. It really is like cutting through butter. Although there is a tactile sensation, the surgeon has to relearn it with the diamond knife.

Dr Waner: That tactile element is very important, so if it has to be relearned, that might be disadvantageous.

Is Skin Cooling a Bunch of Hot Air?

Thermal Imaging and Theoretical Modeling in Skin Cooling

Peter Bjerring, MD, PhD

There are two factors in photothermal light-skin interaction: the heat that goes into the skin and the heat that goes out. Considering the heat that goes in, the important factors are the target structure, wavelength, fluence, spot size, spatial and temporal profiles of the beam, and the pulse duration. The factors important for the heat going out of the anatomical structure that is being targeted would be the thermal relaxation time of the structures, the thermal characteristics of the surrounding tissues, the distance to the surface, and any artificially applied thermal condition. The artificially applied thermal condition of skin cooling is the topic under discussion.

The objectives of artificial cooling are as follows: (1) have no negative impact on the desired physiologic interaction; (2) reduce side effects; (3) give the ability to vary optical parameters, not only laser parameters but also tissue parameters, in order to enhance or improve the treatment effect; and (4) manage side effects to an acceptable level.

TYPES OF SKIN COOLING

There are two types of skin cooling: contact cooling and noncontact cooling. Contact cooling can be either cold objects that reduce the skin surface temperature or heat sinks, which have a high thermal capacity and will extract accumulated heat from the skin surface. Heat sinks do not have to be cold. An example of cold contact cooling could be a cold sapphire tip, or a cooling bracket with circulating ice water. Noncontact skin cooling can be either constant cooling, with continuous-flow cold air, or dynamic cooling, with precisely gated cryogen sprays.

Different contact cooling devices vary considerably, because the temperature and the heat conductivity of the actual cooling device may vary. The duration of the precooling and postcooling, that is, the cooling before and after the laser pulse, is in most cases manually governed and might therefore vary. In

Thermal Imaging
Different surface heating by Dye (left peak) and Ruby (right peak) Lasers

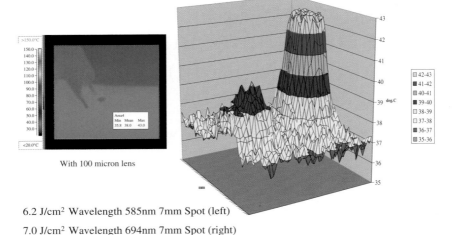

With 100 micron lens

6.2 J/cm^2 Wavelength 585nm 7mm Spot (left)

7.0 J/cm^2 Wavelength 694nm 7mm Spot (right)

F I G U R E 30.1

Thermal imaging demonstrates different surface temperatures of the dye and ruby lasers.

noncontact cooling, the duration of the precooling and postcooling by continuous-flow cold air may vary, and if a large area is cooled, that is, bulk cooling, there might be a better effect of the cooling after the last laser pulse in the area than after the first one. Both the airflow and temperature may change, and the optical properties of the stratum corneum may change as well due to transient freeze-drying. In dynamic cooling, the duration of the spray cooling before and after the laser pulse is very important. Also, ambient humidity may play a role in the forming of the ice coating on the skin surface.

TOOLS FOR MEASURING SKIN SURFACE TEMPERATURES

Two powerful tools are available to help laser surgeons: thermal imaging, which provides dynamic infrared measurements of surface temperature, and theoretical modeling. An example of thermal imaging is shown in Figure 30-1. Two laser pulses are shown with nearly the same energy but with 2 different wavelengths. One was a ruby laser (694 nm), which is moderately absorbed by melanin. The other was a dye laser (585 nm), which has a higher absorption in melanin as well as in hemoglobin. The skin surface temperatures are color-coded on the

Dye Laser with Cryo Spray

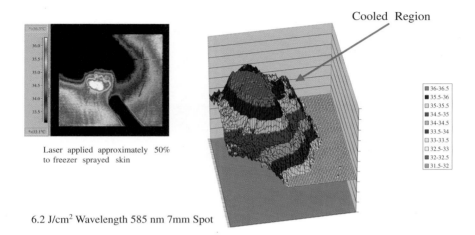

Cooled Region

Laser applied approximately 50% to freezer sprayed skin

6.2 J/cm² Wavelength 585 nm 7mm Spot

■ 36-36.5
■ 35.5-36
□ 35-35.5
■ 34.5-35
□ 34-34.5
■ 33.5-34
□ 33-33.5
□ 32.5-33
■ 32-32.5
■ 31.5-32

FIGURE 30.2

Cooling a portion of the pulsed dye laser treated area shows marked differences in thermal imaging.

figure so it is possible to read which temperatures the skin reaches during the treatments. If, for example, we cool half of the dye laser spot, we can see the decreased skin surface temperatures and directly see how much we have actually cooled the skin surface compared with the noncooled area (Fig 30-2).

In this simple model of the skin (Fig 30-3), the light reaches the skin surface from the left side. Figure 30-4 shows how the energy is distributed after a 1320-nm light pulse. It is apparent that cooling is definitely needed here, as most of the energy is accumulated at the surface and only very little in depth. On the other hand, with a wavelength of 585 nm, only little absorption occurs at the surface, whereas substantial absorption takes place at the level of the capillaries (Fig 30-5).

The conclusion is that skin cooling can be a very useful tool. However, the use of skin cooling when it is not needed introduces a new set of treatment variables, and there is definitely room for closer collaboration between clinicians and physicists to optimize and control the treatment parameters.

I acknowledge Mike Kiernan, PhD, and Marc Clement, PhD, for their assistance with this work.

Theoretical Modeling

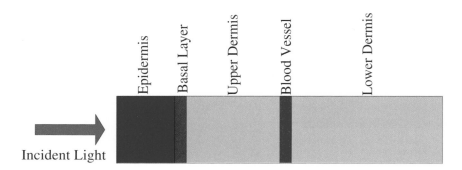

FIGURE 30.3

Thermal model of the skin at incident light impact.

1320 nm Light Distribution in Skin

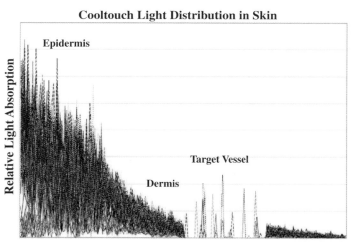

FIGURE 30.4

Energy distribution after a 1320-nm laser pulse.

585 nm Pulsed Dye Laser Light Distribution in Skin

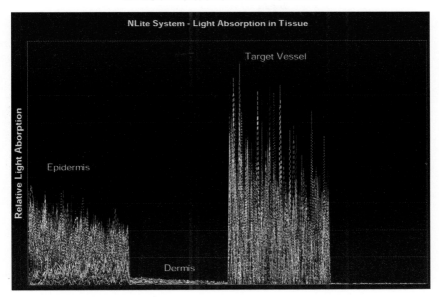

FIGURE 30.5

At 585 nm, there is little surface absorption with substantial absorption at the level of the capillaries.

chapter 31

Practical Implementation of Skin Cooling

J. Stuart Nelson, MD, PhD

The objectives of laser dermatologic surgery are to maximize targeted subsurface chromophore destruction while minimizing damage to the normal overlying epidermis. The problem is that, unfortunately, for many lesions, the threshold for epidermal damage is very close to that for permanent destruction of the targeted chromophore.[1] Therefore, the solution to this dilemma is to selectively cool the epidermal melanin layer while not changing the temperature of the targeted subsurface chromophore[1] (Fig 31-1).

Is skin cooling a bunch of hot air? No. Skin cooling is an excellent idea. It allows clinicians to use much higher doses of incident light by increasing the threshold for epidermal damage. Cooling eliminates heat buildup at the skin surface by conducting heat out of the air-skin interface. Cooling permits patients with darker skin types to receive laser treatment, and it reduces pain and post-treatment edema.

BASIC CONCEPTS OF SKIN COOLING

The question then becomes, How can skin cooling be properly implemented in the clinical management of patients receiving laser therapy? To answer that, let's review the basic concepts of skin cooling. All skin-cooling methods require bringing some kind of medium in contact with the skin surface, and this medium can be a solid, a liquid, or a gas. The rate of heat removal from the skin surface depends on the thermal properties of the cooling medium and the skin, the contact between the cooling medium and the skin, and also the temperature of the cooling medium.

TIMING OF SKIN COOLING

It is important to consider when to apply cooling. Is cooling needed before, during, or after the laser pulse? I think everyone would agree that we want to cool during all of those times, to obtain maximum epidermal protection (Fig 31-2).

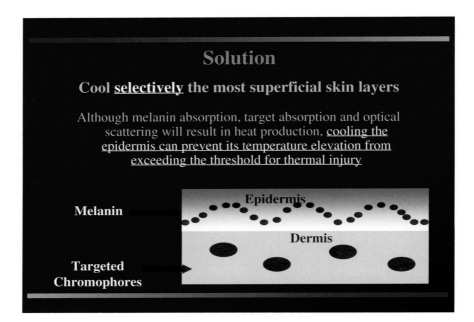

FIGURE 31.1

Selective cooling of superficial skin layers.

SKIN-COOLING METHODS

There are 3 different methods of skin cooling: cryogen spray (dynamic) cooling, contact cooling, and air cooling. Cryogen spray is unique among skin-cooling methods in the fact that it takes advantage of evaporative cooling. After liquid cryogen droplets are sprayed onto the skin surface, the droplets evaporate very quickly, because the temperature of the liquid cryogen layer on the skin surface is approximately −60°C. As the cryogen evaporates, a heat sink is created below the surface, which conducts heat out from the skin. Cryogen spray also allows the opportunity to precool the skin surface before laser irradiation. Cooling is possible during the laser pulse because the cryogen liquid is still on the skin surface. Postcooling recurs after laser exposure as the liquid cryogen continues to evaporate. Therefore, cryogen spray permits cooling to occur before, during, and after laser exposure.

Contact cooling employs either sapphire or quartz plates, which are placed in contact with the skin surface. This method involves heat conduction from the skin surface out into the plate.

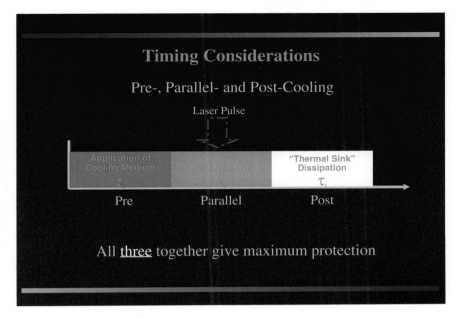

FIGURE 31.2

Timing considerations for cooling skin before, parallel to, and after laser pulse. tc indicates cooling time.

Air cooling uses forced heat convection. A secondary cooling system blows cold air onto the skin surface. As with all 3 techniques, air cooling can use precooling, parallel cooling, and postcooling.

The anatomical depth of cooling depends on the cooling time or the duration that the cold medium is in contact with the skin surface. Generally, the epidermis is cooled in tens of milliseconds. Bulk skin cooling is achieved after several seconds. If the clinician is trying to target chromophores that are close to the skin surface, a very short cooling time is required; for deeper target chromophores, longer cooling times are permissible.

Practical implementation of skin cooling should be determined on an individual basis, taking into consideration epidermal thickness and targeted chromophore depth. Generally, for superficial targeted chromophores, such as blood vessels of port-wine stains or collagen during nonablative laser skin rejuvenation, a large temperature gradient at the skin surface is required with very high spatial selectivity. For deeper targeted structures, for example, hair follicles, prolonged cooling times at lower temperatures are permissible.

Cryogen spray cooling works for treatment of superficial and deep vascular lesions as well as for nonablative skin rejuvenation and hair removal. For treatment of deeper, thicker lesions or for hair removal, cryogen spray cooling, contact cooling, and air cooling work equally well. The air-cooling device provides much more bulk cooling and is not nearly as controllable as either contact cooling or cryogen spray cooling.

REFERENCE

1.   Nelson JS, Majaron B, Kelly KM. Active skin cooling in conjunction with laser dermatologic surgery. *Sem Cutan Med Surg.* 2000;19:253–266.

Is Skin Cooling a Bunch of Hot Air?

R. Rox Anderson, MD

Skin cooling is not a bunch of hot air. However, the type of skin cooling should be matched to the task, the laser, and the individual patient.

PURPOSES OF SKIN COOLING

The reasons for skin cooling vary with different situations. Cooling is not intended just to protect the epidermis. Bulk cooling of the whole dermis also reduces the risk of third-degree burns. With pulse stacking, the laser surgeon is far better off to not do any dynamic cooling but just start with cold tissue. Another objective of skin cooling is to reduce pain. The pain is associated with either unwanted epidermal injury or heating of dermal targets, or both. Dynamic cooling will not help at all with treatment of leg veins, but prolonged, deep cooling of the whole skin will. Another good reason to cool is to reduce post-treatment swelling.

TYPES OF SKIN COOLING

All skin-cooling methods consist of extracting heat from the skin surface, by conduction into an external medium—gas, liquid, or solid. The timing of cooling—before, during, or after the laser pulse—is very important. There are 4 basic types of skin cooling: (1) bulk precooling, which cools the entire skin before light energy is delivered; (2) dynamic precooling, which cools the epidermis before light delivery; (3) parallel cooling, which cools the epidermis during light delivery; and (4) postcooling, which cools the entire skin after light delivery.

The laser surgeon must consider the type of cooling system that is appropriate. The anatomical depth, for the cooling at the time that the laser pulse arrives, is related to the duration of the precooling cycle. Dynamic cryogen spray cooling is a good example of a system that is automated to provide fast and superficial cooling—low temperature but superficial cooling in terms of anatomical depth. I think the Dynamic Cooling Device (DCD) gives the lowest temperatures with the fastest rates of cooling.

The different kinds of skin cooling are best for different purposes. Bulk precooling of the skin, starting with cold skin, reduces the risk for a gross thermal burn. It probably does the best for pain control as well, and, probably the cold-air device is the best for that. Dynamic precooling with the DCD does an excellent job and is the device I would most recommend as an epidermal protectant for short laser pulses. With a pulse duration less than 10 milliseconds or so, dynamic precooling is about the only method that will help. In contrast, parallel cooling is best for epidermal protection for long pulses. With long pulses (30 to 100 milliseconds), which are common for hair removal, the parallel cooling makes a huge difference in the surgeon's ability to treat darker skin types. Postcooling decreases pain and swelling after treatment.

COMPARISON OF SKIN-COOLING DEVICES

Skin-cooling devices have different advantages and disadvantages (Table 32-1). The cryogen spray cooler is the best cooling device available for dynamic precooling. Handpieces with cold windows that move with the handpiece can be used for bulk precooling to some extent, but they are best at parallel cooling. There is no device better than cold-window handpieces for parallel cooling. If cooling is desired during the laser pulse, something must extract heat through a transparent medium. Cooling gels are probably the second best at parallel cooling. Although one can do parallel cooling with a cryogen spray, it is somewhat difficult to have to spray during the laser pulse.

The cold gliding handpiece on the neodymium:YAG laser (CoolGlide, Altus Medical Inc, Burlingame, Calif) does bulk precooling and some dynamic precooling, but this depends on how fast the surgeon glides the handpiece. The

TABLE 32.1

Benefits of Skin-Cooling Devices by Type of Cooling Provided

Type of Cooling	Cryogen Cold-Spray (DCD)	Gliding Window Handpiece	Cold Handpiece	Cold Air	Cooling Gel
Bulk precooling	None	Good	Good	Excellent	Fair
Dynamic precooling	Excellent	Good	Good	None	None
Parallel cooling	Good	Excellent	None	Fair	Good
Postcooling	None	Fair	None	Excellent	Fair

DCD indicates Dynamic Cooling Device.

pulse rate and the glide rate are set appropriately for hair removal in particular. However, there is absolutely no parallel cooling or postcooling in this particular device.

A continuous blast of cold air, I think, is probably the best at bulk precooling. It is a great pain-control technique in some settings. However, it offers no dynamic cooling, and it is not good for parallel cooling, because air is a poor thermal conductor. This method is therefore good mostly for bulk precooling and for postcooling.

CRYOGEN INJURY

One thing to keep in mind during cooling is that it is possible to cause cryogen injury to the skin. Recently I saw a patient from India, who had been treated with a long-pulse alexandrite laser and had arcuate hypopigmented areas resembling doughnuts over almost her entire body. These areas of nearly alabaster-white hypopigmentation where she was treated with the laser were apparently the result of aggressive cooling. I do not know what went wrong, but certainly aggressive cooling can cause cryogen injury to the skin.

Efficacy and Safety of Skin-Cooling Devices

Brian S. Biesman, MD

The last several years have seen tremendous improvements in the quality of cooling devices for laser treatment and the number of options available. However, questions still need to be addressed about optimal skin-cooling parameters.

I herein present the results of 2 recently completed studies (B. S. Biesman, MD, L. Reinisch, PhD, unpublished data, 2001), in which my coworkers and I evaluated the benefits and safety of cooling.

Although cold-air cooling was first reported approximately 4 years ago, there has been little study of this modality. We therefore compared a cold-air cooling device with a widely accepted cooling device, the thermoelectrically (TE) cooled sapphire window, using an 810-nm diode laser.

ANIMALS AND METHODS

We employed a farm piglet model to evaluate the maximum fluence that could be safely used on both light- and dark-skinned animals. The experimental protocol was approved by our institutional animal care committee. We tested the safety of a 60-W diode laser (EpiStar, Nidek Inc, Fremont, Calif) using 2 cooling systems: air cooling and contact cooling. This diode laser can produce pulse durations of up to 700 milliseconds and spot sizes ranging from 1 to 5 mm. We treated 3 light-skinned and 3 dark-brown piglets. Each piglet was treated with a progressively increasing fluence until epidermal changes were noted clinically. Skin cooling was provided with the single-chip, TE-cooled handpiece provided by the laser manufacturer and with the Zimmer cold-air blowing device (Zimmer, Irvine, Calif). The TE-cooled window was set to a temperature of 5°C, while the cold-air blowing device cooled room air to a maximum of −30°C. Immediately after treatment, biopsies were performed.

A second parameter evaluated was the effect of cold-air cooling on the size of the zone of lateral thermal injury created during incisional carbon dioxide (CO_2) laser surgery. A CO_2 laser (UniPulse, Nidek Inc) producing a 0.2-mm diameter beam was used to make incisions in the piglet flank. Half the incisions were created in a standard fashion, and the other half were made as the skin was cooled with the cold-air blowing device.

RESULTS

The results of this study were assessed in terms of maximum tolerated fluence (MTF), defined as the highest fluence that could be delivered without causing epidermal injury. Epidermal injury was evaluated clinically and histopathologically. In the treatment of light-skinned piglets, relatively high fluences could be used safely with both cooling systems. The MTF with both cooling systems was 325 to 350 J/cm^2, well above levels needed to accomplish most clinical objectives. In contrast, when dark-skinned piglets were treated, the MTF achievable with the TE-cooled window was only 75 J/cm^2. Use of the cold air-blowing device doubled the MTF to 150 J/cm^2. This difference was statistically significant ($P < .025$) and most likely is clinically important as well. When the cold air-blowing device was used to cool skin during incisional laser surgery, the amount of lateral thermal injury was reduced by approximately 40%.

COMMENT

In the evaluation of epidermal protection conferred during delivery of 810-nm diode laser energy to skin, the cold-air blowing device offered a statistically significant advantage over a single-chip TE-cooled sapphire window. This advantage was realized only in the treatment of dark-skinned animals. One disadvantage of the diode laser system is the increased risk and discomfort of treating dark-skinned or tanned patients. If the findings from this study translate similarly in human clinical trials, the spectrum of applications and indications for the 810-nm diode laser may be expanded.

With regard to incisional applications, it is difficult to extrapolate the results of this study to clinical applications in humans. The reduction of lateral thermal injury is, of course, important. However, it remains to be seen whether this degree of reduction is great enough to actually decrease the risk of scarring and other complications. Furthermore, it is not possible to assess the relative degree of hemostasis that will be provided when one operates in a vascular area such as the head and neck. When the size of the zone of thermal injury is reduced, it is reasonable to expect that hemostasis may also be less complete. Further study is thus required before a conclusion can be reached about the clinical benefits, if any, of cold-air cooling in conjunction with laser incisional surgery.

Despite the apparent promise of cold-air cooling during cutaneous laser surgery, additional questions remain to be answered. Included among these are the optimal parameters at which the cold air should be delivered. The effect of air temperature, speed, distance from the tissue, and use of adjunctive products such as water or gels all need to be assessed. The cold-air blowing devices currently available do not deliver filtered air. This should not be important when intact skin is treated, but it raises the question of an increased risk of infection in open wounds.

Although the disadvantages of cold-air cooling are few, the units themselves are large and bulky, and generally have awkward handpieces. The risk of air embolism is low, but a case did occur in the early 1980s during surgery performed with a sapphire-tipped neodymium:YAG laser (written communication, L. Reinisch, PhD, August 2001).

Cold-air cooling represents an interesting and apparently effective alternative to cooled sapphire windows. Further refinements of this technique and the delivery systems are needed, as is a comparison to cryogen spray cooling devices.

The study was funded by Nidek Inc, Fremont, Calif.

PART EIGHT DISCUSSION

Kenneth A. Arndt, MD, *Moderator*

> **Emil A. Tanghetti, MD:**   We have been using air cooling since it has was developed, for hair removal and the treatment of leg veins, and we have always used cooling gel. Our belief is that we are converting this air-cooling device into a contact-cooling device, because that gel is being cooled. I think we are combining those 2 methods, and we find it very effective.

I have a question for Dr Nelson. We treated leg veins using a 40-millisecond alexandrite laser. The maximum fluence that the skin could tolerate with the cooling method we used, air cooling plus gel, was approximately 50 J/cm². Another investigator we are aware of gave much higher fluences, 60 to 80 J/cm², with a 3-millisecond alexandrite laser using dynamic cooling. What is really happening with the Dynamic Cooling Device? Is one actually freezing the surface of the skin and changing the optical properties of the skin? In other words, is the surgeon shooting the laser through an optically changed epidermis that makes it like shooting through an ice cube? Also, why are there big discrepancies in maximum fluences between my study and that of the other investigator?

> **J. Stuart Nelson, MD:**   You have to understand the different mechanisms of thermal conduction of heat out of the skin. Evaporative cooling has a heat transfer coefficient of 10,000 to 12,000 W/m²K. Conductive cooling has a heat transfer coefficient of approximately 5000 W/m²K. In terms of efficiency and heat transfer, the evaporative cooling of the cryogen spray cooling device is much more effective in removing a large amount of heat in a very short time than is bulk cooling. Thus, the other investigator who employed cryogen spray cooling could use much higher fluences, because the cooling mechanism was much more efficient.

> **Dr Tanghetti:**   Isn't one shooting through a mist after the cryogen spray is shot? Could it change the penetration of light? Could we be changing the epidermal optical properties? Does that happen, or can it happen?

> **Dr Nelson:**   The clinician is not delivering the laser light through a mist but rather through a liquid layer of cryogen on the skin surface. There is a published report that the liquid cryogen layer on the skin actually has little, if any, absorbance of the wavelengths in the yellow region of the spectrum. If, however, there is frost formation on the skin surface, 10% of the incident light energy might be lost. However, with use of delays ranging from 10 to 30 milliseconds between termination of cryogen spurt and delivery of the laser pulse, frost formation is not an issue An article in a recent issue of *Lasers in Surgery and Medicine* shows that the frost formation is actually a very late phenomenon, which does not occur for 180 to 200 milliseconds after cryogen spurt termination.

> **R. Rox Anderson, MD:**   I think there might also be ice crystals forming in the upper portion of the epidermis, and they will scatter light well. Looking at the transmission of light through a lake of liquid cryogen or the formation of frost, which is the condensation of atmospheric water in solid form and a late event, I would expect substantial light attenuation. I would worry more about light being scattered back from ice crystals inside the tissue. Has this issue been studied, Dr Nelson?

> **Dr Nelson:**   That question has not been specifically addressed.

Dr Anderson: Ice crystals in the skin form the white cryogen frozen-tissue "ball" that all dermatologists are familiar with, and I think it does exist with the cryogen spray, or Dynamic Cooling Device.

Dr Nelson: The white cryogen ball?

Dr Anderson: Yes, during cryosurgery, the tissue becomes alabaster white. That is not frost. That's ice in the tissues.

Dr Nelson: You are speaking about the much longer cooling times associated with cryosurgery, which are not relevant to cryogen spray cooling in conjunction with laser dermatologic surgery. In the latter, ice forms on the skin surface, not in the epidermis.

Dr Anderson: You're absolutely wrong. There is literature from the 1950s that proves the whiteness is ice in the tissues.

Dr Nelson: I do not think that ice formation has been a deleterious issue. Perhaps there are people in the audience who would want to comment that they safely use cryogen spray cooling without adverse effects to the skin. In our laboratory, we have used cryogen spurt durations up to 500 milliseconds and have not noted any deleterious effects.

Dr Anderson: What is the cryogen spurt duration that leads to injury of the skin? There must be an answer to that, because one cannot leave the cryogen spray on the skin forever. Has that been measured?

Dr Nelson: Certainly for cryogen spurt durations up to 500 milliseconds, there has not, to my knowledge, been any report of cryogen-induced injury. In the case that you referred to in your presentation, the woman with the hypopigmentation after laser hair removal, I believe you have the mechanism of injury backward. In the first generation of alexandrite laser devices for hair removal, the cryogen spray did not adequately cover the 12- to 18-mm spot diameter. The damage that you observed in your patient was because the cryogen did not adequately cover the outermost areas of the laser-irradiated spot. Therefore, I believe what you described is laser-induced injury, not cryoinjury.

Dr Anderson: She had arcs of hypopigmentation, which I associated primarily with cryogen injury. It is well known that melanocytes are far more cryogen-sensitive than most other cells, and these hypopigmented areas were far bigger than any laser spot I have ever seen. They were probably 1 inch (2.5 cm) in diameter. Within those areas was a hyperpigmented spot that was perfectly formed and presumably was the laser spot. This is one of the most horrible laser-induced cosmetic side effects I have ever seen. Someone performed a full-body treatment in a very inappropriate way. Her treatment was 2 years ago. I don't know what happened. I would like to get to the bottom of it.

What is your recommendation, Dr Nelson, for the maximum setting of the cryogen spurt duration? If one does not align the spray device perpendicular to the skin and does not pay attention to where one is directing the spray, it is very easy, because of just triangulation, to have the spray hit a spot other than where the laser will hit. So it behooves us to not use a spurt duration that is great enough to cause cryogen injury.

Dr Nelson: I think a cryogen spurt duration up to 100 to 200 milliseconds is certainly very safe.

Dr Arndt: Dr Nelson, you published an article of a study that evaluated the optimal duration of cryogen spray for the pulsed dye laser of 100 milliseconds, with no delay. Would you comment on that?

Dr Nelson: In my practice, for treatment of port-wine stains in infants and young children, I use spurts of 50 to 60 milliseconds with very short delays of 10 to 20 milliseconds. The rationale is that it takes about that long to cool the epidermal basal layer.

Richard Ort, MD: In a recent article in *Lasers in Surgery and Medicine*, the authors commented that the amount of frost obtained was dependent on the humidity of the atmosphere. In a humid area such as Florida, for example, cooling devices cause more frost. So perhaps one might get more interference with the light penetrating into the skin. Also, the condensation of water that occurs, such as from frost, adds heat back to the skin, I believe, so that might help to reduce the risk of cryogen injury.

Robert A. Weiss, MD: I evaluated 3 neodymium (Nd):YAG lasers: one without cooling, the Varia (CoolTouch Corporation, Roseville, Calif) with dynamic cooling, and the CoolGlide (Altus Medical Inc, Burlingame, Calif) with precooling. Whenever we used precooling with the Varia, I had to use much higher fluences to get the same effect on a vein than using the Altus CoolGlide alone, considering similar spot sizes and different pulse durations (Varia, approximately 1 millisecond; Altus, about 10 milliseconds). Could Dr Nelson or Dr Anderson tell me why I had that finding? Was it due to pulse duration differences, or did the precooling maybe diminish the effectiveness of that wavelength?

A physician: What length cryogen spurt durations did you use?

Dr Weiss: We used spurt durations of 10 to 20 milliseconds before the pulse.

A physician: That is very short cryogen precooling. I would not expect that to change the optical properties of the upper dermis or to change the temperature of the blood vessel that you irradiated.

Dr Nelson: I do not have a clear-cut answer to this question. I think it comes back to the issue of whether ice formation occurs in the epidermis. As was just pointed out, water stores a tremendous amount of heat, both in the formation and the melting of ice. If there is indeed water freezing in the upper epidermis after a cryogen spurt, that ice will do the same thing for the skin as ice cubes do for a soft drink. It stays cold a lot longer. The heat that is exchanged with the freezing of ice is several hundred kilocalories per gram. One kilocalorie per gram of water put into the skin raises the skin temperature 1°C. So ice is capable of absorbing laser radiation that would drive the temperature up to several hundred degrees Celsius before the ice even melts. If indeed that is happening in the skin, then a wonderful heat sink is sitting there in the epidermis. Perhaps we should look at that in detail. We just do not know enough about the effects of very cold temperatures being in contact with the skin for very short periods.

Dale Koop, PhD: I am from CoolTouch Corporation. I think duration of the cryogen spurt is the wrong parameter to look at for dynamic cooling. It is the quantity of cryogen the laser surgeon puts on the skin that determines the total amount of kilocalories of heat that are taken out of the skin, so time is an arbitrary parameter. It depends on how big the nozzle of the cryogen spray device is, how big the spray area is, and a lot of other issues. Therefore, 80 milliseconds is a meaningless number without knowing the total quantity of cryogen. A laser system can easily be designed so that the maximum amount of cryogen sprayed into an area does not have enough latent heat evaporation to crystallize the skin or cause any damage. Dr Anderson's case of cryogen damage could have been due to stacking of cryogen, which we have seen, or perhaps something was wrong with the cryogen spray valve.

Cyrus Chess, MD: I want to comment on what Dr Nelson said, that he knows of no reports of blistering. I learned very early in my experience with the cryogen spray cooling that one has to be careful not to stack the cryogen spurts. I created a blister in one of my first patients, because I delivered too much cryogen to the treatment area. One has to learn to work away from the cryogen spray but, more importantly, to not stack the cryogen pulses, to avoid blistering.

Pablo Boixeda, MD: A recent article in *Lasers in Surgery and Medicine* recommended using a cryogen spurt as long as 200 milliseconds for patients with a high concentration of melanin in port-wine stains. Do you have any comment?

Dr Nelson: One of my colleagues, Boris Majaron, has shown that a continuous long spurt is not desirable. It is best to have intermittent, short (10-mm) spurts right before the laser pulse is delivered. When my coworkers and I initially designed the cryogen spray cooling, it was just a simple spray. However, after a closer look at the issues of thermodynamics, I believe that much longer cryogen spurt durations may now be practical based on redesign of nozzle geometry, cryogen delivery, and other factors.

Martin H. Mihm, Jr, MD: I have had the opportunity to study actinic keratoses that we treated with liquid nitrogen in a double-blind study, in which we looked at normal facial skin a given area away from the actual treatment site. For areas of treatment simply for actinic keratoses, superficial dermal fibrosis occurs. Therefore, your injury with liquid nitrogen, I think, goes much deeper than appears, as Dr Anderson mentioned. The dermis is altered by the cryogen in a very superficial way.

PART 9

Lasers and Lights as Diagnostic Tools: Where Are We Now?

Confocal Scanning Laser Microscopy and Optical Coherence Tomography

Thomas E. Rohrer, MD

The answer to the question of where are we now with lasers and lights as diagnostic tools is, We are not quite there yet. However, there are some new technologies that show promise for diagnostic use. I will discuss 2 new laser and light technologies being used for diagnosis: confocal scanning laser microscopy and optical coherence tomography. My primary focus will be on confocal scanning laser microscopy.

CONFOCAL SCANNING LASER MICROSCOPY

A medical imaging device, the confocal laser scanning microscope, has recently become available that may aid surgeons who perform Mohs micrographic surgery in determining the presence or absence of tumor in excised tissue without freezing, sectioning, or staining the tissue first.[1,2] Confocal microscopes use a low-power diode laser that scans across an image area, and then the reflected light gets collected back on a detector and refocused. Because differences in refractive index change signal intensity, it is possible to make a digital, 2-dimensional image from the scan. Confocal microscopes provide magnification up to 1000¥, which gives resolution at a cellular level. These instruments create optical sections of tissue in a horizontal plane. This is similar to what is done in the Mohs technique, and not vertically as seen in traditional sections stained with hematoxylin-eosin (H&E). One limitation of the confocal microscope is that the maximum depth of imaging is only 200 μm, so it does not penetrate very deeply into the tissue. However, it allows for real-time optical sectioning, and the images can be stacked as well. Using this instrument, one can create sort of a miniature computed tomographic (CT) scanner of the skin, and some of the images are quite impressive.

Confocal images compare fairly closely with histologic slides prepared using standard H&E staining of the dermal-epidermal (DE) junction (Fig 34-1), a hair

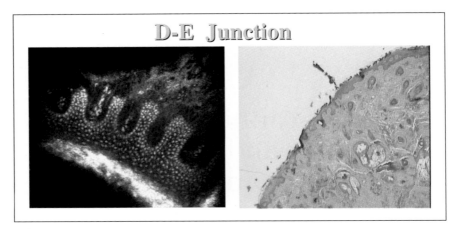

FIGURE 34.1

Comparison of confocal image (left) and histologic slide prepared using standard hematoxylin-eosin (H&E) staining (right) of dermal-epidermal (DE) junction.

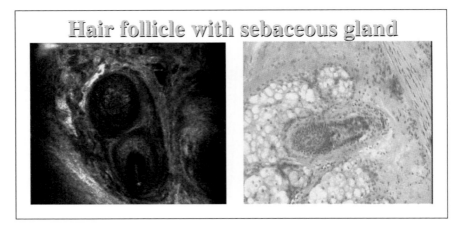

FIGURE 34.2

Comparison of confocal image (left) and image obtained with standard H&E staining techniques (right) of hair follicle with sebaceous gland.

follicle with sebaceous gland (Fig 34-2), and eccrine glands (Fig 34-3). Sections of basal cell tumors also can highlight very well with the confocal microscope.

My coworkers and I designed a study to obtain images, with the ex vivo model of the confocal scanning laser microscope, of tissue samples excised during Mohs micrographic surgery. We compared these images with histologic slides prepared using standard frozen-section H&E techniques. The results of the first phase of the study were previously presented.[3]

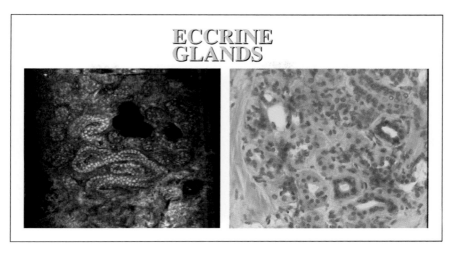

FIGURE 34.3

Confocal image (left) compared with H&E-stained slide (right) of eccrine glands.

MATERIALS AND METHODS

A new-generation confocal scanning laser microscope designed for use with excised tissue samples ex vivo (VivaScope 2000, Lucid Inc, Henrietta, NY) was used for a phase 2 study. Tissue samples were limited to those excised during the first stage of the Mohs procedure.[4] Tissues with dimensions greater than the 1 ¥ 1-cm scanning area of the microscope were excluded from the study.

Fifteen consecutive patients undergoing Mohs micrographic surgery were enrolled in the study under a clinical protocol approved by our institutional review board. Although other tumors were not specifically excluded, all patients in the study had biopsy-proven basal cell or squamous cell carcinoma.

After the usual process of debulking the lesion with light curettage, a small margin was excised around the clinically evident tumor with a standard Mohs micrographic technique. The tissue was marked for orientation, frozen in a cryostat with *optimal cryogenic temperature* (OCT, *Tissue Tek, Miles, Naperville, Ill*), and sectioned. The fresh-frozen sections were placed on a glass slide and processed using standard hematoxylin-eosin staining methods and were then read by the Mohs surgeon for evidence of residual tumor. After the histologic slides had been analyzed and the decision was made to proceed to a second stage or to make a repair, the remaining pieces of frozen tissue were allowed to thaw at room temperature for imaging with the confocal scanning laser microscope. The specimens were rinsed of any residual OCT and immersed for approximately 1 minute in a proprietary solution provided by the manufacturer. The solution serves to enhance the image contrast between the cellular structures of tumor and adjacent cellular structures. Tissue samples were removed from the cellular enhancement solution, blotted dry, placed dermis side down, and secured into a disposable tissue cassette designed for use with the confocal scanning laser microscope. Placement of the tissue dermis side down ensures that the surface of the tissue sample imaged by the confocal scanning laser microscope would be just proximal to the last tissue section sliced with the microtome and mounted on the histologic slide. Care also was taken to maintain consistent orientation between the tissue sample within the cassette and that recorded on the patient records.

Once the tissue cassette was inserted into the confocal scanning laser microscope, the sample was automatically scanned across the objective lens of the system to generate a 10×10 array of individual frames, each of which represents a 1.0-mm (horizontal) × 0.8-mm (vertical) field of view. These individual frames were pieced together by the confocal scanning laser microscope, and a seamless composite map was displayed on the screen. The imaging time of the microscope was approximately 2.5 minutes. We then were able to analyze the tissue maps, as displayed on the monitor of the confocal scanning laser microscope, for the presence or absence of tumor. The results were recorded on a map of the specimen, as is traditionally done in Mohs micrographic surgery.

RESULTS

The imaging time with the confocal scanning laser microscope was approximately 2.5 minutes (Fig 34-4) compared with 15 minutes for H&E processing.

Of the 15 patients enrolled in the study, 4 were excluded because their tissue sections were too large to fit the scanning area. Of the remaining 11 patients, a total of 27 H&E sections and confocal maps were produced, because some patients had more than 2 sections. Eight of the 11 patients had basal cell carcinoma, and 3 had squamous cell carcinoma.

All 16 sections determined to be free of tumor by H&E staining were also read as being free of tumor using the confocal scanning laser microscope. Seven of the 8 sections determined to have tumor by H&E techniques were evaluated as malignant by the confocal microscope (Fig 34-5), an 87.5% correlation. The eighth section, which was indeterminate with the confocal microscope was shown by H&E to be basal cell carcinoma (Fig 34-6). Three sections of squamous cell carcinomas were read by H&E as having inflammation and therefore suggestive of having tumor. The inflammation was seen in only 1 of the confocal maps.

The overall correlation between the H&E and confocal maps was 96% when true-positive and true-negative results were considered. If the specimens with inflammation read as suggestive of malignancy were counted as actually having malignancy, the correlation rate drops to 89%.

COMMENT

In this small pilot study, the confocal scanning laser microscope was shown to be a rapid and fairly accurate method of evaluating tissue margins for cutaneous

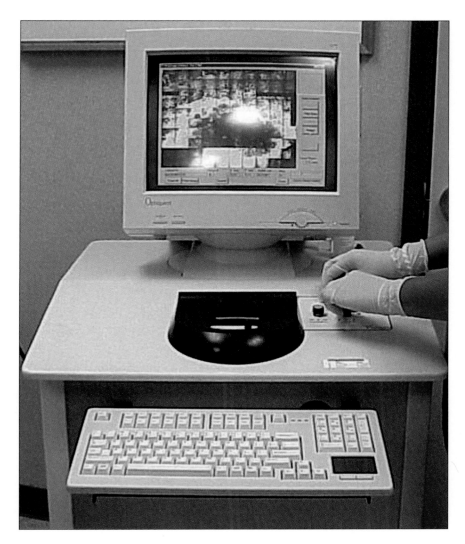

FIGURE 34.4

Confocal scanning. Note: The American Medical Association does not endorse or recommend any particular type or brand of scanner.

malignancy. Whereas the overall correlation with standard H&E staining was between 89% and 96% depending on how the data were evaluated, this new technology is still less accurate than the presumed nearly 100% accuracy of H&E techniques.

Furthermore, our results with the confocal scanning laser microscope in clinical practice are lower than the results obtained in this study, with an accuracy

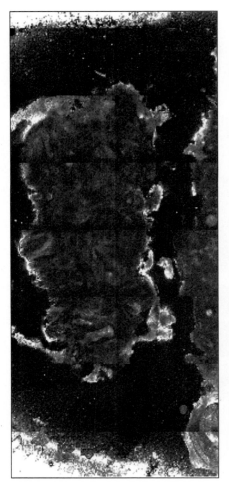 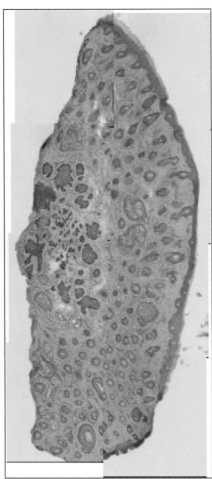

F I G U R E   34.5a   **F I G U R E   34.5b**

True-positives—tissue sections determined to have tumor—detected by confocal
scanning laser microscope (a) and H&E staining (b). Close-up of basal cell carcinoma
with confocal scanning laser microscope (c). Scale bar represents 300 mm in left figure, 100 mm at center, and 400 mm at right.

rate closer to 75%. The instrument has difficulty imaging morpheaform basal
cell carcinomas and many squamous cell carcinomas, so it is not a useful diagnostic tool at this time. The manufacturer is working to address problems with
the device so that it can handle larger tissue sections and have better resolution.
Improved contrast agents are also now available that better highlight tumors and
cellular structures. These changes should help make results more reproducible.
Another problem with the confocal scanning laser microscope, its limited depth
to penetration, may be more difficult to solve.

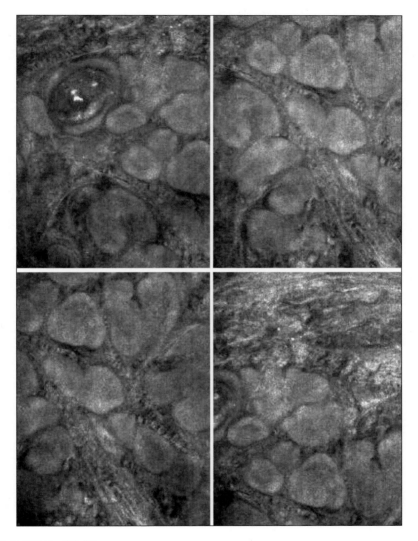

F I G U R E 34.5c

Nevertheless, this technology has already improved rapidly. An initial study that we performed using a first-generation model of the microscope yielded only a 43% correlation between confocal and H&E images (unpublished data, 2000). Other advances in this technology have also been made. Smaller, even handheld devices, with better contrast stains, will soon be available for an in vivo confocal scanning laser microscope. The in vivo model, which is placed on top of the skin to produce a scanned image, may be used in the future to better define the tumor margins. It may be possible to differentiate pigmented lesions and even perform noninvasive "biopsies" for certain cutaneous diseases and malignancies.

With future advances, the confocal scanning laser microscope may soon offer Mohs micrographic surgeons a rapid and accurate diagnostic tool.

OPTICAL COHERENCE TOMOGRAPHY

Another light-based device that may play a role as a diagnostic tool in dermatology is optical coherence tomography. Optical coherence tomography is often used in ophthalmology, and it is basically an optical analog of ultrasound. Optical sonar captures back-reflected light using diode lasers around 1300 nm. It is noninvasive, real-time imaging. The resolution is approximately 15 mm, so it is not as good as confocal microscopy, but it is much better than high-frequency ultrasound. It also produces vertical sections, which dermatologists are used to reading. Detection depth is much deeper than with the confocal microscope, down to 1.5 mm. A lot of this technique involves just figuring out a new language—how to read the images. Although optical coherence tomography is not presently being used in dermatology, it may play a role in the near future. Of the devices we have right now, none is perfect yet.

In summary, none of the laser-based imaging devices are perfectly suited for use in dermatology at present. However, confocal microscopy and optical coherence tomography are both exciting technologies that may be on the verge of becoming very useful in daily practice. Some day in the not-so-distant future, the idea of removing skin and leaving a permanent scar in order to make a diagnosis based on cellular histology may seem barbaric.

REFERENCES

1. Rajadhyaksha M, Grossman M, Esterowitz D, Webb RH, Anderson RR. In vivo confocal laser scanning microscopy of human skin: melanin provides strong contrast. *J Invest Dermatol.* 1995;104:946–952.
2. Rajadhyaksha M, Gonzalez S, Zavislan JM, Anderson RR, Webb RH. In vivo confocal laser scanning microscopy of human skin II: advances in instrumentation and comparison with histology. *J Invest Dermatol.* 1999;113:293–303.
3. Rohrer T. The use of confocal microscopy in Mohs micrographic surgery [abstract]. *Lasers Med Surg.* 2000:3–4.
4. Mohs FE. Chemosurgery, a microscopically controlled method of cancer excision. *Arch Surg.* 1941;42:279–295.

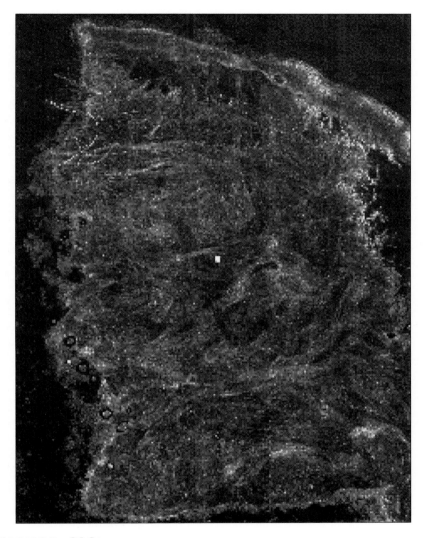

F I G U R E 34.6a

Indeterminate result with confocal scanning laser microscope (a) was found in this
basal cell carcinoma (b).

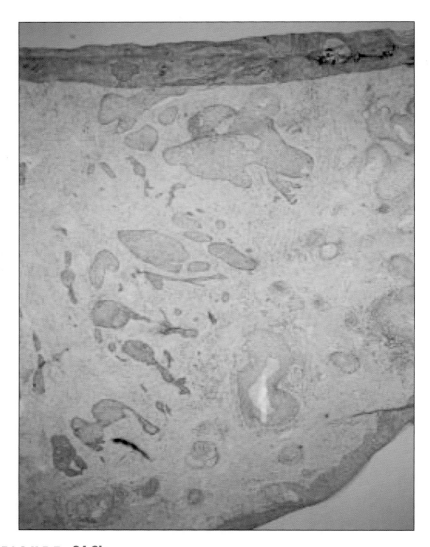

FIGURE 34.6b

Noninvasive Diagnostic Tools for Characterization of Port-wine Stains

J. Stuart Nelson, MD, PhD

A large array of laser devices are now available that allow modification of wavelength, pulse duration, light dose, spot diameter, repetition rate, and skin cooling. To individualize these source parameters, laser surgeons need to understand skin characteristics for each patient. These characteristics include the epidermal melanin content, target absorption, target depth and distribution, target thermal confinement, optical scattering, and how much increase in heat occurs due to optical scattering.

GEOMETRY OF PORT-WINE STAINS

In my practice, I am interested in improving laser therapy for port-wine stains. It is very difficult to estimate how many treatments a child will need for removal of the birthmark. My colleagues and I are attempting to perform diagnostic imaging of port-wine stains, with the goal of optimizing laser parameters. Blanching of port-wine stains is variable and unpredictable. There are several reasons for this. The epidermal melanin concentration changes on an individual patient basis, the depth of the blood vessels in port-wine stains is highly variable (100 μm to 1 mm), and the diameter of these blood vessels also varies widely (10 to 300 μm), based on our histologic measurements. We have found that the geometry of port-wine stains not only varies by patient but also varies from site to site on the same patient.

For example, the optical penetration depth in blood is very steep in the yellow portion of the visible spectrum. With an increase in wavelength from 585 to 595 nm, the optical absorption of blood changes by a factor of 5. Thus, for treatment of port-wine stains with very-small-diameter vessels, the laser surgeon will want to choose the 585-nm wavelength to confine the light absorption into smaller vessels. On the other hand, treatment of much larger blood vessels of port-wine stains or other cutaneous disease will best be accomplished with longer wavelengths, which will penetrate deeper into the vessels.

PULSED PHOTOTHERMAL RADIOMETRY

My colleagues and I at the Beckman Laser Institute in Irvine, Calif, have developed several noninvasive diagnostic tools for characterization of port-wine stains. One tool is based on thermal imaging using pulsed photothermal radiometry. We have adopted 2 approaches. The first uses a single-element detector, with which we measure surface temperature as a function of time. Subsequently, the signal is deconvolved using various heat transfer models to generate the initial space-dependent temperature distribution immediately after laser exposure. It is possible to determine what the rise in temperature, or "temperature jump," of the epidermal melanin was after exposure to pulsed laser. Then, using tomographic reconstruction algorithm techniques, we can determine the depth of the port-wine stain. So from this very simple measurement, one can measure how hot the epidermis gets and how deep the port-wine stain is. This information can help the laser surgeon choose the optimal wavelength, light dose, and cooling parameters to implement. Laser companies could actually incorporate this technology into commercial laser systems for about $1300. There would obviously have to be some software and some algorithm developed to go along with that, but it is feasible.

Our other approach is to image the blood vessels of port-wine stains 3-dimensionally. This image reconstruction is a bit more complicated. It involves taking a time sequence of infrared emission images and then going backward and determining what the temperature distribution was immediately after the laser pulse was delivered. In some port-wine stains, we are now able to resolve individual blood vessels that measure 70 to 100 μm. Certainly, for some pediatric port-wine stains, that is not good enough, but at least resolution of individual blood vessels is beginning to be possible.

OPTICAL DOPPLER TOMOGRAPHY

The last technique I want to mention is optical coherence tomography. Analogous to ultrasound, this technique uses light waves and measures optical backscattering as opposed to acoustic waves. Our group added the Doppler effect, whereby we measure the change in the optical frequency of the light that is backscattered out of human skin containing a port-wine stain. We can actually image these blood vessels in the dermis. After Doppler imaging, we used a very high light dose of the flashlamp-pumped pulsed dye laser (ScleroPLUS, Candela Corporation, Wayland, Mass) to coagulate these blood vessels. A biopsy specimen obtained in the middle of the laser treatment demonstrated good coagulation of the blood vessels. Another Doppler image showed no blood flow after completion of the laser treatment. Our goal is to develop optical Doppler tomography as a noninvasive diagnostic tool and a means to evaluate the efficacy of laser therapy for vascular lesions in situ and in real time.

I think that both optical and thermal techniques have certain roles in optimization of laser treatment parameters. Other research groups around the world also are pursuing these technologies. Higher spatial resolution is still needed, and imaging will be improved with better reconstruction techniques.

chapter 36

New Electro-optic Imaging Tools

R. Rox Anderson, MD

Where are we now in the use of lasers and lights as diagnostic tools? We are in the dark ages, but a renaissance is on the way. As a specialty, dermatology has been slow to adopt diagnostic technology. Most of the current diagnostic tools in the practice of dermatology have been in use a long time. These include magnifiers; microscopy, which was invented in the 1600s; and Wood's light, a fluorescent diagnostic tool that Robert Williams Wood developed in 1908. Epiluminescence microscopy (ELM) is a recent application of ancient technology, using simple magnification. One recent invention that dermatologists use is polarized light to eliminate glare and obtain a better view of the skin, a technique I described in 1991.[1] I cannot think of any other optical diagnostic tools being used in dermatology. I find it amazing that, for the most visible organ of the body, this is all the technology we have for optical diagnostics.

A host of microscopic and macroscopic imaging and spectroscopy techniques are poised to be useful but have not yet found a firm place in diagnosis of skin disease or for guiding procedures such as tumor removal. Among the new electro-optic imaging tools are confocal microscopy (see Chapter 34) and optical coherence tomography (Chapters 34 and 35). I will briefly describe examples of emerging optical diagnostics. There is not time to explain these in detail.

LASER-INDUCED FLUORESCENCE

Another new technique that I think has excellent potential applications for dermatology is femtosecond laser-induced multiphoton fluorescence. In this technique, a couple of infrared photons are absorbed, causing ultraviolet-like excitation transitions and then fluorescence generated by particular molecules. The images are totally different than those obtained with confocal microscopy or optical coherence tomography, because femtosecond laser-induced fluorescence does not use scattered light. Fluorescence is a "fingerprint" for the molecules that fluoresce, such that multiphoton fluorescence microscopy is now the only deep, high-resolution, and specific molecular imaging technique.

Kollias and colleagues[2] studied another technique, called laser-induced fluorescence, which we have not yet used clinically. Skin has 7 distinct fluorophores whereby one can identify an excitation wavelength and the fluorescence emission associated with that molecule. We were able to identify the molecules associated with 5 of those 7 fluorophores. Two of them remain mysterious bands; we do not know what the molecule is.

It is interesting what one could potentially monitor using this method. To my knowledge, no one has tried to image tryptophan fluorescence in the epidermis, whose signal is increased greatly in skin cancer. I think that might be a great way to look for proliferative lesions. NADH is also a fluorescent molecule and could act as a measure of the cell oxidative function. The work by Kollias et al[2] suggests that it is also possible to estimate age by measurement of the skin fluorescent spectra. The cross-links that are formed in photoaged skin are fluorescent molecules, condensation products between elastin and collagen.

Molecular biologists have developed molecules, called molecular beacons, which fluoresce only when they bind to a sequence-specific target. This is done by attaching to the 2 ends of a probe sequence, 1 molecule that fluoresces and another molecule that quenches that fluorescence. Before binding, the quencher and the fluorophore are nearly together, and the molecule does not fluoresce, because the emission is quenched. When the probe binds to a specific sequence, the quencher and fluorophore get separated and the probe becomes fluorescent.

NUCLEAR SCATTERING SPECTROSCOPY

Nuclear scattering spectroscopy is a technique that I think will one day be useful for tumor detection. The size of cell nuclei can be deduced from Mie scattering, as described by Mie around 1900. Cell nuclei are almost perfect spheres, and they scatter light as a group. The theory of Mie scattering suggest that, if one measures the singly scattered light, one can deduce information about the size and index of the particles that are scattering. The inventors of nuclear scattering spectroscopy have clearly shown that it is possible to deduce real morphology of cell nuclei by looking at the singly scattered light. They are doing this using optical polarization.

DIFFUSE OPTICAL TOMOGRAPHY

On the surface of the skin, if one puts light in over here, light scatters all over the place. However, if one measures the light that happens to come out at some distance away from where it went in, one can capture the light that went through a banana-shaped path deep into the tissue. There is a way of doing that over many points—many points of input light and many points of output light. When these points are put into a computer model, the result is a form of tomography, called diffuse optical tomography. Using this technique, researchers have already shown that they can monitor brain function, oxygenation of the brain, and subdural hematomas. To some extent, deep structures such as breast cancer can be imaged using light this way. Nothing has been done in dermatology with diffuse optical tomography.

LASER RAMAN SPECTROSCOPY

When light scatters off molecules, it can exchange a small amount of energy to the vibrational modes of those molecules. One can look at these very weak exchanges between light and the scattering substance and deduce what the vibrational structures of the molecules are. The Harrison Spectroscopy Laboratory at Massachusetts Institute of Technology in Cambridge, Mass, has measured these weak signals from tissue. The technique allows, for example, calculation of glucose and urea levels and so forth in a short time using intact tissue.

Whether and how optical diagnostics enters dermatologic practice depends greatly on a clear definition of what clinicians need to see or diagnose at the bedside. The question we should ask ourselves is, What do we wish we could see or rapidly diagnose?

REFERENCES

1. Anderson RR. Polarized light examination and photography of the skin. *Arch Dermatol.* 1991;127:1000–1005.
2. Gillies R, Zonios G, Anderson RR, Kollias N. Fluorescence excitation spectroscopy provides information about human skin in vivo. *J Invest Dermatol.* 2000;115:704–707.

PART NINE DISCUSSION

Kenneth A. Arndt, MD, *Moderator*

Dr Arndt: Dr Rohrer, how far off do you think we are from being able to perform bedside in vivo visualization of surgical margins, whether for Mohs micrographic surgery or excisions, using confocal laser scanning microscopy?

Thomas E. Rohrer, MD: You would really have to ask the engineers designing the systems, but it is very possible that within 12 to 24 months, something could be developed that actually could be effective and useful.

Dr Arndt: Dr Anderson, the first confocal microscopic images I saw emanating from your laboratory almost a decade ago were fuzzy, but they are getting much clearer now, and Dr Rohrer is using confocal microscopy clinically. At some point, are we going to stop using hematoxylin-eosin (H&E) sections? Is confocal microscopy actually what we are going to be doing?

Dr Anderson: I don't know the answer. It actually has been only 5 or 6 years since reflectance confocal microscopy was first used for the skin. We need good stains, and I don't think this technique has any accepted use right now in standard pathology. The real challenge is to get it into the clinical arena and be minimally invasive. I think we will get there, but I don't know when. The early ultrasound images were poor, and it took 20 years for ultrasonography to be used routinely, as it is now. I don't know how long it will take for confocal microscopy to enter the clinical arena.

Melanie C. Grossman, MD: Dr Anderson, I am intrigued by the proposal of being able to measure the age of skin using a fluorescence device. I'm wondering whether it is possible to obtain some sort of simple device to study various topical antiaging creams.

Dr Anderson: The answer is yes.

Dr Grossman: How expensive is the device?

Dr Anderson: It is not very expensive. A fiberoptic-coupled skin fluorometer costs probably about $10,000. I think Ocean Optics Inc (Dunedin, Fla) makes one that uses a card that plugs into the back of a personal computer. It has been used to look at photoaged skin. In a mouse study, we found that the accumulation of what one thinks of as solar elastosis is linked to a specific fluorophore, excited at about 370 nm and emitting around 420 nm. It was possible to figure out what the cumulative dose of the ultraviolet (UV) exposure in these mice was based on skin fluorescence measurements. Other investigators have conducted a study in humans of sun-exposed and non–sun-exposed fluorescence and independently reported the same type of fluorescent spectral signature. I think that such a device might be useful, perhaps for measuring the efficacy of nonablative rejuvenation. We clearly need better end points for that procedure, which often causes only subtle effects clinically.

Roland Kaufmann, MD: I have a question for Dr Waner concerning phlebosurgery and your venous visualizer—your infrared visualizing system. We perform many phlebectomies of very fine veins using tumescent anesthesia or local anesthesia. It must be much faster to remove the veins using your system. Have you any experience with it in phlebology?

Milton Waner, MD: Yes, in fact, that was one of the applications we considered. A vascular surgeon who works with this device in my institution finds it very useful to visualize some of the veins. The infrared visualizing system can visualize the saphenous vein on just about everybody, so it is extremely helpful. It also is being used with intravascular coagulation devices, such as the radiofrequency device. Laser surgeons are interested in using the vein finder for access and for localizing veins. Certainly, it is very useful in phlebology.

There is another application that I did not mention, and that is in forensic medicine. The infrared vein finder can help detect subsurface bruising, which cannot be seen with the naked eye, especially early after trauma. So it also has applications for detecting signs of child abuse and in forensic medicine.

Roy Geronemus, MD: Dr Waner, I would think there would be numerous cosmetic indications as well, including localizing the needle for botulinum toxin injections to avoid hitting a vein and the subsequent bruising. It might also help define how to treat vascular lesions, particularly of the venous type. I think there could be some real value, and I would like to see you pursue the study of those applications.

Martin H. Mihm, Jr, MD: I think that there is great hope for use of the ex vivo confocal scanning laser microscope (VivaScope 2000, Lucid Inc, Henrietta, NY). As long as one looks above the basement membranes, there is great detail available with this technique, even in a case of Darier disease that I saw, in which I could clearly see and appreciate keratin clumps. I think this technique is very useful for appreciation of melanocytic lesions—benign vs atypical intraepidermal proliferations and superficial invasion. Once one scans through the basement membrane, images become quite blurred. However, in the dermis one can appreciate, for example, lymphocyte trafficking. One of the things that other investigators are attempting with this technique is to see the difference between graft-vs-host reaction lymphocytes and drug reactions. I think there is very much to be gained from this technique.

Lasers and Psoriasis: An Illuminating Combination

Rationale for Vascular-Specific Laser Treatment of Psoriasis

Brian D. Zelickson, MD

Psoriasis is a common chronic skin disorder whose etiology is unknown. There are many different factors that have a role in the development of prop-agation of psoriasis, and there are many different treatment modalities that affect various potential etiologic factors to enhance clinical improvement. This article will review the use of vascular-specific lasers for further defining the role of the blood vessel in the psoriatic process and as a possible treatment device.

A review of the literature shows that the blood vessel is not the main etiologic factor of psoriasis, but it certainly plays a major role in the propagation of a pso-riatic plaque.[1-5] The prominent vasculature in a psoriatic plaque can be seen in images of the skin obtained with the ex vivo confocal scanning laser microscope. Figure 37-1 shows the top of the epidermis stained with a CD-31 stain, which stains blood vessels, and with a PG-9.5 stain, which stains nerves green. In the psoriatic plaque, one can see large, dilated loops that transfer into the dermal papillae. This figure shows that there is a lot of chromophore that can be at-tacked with a pulsed dye laser.

Almost all the available lasers have been used to treat psoriasis, and several have clearance from the US Food and Drug Administration (FDA) for the treat-ment of psoriasis. In this article, I will primarily discuss the pulsed dye laser and will summarize the previously reported studies that used the pulsed dye laser for the treatment of psoriasis.

REVIEW OF THE LITERATURE

A total of 191 plaques (94 patients) treated with the pulsed dye laser have been reported in the literature.[1-5] The number of treatments ranged from 1 to 5. Fol-low-up ranged from 2 to 13 months, with an average of 5 months. In general, 50% to 60% of treated patients had a good to excellent response, and 18% of

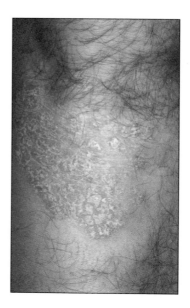

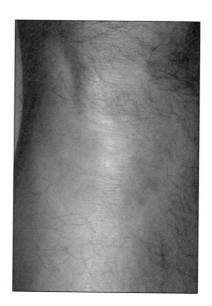

FIGURE 37.1

Pre-treatment (top); Treatment with pulsed dye laser (585 nm, 0.45 milliseconds) obtained good clearing (bottom) of psoriasis, although some dyspigmentation is seen.

the patients had complete clearing of their treated psoriatic plaques. Treatment parameters used in these studies were a 5-mm spot size; wavelength of 585 nm; fluences of 2 to 9 J/cm²; and pulse duration of 0.2, 0.45, or 1.5 milliseconds. Treatment intervals of 2 to 4 weeks generally were used. The best treatment parameters, based on a review of the literature and my own observations (unpublished data, 1996 to 2000), appeared to be fluences of 7 to 9 J/cm², a pulse duration of 0.45 milliseconds, and multiple treatments at 2- to 4-week intervals. My coworkers and I[4] produced purpura using fluences anywhere from 5 to 7 J/cm², sometimes up to 8 J/cm², and treating at 3-week intervals. Usually, in my clinical experience (unpublished data, 1996 to 2000), if patients responded, they would respond in about 2 treatments, and it usually took 4 to 6 treatments for the patients who did not respond in 2 treatments to respond. Remissions of up to 9 months have been published,[6] and my colleagues and I have seen complete remission in some patients lasting as long as 5 years at final follow-up (unpublished data, 1996 to 2000).

A study from the Netherlands using the pulsed dye laser (585 nm, 0.45 milliseconds) obtained good clearing of psoriasis, although some hyperpigmentation was seen after treatment (Fig 37-1). Confocal imaging of psoriatic plaques before and after treatment with the pulsed dye laser has been useful in showing the efficacy of treatment[4] (Fig 37-2).

PULSE DURATION

We tested different pulse durations with a 585-nm pulsed dye laser for the treatment of psoriatic plaques (unpublished data, 1998). The 0.45-millisecond pulse duration worked a little better than some of the longer pulse durations (1.5, 6, and 10 milliseconds). We also found that the epidermal injury with pulse durations shorter than 0.45 milliseconds was too great, with ulceration occurring.

ADVANTAGES AND DISADVANTAGES

The advantages of the pulsed dye laser are that it is simple to operate and nontoxic, and potentially can provide long-term remission. The disadvantages of this laser treatment are that it is relatively painful, can treat only limited disease, and has a response rate of only 50% to 60%. It also has a risk of causing scarring, hyperpigmentation, and depigmentation. This laser treatment has a 2- to 3-week healing time. For that reason, we wait 3 or 4 weeks between treatment sessions, because patients do get some ulceration and scabbing as a result of the treatment. A final drawback is that there is no standard reimbursement for this particular procedure.

In conclusion, the indication for pulsed dye laser treatment in psoriasis is localized disease that is unresponsive to other therapies.

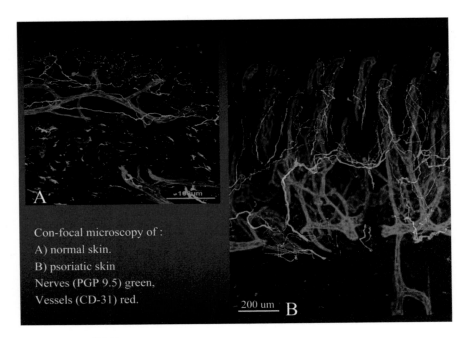

Con-focal microscopy of :
A) normal skin.
B) psoriatic skin
Nerves (PGP 9.5) green,
Vessels (CD-31) red.

FIGURE 37.2

Prominent vasculature in psoriatic plaque in images of skin obtained with ex vivo confocal scanning laser microscope. Blood vessels are stained with CD-31 stain, and nerves are stained with PG-9.5 stain. Left, Ex vivo confocal microscopic images show large, dilated loops before treatment of psoriasis with pulsed dye laser. Right, After treatment, results are not completely normal, but diameter of loops is smaller and number of vessels is smaller in treated plaque.

REFERENCES

1. Hacker SM, Rasmussen JE. The effect of flash lamp-pulsed dye laser on psoriasis [letter]. *Arch Dermatol.* 1992;128:853–855.
2. Katugampola GA, Rees AM, Lanigan SW. Laser treatment of psoriasis. *Br J Dermatol.* 1995;133:909–913.
3. Ros AM, Garden JM, Bakus AD, Hedblad MA. Psoriasis response to the pulsed dye laser. *Lasers Surg Med.* 1996;19:331–335.
4. Zelickson BD, Mehregan DA, Wendelschfer-Crabb G, et al. Clinical and histologic evaluation of psoriatic plaques treated with a flashlamp pulsed dye laser. *J Am Acad Dermatol.* 1996;35:64–68.
5. Lanigan SW, Katugampola GA. Treatment of psoriasis with the pulsed dye laser. *J Am Acad Dermatol.* 1997;37:288–289.
6. Bjerring P, Zachariae H, Sogaard H. The flashlamp-pumped dye laser and dermabrasion in psoriasis: further studies on the reversed Koebner phenomenon. *Acta Derm Venereol.* 1997;77:59–61.

Treatment of Psoriasis With the 308-nm Excimer Laser

Roy Geronemus, MD

The treatment of psoriasis has challenged dermatologists for many years. One of the most effective treatments has been ultraviolet light phototherapy using a wavelength in the 300- to 313-nm range. This treatment has not generally been used for localized psoriasis, which can now be effectively treated with the 308-nm excimer laser using a xenon chloride lasing medium. The rationale for this treatment is that the laser may provide a relatively convenient treatment and spare uninvolved skin while avoiding the unwanted effects of topical treatments.

With others, I participated in a multicenter study to establish the efficacy and safety of the 308-nm excimer laser for treatment of psoriasis. The results were published in the *Journal of the American Academy of Dermatology*.[1]

PATIENTS AND METHODS

In a multicenter study involving 5 dermatologic practices, 124 patients were enrolled for treatment with the 308-nm excimer laser using a xenon chloride lasing medium (XTRAC, PhotoMedex Inc, Radnor, Pa). This laser employs directed ultraviolet light. The parameters used were a 30-nanosecond pulse width, spot size 3.2 cm^2, and fluences ranging between 100 and 350 mJ/cm^2, which is usually 3 times the minimal erythema dose (MED). Ninety-four (76%) of the patients in this study had skin types II or III. All patients had stable plaque psoriasis covering less than 10% of their body surface area. Generally, previous therapy, including phototherapy, had been discontinued. Systemic therapy had been discontinued for at least 2 months before treatment, and topical therapy had been stopped at least 1 month earlier.

Typically, we performed an MED test before the laser treatment, and the results of this test served as an initial parameter for the treatment. Treatments took place twice weekly, and we made adjustments in dosimetry depending on the clinical response that we saw after the first treatments and the presence of side effects. The end point was 10 treatments or clearing of plaques. Clearing was considered to be greater than 90% improvement at the end of the study.

RESULTS

Of the 124 patients enrolled, 92 completed the entire protocol. None of the patients who discontinued treatment early did so because of dissatisfaction with the results. Most of these patients had logistical reasons why they discontinued treatments. Of the 92 patients who met the protocol requirements of 10 treatments, 66 (72%) had at least 75% improvement of plaques in an average of 6.2 treatments. In 10 treatments, there was greater than 75% improvement in 77 (84%) of the patients and greater than 90% improvement (clearing) in 46 (50%) of the patients. Two patients achieved clearing in 1 treatment alone.

Patients generally did not experience substantial discomfort during the treatments. Other side effects were generally high. Common side effects included erythema (in 50% of 92 patients), blistering of no clinical significance (45%), and hyperpigmentation (38%). Subsequent to the study, we have been able to greatly diminish the number of patients with the side effect of blistering, based on improved parameters and improved fiberoptics of the laser.

COMMENT

The 308-nm excimer laser appears to be safe and effective for the treatment of chronic plaque psoriasis. Although inverse psoriasis was not included in the study, it is another indication for excimer laser therapy.

Treatment with the 308-nm excimer laser has several advantages over conventional therapy. It requires fewer patient visits than does conventional therapy, which can exceed 30 treatments. Unlike conventional treatment, the excimer laser targets only the affected areas of the skin, sparing the surrounding uninvolved skin.

Treatment of the scalp, nails, or diffuse body involvement has not yet been studied. Future applications of this treatment may include vitiligo, hypopigmentation, cutaneous T-cell lymphoma, lichen planus, and atopic dermatitis.

REFERENCE

1.   Feldman S, Mellen B, Housman TS, et al. Efficacy of 308-nm laser treatment of psoriasis: results of a multicenter study. *J Am Acad Dermatol.* 2002;46:900–906.

chapter 39

Comparison of Lasers Used in Treatment of Psoriasis

Richard E. Fitzpatrick, MD

Psoriasis occurs in approximately 2% of the population, and 80% to 85% of these individuals have mild to moderate psoriasis, according to the National Psoriasis Foundation. The severity of psoriasis is defined by the amount of skin area that the disease covers. If the area of involvement is greater than 10%, the psoriasis is considered severe. If involvement is less than 2% of the body surface, the disease is considered mild. The severity does not refer to the activity of the disease but to the area of involvement. Patients who have localized disease have difficulty receiving effective treatment, because usually they use only topical agents. Topical treatments have a clearance rate of probably approximately 20%, and when there is clearing, it lasts no longer than 3 months at a time. Only a small percentage of affected individuals see dermatologists for treatment of the condition. In the United States, approximately 750,000 people with mild psoriasis and 460,000 people with moderate to severe psoriasis are under the care of dermatologists, according to the National Psoriasis Foundation.

Phototherapy is considered the gold standard for treatment of psoriasis and usually requires 30 or more treatments to produce clearance. A study performed by Parrish and Jaenicke[1] approximately 20 years ago showed that the action spectrum of ultraviolet B (UV-B) light for psoriasis is in the 300- to 313-nm range; outside that range, there is no activity toward clearing psoriasis. A narrow-band UV-B is far more effective.[2] The excimer laser has a wavelength of 308 nm, which is in the spectrum for effective phototherapy.

Lasers that have been used in psoriasis include the argon, carbon dioxide (CO_2), neodymium:YAG, pulsed dye, and excimer lasers. According to reported studies with the argon laser, 19 patients with psoriasis were treated.[3] The cases that cleared had no recurrence in a year, but there was a problem of scar formation using the argon laser.

CARBON DIOXIDE AND NEODYMIUM:YAG LASERS

With the CO_2 laser (10,600 nm), there have been a total of 25 patients reported in the literature, and the results have been disappointing.[4-6] Patients had primarily stable plaque psoriasis but experienced only short-term benefits, with subsequent recurrence of the plaques.

Ruiz-Esparza[7] treated 3 patients using the low-energy (1064-nm) neodymium:YAG laser and found only a partial response.

PULSED DYE LASER

In Chapter 37, Dr Zelickson reported the results of the pulsed dye laser (585 nm) involving 94 patients described in 5 articles.[8-12] There was a definite positive response, with some remissions lasting more than 1 year. However, the treatment was not uniformly beneficial, pain and purpura were side effects, and, from a practical viewpoint, it has not been an easy treatment to give because of the small spot size and low pulse repetition rate.

EXCIMER LASER

I think the excimer laser is quite different from all of these other laser treatments of psoriasis because it is a proven treatment. In a clinical study involving 124 patients, there was greater than 75% clearance in 72% of patients in 6.2 treatments (see Chapter 38). The excimer laser uses an ultraviolet wavelength and one of its major benefits is its ability to target the psoriatic plaques specifically and avoid getting excessive ultraviolet light exposure in nonpsoriatic areas of the skin.[13-15] It is appropriate for the 80% to 85% of patients who are difficult to treat with phototherapy, because full-body exposure to the ultraviolet radiation of phototherapy would increase their risk of skin cancer. Treatment with the excimer laser has decreased side effects. It also has increased effectiveness, requiring 6 to 10 treatments vs 30 or more treatments with conventional therapy.

REFERENCES

1. Parrish JA, Jaenicke KF. Action spectrum for phototherapy of psoriasis. *J Invest Dermatol.* 1981;76:359–362.
2. Coven TR, Burback LH, Gilleaudeau P, et al. Narrowband UVB produces superior clinical and histopathologic resolution of moderate to severe psoriasis in patients compared with broadband UVB. *Arch Dermatol.* 1997;133:1514–1522.
3. Harrison PB, Walker GB, Davis JE. Trauma for psoriasis [letter]. *Lancet.* 1985;2:1063–1064.
4. Bekassy Z, Astedt B. Carbon dioxide laser vaporization of plaque psoriasis. *Br J Dermatol.* 1986;114:489–492.
5. Alora MB, Anderson RR, Quinn TR, Taylor CR. CO_2 laser resurfacing of psoriatic plaques: a pilot study. *Lasers Surg Med.* 1998;22:165–170.
6. Asawanonda P, Anderson RR, Taylor CR. Pendulaser carbon dioxide resurfacing laser versus electrodesiccation with curettage in the treatment of isolated, recalcitrant psoriatic plaques. *J Am Acad Dermatol.* 2000;42:660–666.
7. Ruiz-Esparza J. Clinical response of psoriasis to low-energy irradiance with the Nd:YAG laser at 1320 nm: report of an observation in three cases. *Dermatol Surg.* 1999;25:403–407.

8. Hacker SM, Rasmussen JE. The effect of flashlamp-pulsed dye laser on psoriasis [letter]. *Arch Dermatol.* 1992;128:853–855.

9. Katugampola GA, Rees AM, Lanigan SW. Laser treatment of psoriasis. *Br J Dermatol.* 1995;133:909–913.

10. Ros AM, Garden JM, Bakus AD, Hedblad MA. Psoriasis response to the pulsed dye laser. *Lasers Surg Med.* 1996;19:331–335.

11. Zelickson BD, Mehregan DA, Wendelschfer-Crabb G, et al. Clinical and histologic evaluation of psoriatic plaques treated with a flashlamp pulsed dye laser. *J Am Acad Dermatol.* 1996;35:64–68.

12. Bjerring P, Zachariae H, Sogaard H. The flashlamp-pumped dye laser and dermabrasion in psoriasis: further studies on the reversed Koebner phenomenon. *Acta Derm Venereol.* 1997;77:59–61.

13. Asawanonda P, Anderson RR, Chang Y, Taylor CR. 308-nm excimer laser for the treatment of psoriasis: a dose-response study. *Arch Dermatol.* 2000;136:619–624.

14. Bonis B, Kemeny L, Dobozy A, Bor Z, Szabo G, Ignacz F. 308 nm UBV excimer laser for psoriasis [letter]. *Lancet.* 1997;350:1522.

15. Kemeny L, Bonis B, Dobozy A, Bor Z, Szabo G, Ignacz F. 308-nm excimer laser therapy for psoriasis. *Arch Dermatol.* 2001;137:95–96.

PART TEN DISCUSSION

Jeffrey S. Dover, MD, FRCPC, *Moderator*

Klaus Fritz, MD: I wish to add some information to the data presented on the excimer laser. I have treated approximately 150 patients with the excimer laser, and we evaluated 40 patients by means of a psoriasis area severity index (PASI) score, and I can confirm the data that Dr Geronemus presented. We had clearance of 40% after 3.9 treatment sessions and more than 75% clearance after 6 to 10 sessions using the same parameters he showed. In my practice, my patients often want local treatment or combination treatment, and so one of the most popular treatments is calcipotriene. A report in the literature showed that there is a benefit of combination treatment with calcipotriene cream and narrow-band ultraviolet B (UV-B) light therapy. We therefore used this combination therapy in 12 patients. Instead of the 3.9 treatment sessions required with the excimer laser only, we achieved a 40% clearance in just 2.2 sessions with the combination treatment, and a 75% reduction was reached after 5 to 8 sessions.

Dr Dover: How often did your patients apply the calcipotriene? Was it twice a day?

Dr Fritz: Twice a day. We started the treatment 0 to 3 days before we treated with the excimer laser, so the plaques were less scaly and a little thinner. Maybe the laser light penetrated better after application of calcipotriene, or there was another combination effect.

Dr Dover: After how many treatments with the calcipotriene did you achieve 75% clearing?

Dr Fritz: Five to 8 sessions if I combined the cream with the excimer laser and 6 to 10 sessions if I did not combine it. The main thing is that the psoriasis cleared much faster with the addition of calcipotriene treatment before laser therapy. After 2 treatment sessions, patients saw a noticeable improvement, and these are patients who are not used to getting a fast improvement in their psoriasis plaques.

Dr Dover: How long have your patients stayed in remission?

Dr Fritz: I have used this treatment for 4 to 5 months, but I cannot tell you remission rates. As far as we know from high-dose UV-B treatment, usually one sees a better response and longer remission if a high dose is given. I imagine that the combination therapy with calcipotriene will enhance the remission rate.

Harvey Jay, MD: There are 2 questions that come to mind regarding excimer laser treatment of psoriasis. First, what is the advantage, in this particular situation, of a laser over a smaller light source? Second, I think the oncogenic potential of the 308-nm excimer laser needs to be addressed. It has not been associated specifically with 308 nm, but it has with UV-A.

Dr Dover: Let's address your first question.

Dr Jay: What would be the advantage of a laser? Fluorescent bulbs are used now for treatment of psoriasis. The advantage of the excimer laser is simply that it can deal with a smaller targeted area.

Richard E. Fitzpatrick, MD: The advantage is that a laser gives a high-intensity, uniform output that can be targeted specifically to the lesions. It is very hard to do that with an ultraviolet light source. I have not seen an ultraviolet light source that is capable of doing that. Is there one?

R. Rox Anderson, MD: I do not think there is anything special about the laser in this setting. The excimer laser is a decent tool to generate a lot of narrow-band UV-B, and it happens to go through a fiber rather easily, but conventional light sources can do this, too. This is not new. Handheld mercury lamps that can clear psoriasis have been around for decades. I cannot remember the specifications of the excimer laser, but I think the clinical model is capable of transmitting about 10 W through a fiber, and if one wants to cover a lot of ground, one can. It is difficult to do that with conventional light sources.

Dr Dover: What about the potential carcinogenicity of the 308-nm laser?

Dr Anderson: That's a great question. It comes up all the time. If a researcher wants to produce cancer in a mouse with UV light, the best way is to give many small doses spread out over time on the whole body, which is the way we currently do phototherapy. So, yes, UV is carcinogenic. There is always a risk. Most patients with psoriasis, however, are not that worried about carcinogenicity. I think high-dose local therapy is much less of a total-body lifetime risk for UV-induced carcinogenesis than small-dose generalized therapy.

Dr Jay: Many new immunologic agents are being used, and clearly there are, in this area, easy ways of evaluating the effect on the skin. I wonder whether any studies have been done in terms of tumor necrosis factor or other factors. That would be an obvious way to see exactly where the mechanism of action of these lasers is. Has any of that been done at all?

Brian D. Zelickson, MD: We have done a little of that type of research. An article by other investigators was recently published in the *British Journal of Dermatology* that examined cell mediators of inflammation using the pulsed dye laser to treat psoriasis. It appeared as if the vascular response did not necessarily correlate with a decrease or increase of the specific markers that were studied, so it was an independent phenomenon.

Emil A. Tanghetti, MD: We have some experience with the excimer laser using combination therapies. In one subset of patients who were receiving UV-B light therapy just before the initiation of laser therapy, we performed a test for minimal erythema dose (MED) and found that there was no MED even seen. We therefore started with a rather conservative dose, such as a 5 MED with a multiplier of 3, and every patient blistered substantially, because the MED of a psoriatic plaque is different from the MED of normal skin. Despite the blistering, most of the patients cleared in one treatment. I caution anyone who is determining an MED based on normal skin. With psoriatic skin, especially skin that has been treated with a topical retinoid, such as topical vitamin D, the MED of a psoriatic plaque is going to change. Fortunately, when that does happen, patients do very well.

Roy Geronemus, MD: I think Dr Anderson showed that. Your study was a dose-response study, and those patients who did blister did very well. We have found that as well, but a number of our patients really do not want a long downtime. They are looking for some intermediary type of response, so they will tolerate a few side effects, maybe minor blistering or minor discomfort, but in most cases, they do not want the severe blistering.

Dr Tanghetti: Another thing is that the duration of remission really depends on the time of year that the study is performed. In our psoriatic population, the length of remission can be very different depending on the season.

Dr Anderson: I have a clinical point. I think the optimal dose is inversely related to the size of the psoriatic plaque. For a patient with large plaques, I recommend starting off with a dose around 3 times the MED, so as not to cause blisters. I have yet to see anybody blister at 3 times the MED, and MED is measured on normal skin, not plaque-affected skin. I am aware of a soon-to-be-published study performed by other investigators, who gave blistering doses (10 times the MED). All the patients blistered, but the plaques in more than 50% of the patients cleared in a single treatment. Those results cannot be ignored. I have patients who hate the little plaques on their elbows and knees and who do not respond to phototherapy, and I think to achieve clearing in half of those patients in a single treatment would be remarkable.

Maria I. Martinez, MD: How practical is it to treat patients with the excimer laser, since I understand this laser is very expensive?

Dr Geronemus: Cost is a major issue now. We do not yet have the specific acceptance of a *Current Procedural Terminology®* (*CPT*) code by many of the insurance companies for this procedure, and therefore many patients do not want to pay out of pocket for it. Those who are willing to do so generally have been very happy with the results. I think many people are used to psoriasis treatments being covered by third-party payers, and the lack of coverage for excimer laser treatment has certainly limited the acceptance of this procedure. It is my understanding, though, that the manufacturer of the excimer laser, PhotoMedex Inc (Radnor, Pa), has now obtained approval from 16 different insurance companies for acceptance of this treatment as a separate and distinct procedure from phototherapy.

Whitney D. Tope, MPhil, MD: I just want to add, in terms of laser treatment of psoriasis, we should think about photodynamic therapy (PDT) for treatment of psoriasis. It is possible to clear psoriatic plaques with a single dose of PDT. A couple of companies are developing topical formulations of previously intravenously administered photosensitizers, and psoriasis is one of the indications at the top of their list.

Dr Anderson: I also am aware of a trial whose results clearly showed that intravenous administration of a benzoporphyrin derivative as a photosensitizer for PDT can clear psoriasis in a single treatment. Regarding the topical studies you mentioned, I can tell you that PDT is an exercise in pain control, and it really hurts. I have tried to figure out how to make PDT work without pain, and I just don't have a good way around it. I think there are some issues that need to be addressed about PDT.

Lisa Kellett, MD: I have 2 questions for anyone on the panel. First, would you be comfortable treating children with the excimer laser, either for psoriasis or potentially for atopic dermatitis? Second, why isn't koebnerization more common after treatment with the excimer laser? Is a cytokine or growth factor or something else being suppressed?

Dr Geronemus: I was just going to address the pediatric aspect. I think that phototherapy in children can be done, but, again, it's all a question of the cumulative dose. I certainly would not want to be treating a child with photo-therapy on a regular basis year after year, but I think it can be used in appropriate situations intermittently.

Dr Anderson: I would stay away from it in children if at all possible. There now is an effective drug, tacrolimus, to treat atopic dermatitis, and I don't see any reason to use an excimer laser on a child with that disease. I will mention another indication for the excimer laser. We have treated oral lichen planus and had excellent results after 6 treatments in people with erosive lesions who could not even eat. I am interested in whether lichen simplex chronicus, which responds poorly to conventional treatment, will respond to the excimer laser. We have not yet tried that. I encourage people who have this laser in their practice to use it for that purpose and see what the response is.

Christian Raulin, MD: My assistant doctor asked me, if we work 1 hour every day with the excimer laser, whether there would be a risk to his hands because of the scattering light. Should he use gloves, or are sunblocks enough? What do you think about this?

Dr Anderson: The laser has a plastic shield that absorbs the scattered light. When it is in use, the bright blue light seen is fluorescence. The operator's exposure to the UV radiation is nil. It is not an issue.

Dr Fritz: I have 3 comments about the discussion. First, I do not want the audience to believe that blistering is normal. I tell my patients about the potential for blistering, and some ask me to produce blistering because it is possible to clear the psoriasis plaques with only 2 sessions. Other patients do not want the treatment administered that way, so we combine excimer laser therapy with the cal-cipotriene, which, according to the medical literature, is photoprotective, or protective against carcinogenic effects. Second, the carcinogenicity of excimer laser treatment is not as great as if you do 30 to 40 psoralen–UV-A (PUVA) or narrow-band UV-B treatments, if one sums up the dosage. Third, as long as patients pay all psoriasis treatment expenses out of their pocket, the costs are tremendously lowered with the laser. The cost of traditional phototherapy for psoriasis of 10% to 20% of the body is about $4000 to $6000 for 6 months. The excimer laser cuts down the cost tremendously, maybe by one third or one half.

The Role of Lasers in the Treatment of Scars, Hypopigmentation, and Depigmentation

chapter 40

Acne Scars: Classification and Treatment

Michael S. Kaminer, MD

Ten years ago, there was no laser skin resurfacing of acne scars, only surgical treatment, and most physicians thought that was somewhat inadequate. Then 5 or 6 years ago, laser resurfacing began to be used and became the most common way to treat acne scars, and many investigators reported a statistically significant improvement of approximately 50%. Today my opinion, based on my experience, is that resurfacing alone is not enough to treat acne scars. Perhaps we need to use a different approach in the treatment of acne scars.

CLASSIFICATION

To guide in the treatment of acne scarring, Jacob, Dover, and I[1] devised a classification of acne scars. I have been using this classification for 2 years, and it is fairly reproducible. The 3 types of scars are: ice-pick scars, rolling scars, and boxcar scars (Fig 40-1). Ice-pick scars are the traditional, very deep scars, which are somewhat narrow and shallow. Rolling scars are what I like to think of as wavy, undulating scars that do not appear discrete (Figs 40-2 and 40-3). They have what I call dermal "tethers," which are attached to a fibrous mass or something else in the dermis, but they seem to be bound down. Boxcar scars are round to oval, have sharply demarcated vertical edges, and look like chickenpox scars (Figs 40-4 and 40-5). They have 2 subtypes: superficial and deep.

The diagram in Figure 40-1 shows an arbitrary depth to which laser resurfacing can reach (not nonablative lasers but resurfacing). It is apparent that ice-pick scars and the deep boxcar scars are deeper than that. Therefore, laser resurfacing performed in a patient with predominantly deep boxcar and ice-pick scarring would fail. Resurfacing of the dermal tethers of rolling scars down to the reference line shown in Figure 40-1 may improve the scars, but some of the scar tends to come back. More appropriate resurfacing in a patient with rolling scars would involve treating to the depth of the scar and to these little fibrous bands.

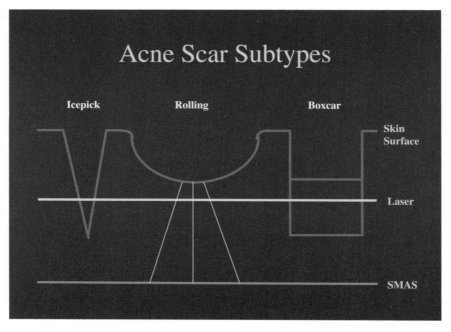

FIGURE 40.1

Acne scar subtypes. Yellow reference line indicates depth of ablation and resurfacing capability of carbon dioxide laser; green line, superficial musculoaponeurotic system to which fibrous bands adhere, creating rolling scars.

In my opinion, the superficial boxcar scar is the only type of acne scar that responds completely to resurfacing.

TREATMENT

Ice-pick scars can be treated surgically by punch excision or punch grafting. I prefer excision because of the potential for color mismatch with punch grafting. The dermal tethers of rolling scars can be cut using a subdermal undermining procedure described in 1995, which Orentreich and Orentreich[2] called Subcision. It is debatable whether subdermal undermining can be performed under boxcar scars. Surgical options for boxcar scars include punch excision for smaller scars, punch grafting, or punch elevation. For treatment of acne scars 3.5 to 4 mm in diameter, I obtain a punch biopsy so that it matches the diameter of the scar, raise the scar to get it flat, and then put a small amount of glue (Dermabond) right over the scar and hold it in place with a tape bandage (Steri-Strip). That treatment seems to work well. Because people with acne scarring tend to not heal well, when I perform a punch excision of the scar, I use a single 6-0 plain gut suture and put a drop of Dermabond glue over it. The sutures

Rolling Scars

- Dermal tethering
- Shadowing

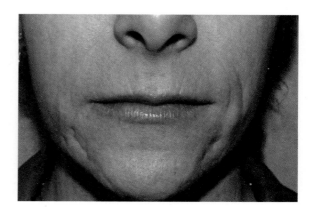

FIGURE 40.2

Rolling scars on woman's chin.

Rolling Scars

- How to treat?
  - Subcision
  - Injectables
  - Cool Touch 2
  - Resurfacing

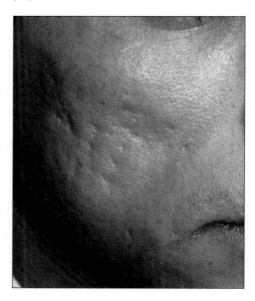

FIGURE 40.3

Rolling scars on patient's cheek.

Boxcar Scars

- How to treat?
  - Punch excision
    - Dermabond plus gut
  - Punch grafting
  - Resurfacing

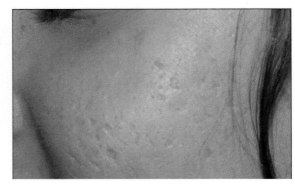

FIGURE 40.4

Boxcar scars.

Q: How do you handle the patient with extensive scarring?

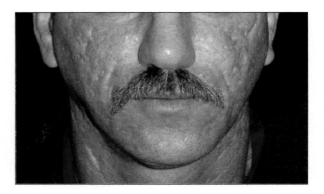

FIGURE 40.5

Extensive acne scarring by boxcar scars.

absorb fairly quickly—in about 5 days—so track marks do not develop, and the glue tends to hold things together for about 7 to 10 days. Our results have seemed to improve a lot with the use of both suture and glue.

Nonsurgical treatments of acne scars include subcutaneous or dermal fillers, chemical peels, and microdermabrasion. I think that microdermabrasion does not do a whole lot for improving scarring. Dermabrasion, on the other hand, may still be one of the gold standards for treatment of acne scars, because it can go a little bit deeper than laser resurfacing. More aggressive chemical peels sometimes decrease acne scarring a little.

Combining Treatments

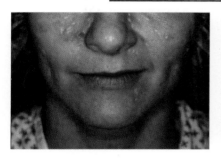 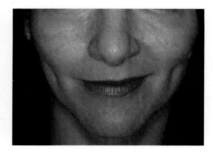

FIGURE 40.6

Left, Before treatment by punch excision, elevation, and subdermal undermining (Subcision). Right, Six months after laser skin resurfacing.

For laser skin resurfacing of acne scars, the carbon dioxide (CO_2) and erbium:YAG lasers are used. Laser resurfacing is best used for shallow boxcar scars, superficial rolling scars, and residual scars after excisions.

COMBINATION TREATMENTS

The patient with extensive acne scarring, in my opinion, is best treated with a combination of surgical and laser treatments. I treated the patient shown in Figure 40-6 for approximately 1 year with punch excision and closure of her many sinus tracts. I also used Subcision on some of the scars at the same time. Then the patient underwent laser skin resurfacing 6 months later, and good results were finally achieved. Therefore, I think there is a benefit to combining treatments.

I have some unresolved questions about treatment of acne scars. What is the optimal time frame between excision (or Subcision or any other treatment) and resurfacing? What is the role of nonablative lasers for treatment of some of the subtypes of scars? Why do some people with acne scarring scar, whereas others who get acne as an adolescent do not scar? I think that last question is important for two reasons. First, the people who get the scarring might like to know how they can prevent it. Second, people who scar do not seem to respond quite as well to surgery or other invasive treatments as do people without a history of acne scarring, and that is one reason why these patients are a challenge to treat.

REFERENCES

1. Jacob CI, Dover JS, Kaminer MS. Acne scarring: a classification system and review of treatment options. *J Am Acad Dermatol.* 2001;45:109–117.
2. Orentreich DS, Orentreich N. Subcutaneous incisionless (Subcision) surgery for the correction of depressed scars and wrinkles. *Dermatol Surg.* 1995;21:543–549.

chapter 41

Laser Treatment of Hypertrophic Scars

Whitney D. Tope, MPhil, MD

I will discuss another major group of scars that laser surgeons treat: hypertrophic scars. Lasers can smooth a hypertrophic scar and make a noticeable improvement in skin color, texture, and symptoms. Although pulsed dye lasers are commonly used to treat hypertrophic scars, there is much we do not know that would optimize treatment.

OPTIMAL LASER PARAMETERS

Attempts have been made to determine the optimal parameters for laser treatment of hypertrophic scars. Reiken et al[1] transplanted human keloidal scar tissue into athymic nude mice ($1 \times 1 \times 1$ mm transplants) and performed 2 sets of experiments. The first experiment employed a fixed wavelength of 585 nm, a pulse duration of 450 microseconds, and varied fluence. They looked at changes in the volume of the laser-treated scar tissue. At 2 J/cm^2, there was no change in volume compared with untreated controls, and there were no vascular effects noted in implants excised at 24 hours. At 6 J/cm^2, transplanted scars were 70% smaller 17 days after treatment. Specimens obtained at 24 hours showed endothelial cell changes only. At 10 J/cm^2, scar implants were 92% smaller, and specimens demonstrated endothelial cell changes and thermal collagen damage in the perivascular stroma. The next experiment used a fixed fluence (6 J/cm^2) and a fixed pulse duration (450 microseconds), but Reiken et al varied the wavelength, 585 through 600 nm. At 585 nm, implants excised 17 days later were 81% smaller vs untreated controls; at 590 nm, 72% smaller; at 595 nm, 65% smaller; and at 600 nm, the volume change was minimal, similar to controls.

This study showed clear superiority of a 585-nm wavelength and a 450-microsecond pulse duration in the treatment of hypertrophic scars; however, it did not establish the effects of longer pulse durations that are available now or higher fluences at longer wavelengths, such as 595 or 600 nm. It also did not examine the effect of current cooling mechanisms. I think this study should be used as a basis that directs experimental treatment of hypertrophic scars at higher fluences with longer wavelengths. If the scar's target chromophore is really the vasculature, one should be able to affect scar vasculature with the diode (800 nm), long-pulse alexandrite (755 nm), and long-pulse neodymium (Nd):YAG (1064 nm) lasers. The wavelengths of these lasers are absorbed to some degree by hemoglobin and penetrate more deeply in tissue than do shorter pulsed dye laser wavelengths. Laser surgeons should try some longer wavelengths at higher fluences, to overcome a lower absorption coefficient for hemoglobin, and protect the epidermis to achieve a better effect on hypertrophic scars, particularly in darker skin types.

PREVENTION OF HYPERTROPHIC SCARS

There has been some effort to prevent hypertrophic scars. Although results are difficult to interpret, studies reported in the literature suggest that treatment with the pulsed dye laser immediately after reconstruction may assist in preventing these scars.[2,3] Many investigators have begun to use topical imiquimod on hypertrophic scars with and without laser treatment, in an attempt to produce a better treatment response. I have seen no published objective data demonstrating that imiquimod alone or combined treatment significantly improves hypertrophic scars vs pulsed dye laser treatment alone.

TREATMENT

Hypertrophic scars require persistent treatment. A patient of mine who had symptomatic keloidal scars on the center of his chest obtained good results from pulsed dye laser and, in about half of his treatments, intralesional steroids, but treatment took 3 years (Fig 41-1). My first line of therapy for hypertrophic scars in patients who have Fitzpatrick phototypes I through III is monthly pulsed dye laser with immediate postirradiation triamcinolone acetonide injections. I use high concentrations (40 mg/mL) but tiny volumes of the steroid placed carefully to get the steroid precisely where I want it. I perform a minimum of 6 treatment sessions. If I see improvement, I continue laser treatment; if I do not see improvement, I consider other treatments.

Patients with Fitzpatrick phototypes IV through VI are a difficult group to treat with lasers, particularly the pulsed dye laser, because moderate fluences, which would be expected to improve the scar, can ablate the epidermis. Lasers equipped with cooling technology may prevent this unwanted effect. Because of the increased risk of epidermal injury, at this time I tend not to choose to treat hypertrophic scars with laser in individuals with higher phototypes.

A long-standing question in the laser treatment of scars has yet to be answered. Why is there an apparent bimodal response of scar tissue treated by pulsed dye laser? Low-fluence treatment has been reported to improve atrophic scars by improving collagen production,[4] yet higher fluences appear to improve hypertrophic scars by enhancing collagen degradation. As Zelickson and Kist[5]

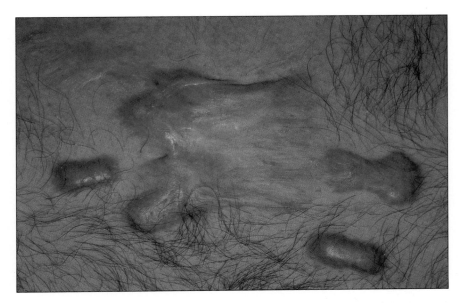

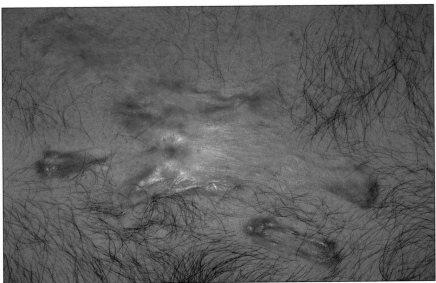

FIGURE 41.1

Top, Multiple keloidal chest scars recalcitrant to treatment before pulsed dye laser treatment. Bottom, Clinical improvement (flattening, softening, decreased erythema, and decreased symptoms) 3 years later. Treatment consisted of more than 24 pulsed dye laser treatments, half of which were immediately followed by intralesional injections of triamcinolone acetonide.

have shown, almost any visible to near-infrared light source can injure "normal" photodamaged dermis and enhance collagen production. A much greater understanding is needed of all these effects and of scar tissue metabolism in general to optimize the treatment of scars with lasers or any other modality.

REFERENCES

1. Reiken SR, Wolfart SF, Berthiaume F, Compton C, Tompkins RG, Yarmush MI. Control of hypertrophic scar growth using selective photothermolysis. *Lasers Surg Med.* 1997;21:7–12.

2. McCraw JB, McCraw JA, McMellin A, Bettencourt N. Prevention of unfavorable scars using early pulsed dye laser treatments: a preliminary report. *Ann Plast Surg.* 1999;42:7–14.

3. Shakespeare PG, Tiernan E, Dewar AE, Hambleton J. Using the pulsed dye laser to influence scar formation after breast reduction surgery: a preliminary report. *Ann Plast Surg.* 2000;45:357–368.

4. McDaniel DH, Ash K, Zukowski M. Treatment of stretch marks with the 585 nm flashlamp pumped dye laser. *Dermatol Surg.* 1996;22:332–337.

5. Zelickson BD, Kist DA. Pulsed dye laser and Photoderm treatment stimulates production of type-I collagen and collagenase transcripts in papillary dermis fibroblasts. *Lasers Surg Med.* 2001;(suppl 13):33.

Laser Treatment of Scars

George J. Hruza, MD

R esults of laser treatment of scars have varied. Alster et al[1] treated half of a sternotomy scar with laser, and, compared with the half that did not receive laser treatment, results were impressive. However, not everyone has had results as successful as the initial results of Alster and colleagues. More recent studies suggest that laser treatment is perhaps not as helpful for hypertrophic scars as originally thought. In a study published in the *Archives of Dermatology*, 20 patients with hypertrophic scars were treated with the pulsed dye laser, and results were compared with those of silicone gel treatment and control.[2] The authors found no benefit of the pulsed dye laser; results were the same as the control. There were some differences, however, from the study by Alster et al. The investigators used higher fluences and smaller spot sizes. They overlapped the pulses, and most of their patients had darker skin types, in which laser seems to be not quite as effective.

I believe there is a definite role for the laser in treatment of hypertrophic scars, but I think lower fluences are required. For hypertrophic scars, I find that lower fluences and bigger spot sizes work better than do higher fluences. A hypertrophic scar can be dramatically improved (Fig 42-1) but, more often, the results are less impressive (Fig 42-2, left). The patient shown in Figure 42-2 underwent 4 pulsed dye laser treatments without corticosteroid injections. There was improvement in the scar after treatment (Fig 42-2, right), although it did not completely disappear.

Another use for the pulsed dye laser that I find helpful is to decrease shininess of scars. A patient referred to me for treatment of moderate scarring after carbon dioxide (CO_2) laser resurfacing had a hypertrophic scar on the cheek, which was red, shiny, and very hard (Fig 42-3, left). After treatment with the pulsed dye laser, the treated area was depigmented, as expected, but the skin also was supple and had lost its shininess (Fig 42-3, right). Scars can be resolved as long as treatment is performed very early, as the scar is about to develop. I think this laser is best for recent scars and red scars and maybe as prevention of surgical scars.

With the pulsed dye laser, I like to use a 585-nm wavelength, 0.5-millisecond pulse duration, 10-mm spot size, and fluence of 3 to 5 J/cm² (usually about 4 J/cm²). I repeat treatment every 4 to 6 weeks. Usually for the thicker scars, I

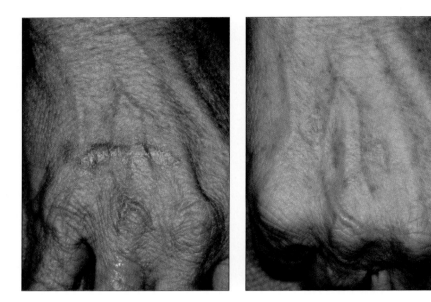

FIGURE 42.1

Hypertrophic scar before (left) and 6 months after (right) 1 pulsed dye laser treatment, with almost complete resolution of scar.

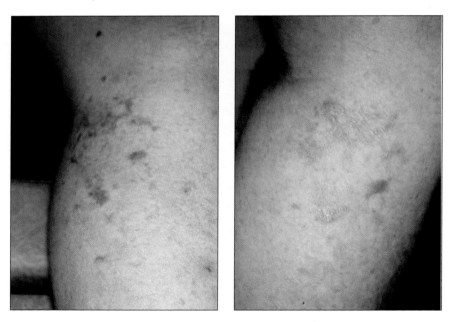

FIGURE 42.2

Dog bite–related hypertrophic scars before (left) and 2 months after (right) 4 pulsed dye laser treatments, with modest improvement of scars.

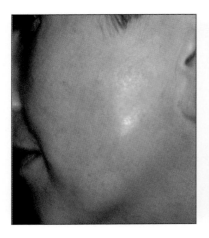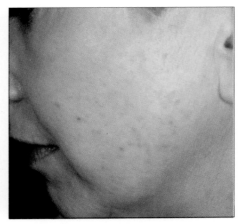

FIGURE 42.3

Left, incipient hypertrophic scars after carbon dioxide laser resurfacing. Right, Six months after 6 pulsed dye laser treatments, with normalization of skin texture. Hypopigmentation has persisted.

combine laser treatment with corticosteroid injections. I like to use 40 mg/mL of triamcinolone acetonide and occasionally 5-fluorouracil injections. I apply occlusive dressings as soon as evidence of hypertrophy becomes apparent. The dressings do not have to contain silicone. If the scar is old, the laser surgeon can resurface it and basically make a new scar, which can then be treated with the pulsed dye laser.

PROPHYLAXIS

An uncontrolled study showed improvement in the incidence of postoperative scars using multiple treatments with the pulsed dye laser soon after surgery.[3] Another study, which was better controlled, also showed protection against hypertrophic scars with postoperative laser treatment.[4] The problem with using the laser prophylactically is that insurance may not pay for it. However, if patients are willing to pay out of pocket, I think it is helpful to treat a few times in areas at high risk for hypertrophic scarring.

KELOIDAL SCARS

For treatment of keloids, the CO_2 laser is not helpful, and the pulsed dye laser also cannot improve appearance of the scars. A recent study compared treatment of keloids with the pulsed dye laser vs silicone gel, and there was no improvement with the laser.[5] The laser sometimes can reduce the pruritus symptoms

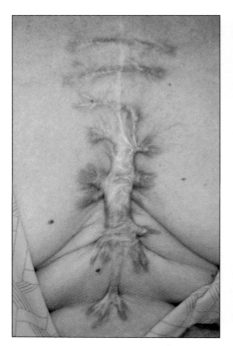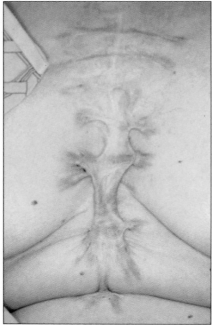

FIGURE 42.4

Left, Extensive keloids on chest secondary to sternotomy. Right, Six weeks after 4 pulsed dye laser treatments and multiple intralesional corticosteroid injections with scar flattening, elimination of pain and tenderness, and reduction of erythema.

that patients with keloids have, but the scar does not usually change in appearance except for reduction of erythema. A woman's contracted keloidal scar, after multiple treatments with pulsed dye laser and intralesional corticosteroids, still looked unattractive, but it was flatter from the injections and the redness disappeared from the laser (Fig 42-4). The symptoms also were much better, so the pulsed dye laser can have some benefit for these patients with keloidal scarring.

OTHER SCARS

Laser treatment can benefit other types of scars. For treating nonhypertrophic surgical scars on the face, I now use a variable-pulse erbium:YAG laser. Treatment should occur 6 to 10 weeks postoperatively. The erbium:YAG laser also can smooth skin grafts (Fig 42-5) and skin flaps that have a thickened area (Fig 42-6).

Varicella scars, if they are fresh, can improve greatly with laser resurfacing. If the scars are old, however, they can be very difficult to decrease.

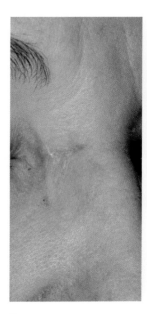
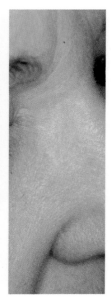

FIGURE 42.5

Left, Six weeks after graft placement. Right, Three months after carbon dioxide laser resurfacing, with smoothing of skin contour and improvement in skin color match.

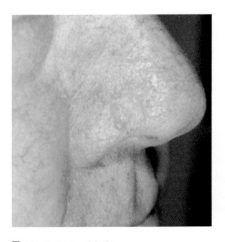
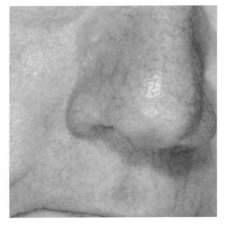

FIGURE 42.6

Left, Six weeks after 2-stage nasolabial flap. Right, Six weeks after variable-pulse erbium:YAG laser resurfacing, with flattening of trapdoor deformity.

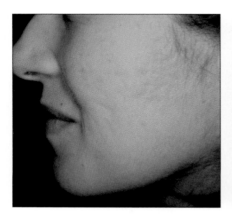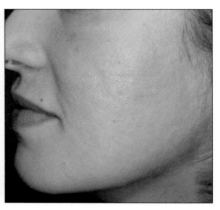

FIGURE 42.7

Left, Mild saucer-shaped acne scars. Right, Two months after variable-pulse erbium:YAG laser resurfacing, with noticeable effacement of acne scars.

On superficial acne scars, the laser alone can usually achieve good results (Fig 42-7), but multiple combination treatments are better, such as punch excision, punch grafting, subdermal undermining (Subcision), and punch elevations. I prefer to perform these surgical procedures 2 to 3 months before laser resurfacing.

REFERENCES

1. Alster TS, Williams CM. Treatment of sternotomy scars with 585 nm flashlamp-pumped pulsed dye laser. *Lancet.* 1995;345:1198–2000.

2. Wittenberg GP, Fabian BG, Bogomilsky JL, et al. Prospective, single-blind, randomized, controlled study to assess the efficacy of the 585-nm flashlamp-pumped pulsed dye laser and silicone gel sheeting in hypertrophic scar treatment. *Arch Dermatol.* 1999;135:1049–1055.

3. McCraw JB, McCraw JA, McMellin A, Bettencourt N. Prevention of unfavorable scars using early pulse dye laser treatments: a preliminary report. *Ann Plast Surg.* 1999;42:7–14.

4. Nouri K, Jimenez G. 585 nm pulse dye laser in the treatment of surgical scar starting on the suture removal day. *Lasers Surg Med.* 2001;28(suppl 13):32.

5. Paquet P, Hermanns JF, Pierard GE. Effect of the 585 nm flashlamp-pumped pulsed dye laser for the treatment of keloids. *Dermatol Surg.* 2001;27:171–174.

chapter 43

Excimer Laser for Repigmentation of Laser-Induced and Surgically Induced Depigmentation

Roy Geronemus, MD

Lasers are effective therapy for a wide variety of scars. For hypertrophic scars, I believe the pulsed dye laser makes a difference not only in new scars but also in long-term scars. Kilmer and Chotzen[1] demonstrated this. My group also has effectively treated long-term burn scars (scars 20 to 40 years old) that are not overly thick or keloidal, using pulsed dye laser alone without injections. Only the thinnest of keloids will respond to pulsed dye laser therapy. Erythematous scars, however, respond very well to the pulsed dye laser. Atrophic scars, unless they are very deep, fibrotic scars, can benefit greatly from nonablative techniques, particularly with the 1320-nm neodymium (Nd):YAG laser (CoolTouch II, CoolTouch Corporation, Roseville, Calif). I do not resurface acne scars very often. In these cases, I have switched over to nonablative techniques, particularly with the CoolTouch II, often in combination with a 1064-nm Nd:YAG laser, and have had surprisingly good results. Leukoderma can now also be treated with laser.

Hypopigmentation is now recognized as a common delayed complication of laser resurfacing as well as surgical procedures. In a study by Bernstein and my group,[2] we found that approximately 16% of patients experienced hypopigmentation subsequent to carbon dioxide (CO_2) laser resurfacing. Other studies show an incidence of 8% to 26% of leukoderma as a complication of CO_2 laser resurfacing.

Histologically, it has been demonstrated that a decrease in epidermal melanin occurs after laser resurfacing. Irreversible melanocytic injury results from thermal damage. Grimes et al[3] demonstrated that epidermal melanin and residual epidermal melanocytes are present after laser resurfacing but do not transfer melanin to the epidermis. The authors also demonstrated the use of topical psoralen–UV-A (PUVA) therapy in patients with hypopigmentation, with 71% of patients achieving moderate to excellent repigmentation. Unfortunately, repigmentation required an average of 25 PUVA treatments with a mean cumulative energy of 46 J.

Ultraviolet B (UV-B) has also been found to be helpful for vitiligo, increasing the melanocytes stimulated so one sees increased pigmentation in the epidermis on biopsy. There is a concern about the cumulative dose of UV-B radiation in these types of patients. Spencer and colleagues[4] have demonstrated that vitiligo can respond to the use of the excimer laser using a 308-nm source, which was recently approved by the Food and Drug Administration (FDA).

REPIGMENTATION OF LEUKODERMA

In a pilot study, my coworkers and I (unpublished data) evaluated the 308-nm excimer laser (PhotoMedex, Radnor, Pa) for treatment of depigmentation after surgery and laser resurfacing.[5] We have since studied 5 patients, all women, aged 37 to 61 years, with a leukoderma history of 3 to 10 years. We used a pulse width of 20 to 40 nanoseconds, a 3.2-cm^2 spot size, and treatment doses of 100 and 350 mJ/cm^2. The clinical end point was erythema. There was no pain or downtime associated with this procedure. Generally, we offered 10 treatment sessions, twice weekly for approximately 5 weeks. We evaluated these patients by photography, and we used the quartile system to evaluate their response.

The clinical response varied from only 25% to more than 75%. After 8 excimer laser treatments in 1 patient who had undergone resurfacing of a small lesion on the cheek and had leukoderma, repigmentation occurred. Another patient with leukoderma following laser resurfacing of the upper lip underwent excimer laser treatments and experienced substantial repigmentation. The patient was very happy with the result. The only side effect was mild erythema. A patient who had postdermabrasion hypopigmentation had a substantial return of pigmentation after excimer laser treatments. Another patient, who underwent Q-switched laser treatment of multiple lentigines on her back, had repigmentation to a large degree with a series of treatments using this technique.

Histochemical analysis showed the relative absence of melanocytes and posttreatment return of pigmentation in a patient from the leukoderma study.

REPIGMENTATION OF SCARS

We have also studied this laser for the treatment of postsurgical scars, using the same technique of 2 treatments per week, in 10 patients and achieved a rather substantial response in terms of repigmentation. A patient had a preauricular scar in front of the right ear following a face-lift, and after excimer laser treatments there was increased pigmentation (Fig 43-1). Histologically, the increased pigmentation could be seen using a Fontana-Masson stain in the area that had had a relative absence of melanocytes. In a patient who had a port-wine stain that had been excised many years earlier, we were able to repigment the scar to some degree. A blepharoplasty scar had repigmentation after only 6 laser treatments, an acceptable cosmetic result. Repigmentation occurred to a large degree

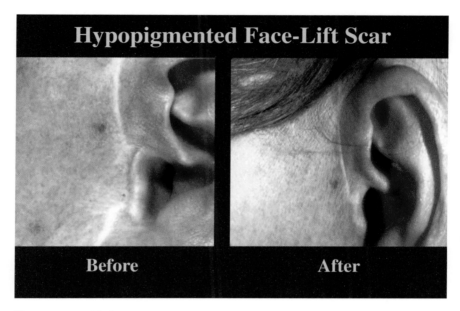

Hypopigmented Face-Lift Scar

Before

After

FIGURE 43.1

Hypopigmented face-lift scar before (left) and after (right) excimer laser treatments.

after treatment of a linear scar just above the vermilion border of the lip. There was an absence of side effects, such as pain, associated with this treatment, and there was no need for postoperative care.

LONG-TERM EFFECTS

A longer follow-up is needed. It is unclear from the results of these pilot studies whether we are inducing permanent repigmentation or just a suntan. We have seen some loss of pigment in some patients after several months, so it is possible that some patients will require maintenance therapy to maintain the repigmentation long term.

REFERENCES

1. Kilmer SL, Chotzen V. Pulsed dye laser treatment of old burn scars. *Lasers Surg Med.* 1997;9(suppl):34.
2. Bernstein L, Kauvar A, Grossman M, Geronemus R. Short and long term side effects following CO_2 laser resurfacing of rhytides. *Dermatol Surg.* 1997;23:519–525.
3. Grimes PE, Bhawan J, Kim J, Chiu M, Lask G. Laser resurfacing-induced hypopigmentation: histologic alterations and repigmentation with topical photochemotherapy. *Dermatol Surg.* 2001;27:515–520.
4. Spencer JM, Nossa R, Ajmeri J. Treatment of Vitiglio with the 308-nm excimer laser: a pilot study. *J Am Acad Dermatol.* 2002; 46:727–731.
5. Friedman J, Geronemus RG. Use of the 308-nm laser for postresurfacing leukoderma. *Arch Dermatol.* 2001; 137:824–825.

PART ELEVEN DISCUSSION

Jeffrey S. Dover, MD, FRCPC, *Moderator*

Richard E. Fitzpatrick, MD: I have 3 comments. First, we conducted a study of treatment of sternotomy scars with different fluences of the pulsed dye laser. The intent of the study was to show that the higher fluences worked better, but, to my surprise, the lower fluences actually worked better. For example, 3 J/cm^2 was better than 5 or 7 J/cm^2, so I agree with Dr Hruza that the lower fluences seem to be better. Second, we found that carbon dioxide (CO_2) laser works really well for the treatment of hypertrophic scars (not keloids). It "melts" them away. Third, as far as timing of the excision of boxcar acne scars, we found that intraoperative excision works much better—dramatically better—than excision either before or after carbon dioxide (CO_2) resurfacing. I invite comments about that.

George Hruza, MD: I totally agree. For the ice-pick scars, I routinely perform intraoperative excision at the time of the resurfacing. I punch out the scar first, then perform resurfacing, and then I sew up the wound. This technique works very well. Of course, if I perform subdermal undermining (Subcision) in these patients, I like to do it ahead of time, not at the time of the procedure.

Dr Dover: Dr Hruza, how do you stop the hemorrhage obtained from the punch before you perform the resurfacing?

Dr Hruza: That is generally not a big problem. With pressure, the bleeding stops within a couple of minutes.

Dr Dover: But no electrocautery, presumably, or chemical cautery?

Dr Hruza: I do not use form of cautery.

Dr Dover: I raise this point, because one should never use chemical cautery on the lesion of a punch excision or excision. Doing so will extend the depth of the CO_2 or erbium:YAG laser-induced burn greatly and cause focal scarring, which we have seen.

Dr Hruza: I just saw a patient referred from another physician, who had used Monsel's (ferric subsulfate) solution to stop the bleeding after resurfacing, and the patient had big streaks of hyperpigmented tattoo. The tattoo was pretty fresh, so we resurfaced those areas with the erbium:YAG laser and were able to get it all out, because it was pretty superficial.

Dr Dover: Has anyone tried performing Subcision, as Dr Kaminer described, intraoperatively? Our problem is that we get so much edema immediately after resurfacing that we can no longer see the undulation, and we cannot target many of the rolling scars. As a result, we have not been able to do so.

Dr Fitzpatrick: I don't know if I can perform Subcision in such a targeted way, but I do undermine around the area where I am doing the punch excision. If I perform multiple punch excisions or, sometimes, relatively large linear excisions, I will undermine widely, even with the punch excisions, just to pick up the connections in the dermis around the excision.

Michael S. Kaminer, MD: It seems that many people believe it helps to perform the punch excisions during laser resurfacing. In my mind, there are 2 limitations with doing that. The first one is a practical issue. If you want to perform 30 or 40 punch excisions and get down to the point at which you are doing some punch elevations, putting sutures and glue in, whatever you decide you want to do, and then perform Subcision at the same time, it makes it a lot harder to approach each scar in a more targeted way. The second issue is a bigger one for me. Many of my patients with acne scars do not want to undergo resurfacing. I have found in many patients that these scar-reduction procedures can produce a substantial amount of improvement without the resurfacing. A lot of my patients will have resurfacing later, and most of them will benefit from resurfacing. I offer patients a staged treatment algorithm, which gives them a lot of improvement and still leaves them the option of resurfacing at a later stage.

Dr Fitzpatrick: I used to think that way, but I think that patients with acne scars much prefer to get things done in a single treatment. The multiple treatment approach, which has kind of been the traditional approach, turns off a lot of patients. Many of them do not come back for the second or third treatment. My patients have been far happier doing everything in 1 procedure.

Dr Kaminer: I think it gets down to one very unquantifiable thing, which is practice style. If I were to tell all my patients with acne scars that the only way they could get improvement of their scars was to have 1 procedure of excision, Subcision, and resurfacing, then my patients would probably do the same. However, I tell them differently, so my patient return rate for reexcisions or subsequent treatments is virtually 100%, because the patients have bought into the concept of multiple treatments. I think both approaches are excellent ways of getting the results. The choice sometimes comes down to the individual patient, too. Some patients might not want the all-in-one-style, and others might not want my approach.

Whitney D. Tope, MPhil, MD: Like Dr Kaminer, I treat scars in a staged fashion. My patients always seem to return, because they really want to deal with the scarring. Roughly 50% of the patients in whom I perform punch excision are happy with the results and say they do not need any more treatment.

Jerome M. Garden, MD: I have a few comments. First, I agree with the approach of using the pulsed dye laser at the lower fluences for the hypertrophic scars. However, in scars that are fairly thick, sometimes the low doses, even after multiple treatments, do not seem to reduce the scars. I have then used high fluences and have seen some positive responses. Second, using the pulsed dye laser, I treated a patient for some acne-induced scars on the chest with the low-fluence approach, and she had an inflammatory response, in which the hypertrophic scar became thicker.

My third comment is to Dr Geronemus. When we use the 308-nm excimer laser on hyperplastic epidermis, as seen in psoriasis, the epidermis is thick, but when we use this laser on scars, the epidermis may not have the same integrity. Will these scars, especially if maintenance therapy is required, become more susceptible to ultraviolet (UV) damage and ultimately, perhaps, DNA changes?

Roy Geronemus, MD: I think the cumulative dose from this UV-B laser at 308 nm is relatively small. It is in the millijoule range per treatment session, so the cumulative dose is still dramatically lower than from UV-B phototherapy. I don't think cumulative UV exposure will be a major problem.

Harvey Jay, MD: Dr Geronemus, I had a question in regard to the relative response of vitiligo vs postresurfacing hypopigmentation. In these 2 conditions, I think one is dealing histologically with different circumstances, a complete lack of pigment, and perhaps a lack of melanocytes. Is there any mechanism postulated as to how excimer laser light would work for vitiligo, as opposed to hypopigmentation?

Dr Geronemus: Both conditions seem to respond to the excimer laser. We have much less experience treating vitiligo, so I am relaying information from another group, which saw very good responses in patients with that disease. Also, they are seeing long-term benefit, and very few of their patients have lost repigmentation over time. So the mechanism is apparently the same, the treatment is almost identical, and responses are good for both.

R. Rox Anderson, MD: The responsiveness in vitiligo depends very much on the body site. The response of facial vitiligo is far better than the "egg roll" sort of vitiligo plaques—macules of vitiligo that are tougher to treat with conventional psoralen–UVA (PUVA) therapy.

Melanie C. Grossman, MD: I think that nonablative techniques should be studied for treatment of atrophic scars of acne. I have been pleasantly surprised by great responses to a series of treatments using the Q-switched neodymium (Nd):YAG laser. There is no downtime; patients can go right back to work or school. This laser also is helpful in treating old varicella scars. Results have been pretty dramatic with the Q-switched Nd:YAG laser. I encourage everybody to try it.

Emil A. Tanghetti, MD: Because vitiligo is essentially an immunologic process, we have been prescribing tacrolimus in a number of patients in conjunction with their going out in the sun. We have seen partial repigmentation in at least 6 patients. Tacrolimus is something to consider in patients who have vitiligo, to use in conjunction with other treatments.

Arielle N. B. Kauvar, MD: For years I treated hypertrophic scarring with the 0.45-millisecond pulsed dye laser, and now I am routinely using a pulse duration of 1.5 milliseconds and getting the same results. I wonder if anyone has experience with longer pulse durations. I do not see a difference with longer pulse durations.

Dr Tope: With or without cooling?

Dr Kauvar: With cooling.

Dr Tope: I did a paired comparison in 5 patients using 1.5- and 0.45-millisecond pulse durations with the 585-nm pulsed dye laser, and every patient thought that the side of the scar treated at 0.45 milliseconds had much better results than at 1.5 milliseconds. I gave 4 to 5 treatments, so that is why I have stuck with 585 nm and 0.45 milliseconds in treating hypertrophic scars. Now that cooling is available to protect the epidermis, I think we need to investigate longer wavelengths and higher fluences with cooling to see whether we can achieve better responses.

Dr Dover: We no longer have a 0.45-millisecond pulsed dye laser. We treat all the scars at 1.5 milliseconds with purpura doses, not very high fluences, and results appear to be at least as good as what we used to get with the shorter-pulse dye laser, if not maybe better. We use cooling, a 595-nm wavelength, 1.5-millisecond pulse duration, and 7-mm spot at 7 to 7.5 J/cm^2, which induces pretty good purpura, or for a 10-mm spot, 6.5 to 7 J/cm^2.

Dr Kauvar: I actually did a paired comparison before I switched over to the 1.5-millisecond laser, and I don't see a difference in results at all.

Dr Dover: That's what we did when we had both lasers. It would be nice for someone to perform a definitive paired comparison with slightly larger numbers of patients than Dr Tope had.

Dr Geronemus: I disagree with Dr Tope, in that I think it is possible to treat dark-skinned patients with hypertrophic scars, particularly with the use of cooling. I can treat skin types IV through VI. It can be done safely. One just needs to be more conservative, and I think the cooling is helpful.

Dr Dover: Cooling has changed the way we practice medicine, and nobody here would like to treat any of these scars without using cooling. We probably could not use 1.5 milliseconds at the fluences we use without cooling.

Dr Kauvar: I have another point. Dr Hruza showed that resurfacing with the CO_2 laser after Mohs surgical defects may reepithelialize these defects very well. Dr Geronemus and I had a series of patients with superficial Mohs defects treated with the erbium:YAG laser. We obtained incredible results, especially on the nose and medial aspect of the cheeks, where it appears as if there has been no procedure at all. I think that erbium:YAG laser resurfacing is a wonderful technique for treating Mohs defects.

Dr Dover: Dr Hruza has actually performed hundreds of these cases and had al-most scarless results. His work was published in *Dermatologic Surgery* (Ammirati CT, Cottingham TJ, Hruza GJ. Immediate postoperative laser resurfacing improves second intention healing on the nose: 5-year experience. *Dermatolog Surg.* 2001;27:324–325). You are now getting reimbursement from some insurance carriers for doing this procedure, isn't that correct, Dr Hruza?

Dr Hruza: Yes, I get reimbursed if I do immediate resurfacing. We now use the variable-pulse erbium:YAG laser for the procedure to avoid the problem of hy-popigmentation that we saw with the CO_2 laser. Medicare routinely will reimburse for the procedure. Most often I do the procedure in patients for whom the alterna-tive is a skin graft, so I don't think it is unreasonable for the insurance companies to reimburse a modest amount of money compared with hundreds of dollars for a skin graft. Medicare, as I said, routinely reimburses for the procedure, certainly af-ter the Mohs surgery. The other insurance plans will reimburse for it, but generally an appeal is needed at least half of the time. They are much more likely to reim-burse the immediate resurfacing type of procedure than when we do the spot laser abrasion (*Current Procedural Terminology*® *[CPT]* code 15786) at 6 to 8 weeks to enhance the scar. Some of those plans will never pay for delayed resurfacing.

Robert A. Weiss, MD: I wanted to mention the value of intense pulsed light (IPL) in hypertrophic scarring. We had approximately 80 cases and used very different parameters for the photorejuvenation. We obtained good results. We have switched over to the 2-millisecond long-pulse dye laser and are conducting a study treating half of the scars with the IPL and half with the long-pulse dye laser. So far, statistical analysis shows that results with both are about the same.

Dr Dover: What parameters do you use for the IPL?

Dr Weiss: We usually will use a triple pulse of 3 to 4 milliseconds with a 20-millisecond delay between pulses, and the fluence typically ranges from 38 to 48 J/cm².

We also find that there are 2 groups of patients. For those with acne who want immediate results, we do everything at one time: Subcision and the erbium:YAG laser resurfacing over that. Then for the patients who want to do treatment really slowly, we use the nonablative techniques, such as the 1320-nm Nd:YAG laser and microdermabrasion, and get great results. Sometimes results are influenced by the extent of scarring and the skin color and ethnic background as well.

Carolyn Jacob, MD: I agree with Drs Tope and Kaminer regarding the multistep approach to treating acne-scarred patients. I would be interested to hear anybody else's experience with using some of the lasers or nonablative lasers for the treatment of active acne. Some of the laser companies are now touting their lasers for treatment of active acne. We have had a small amount of success using the pulsed dye laser (NLite, ICN Pharmaceuticals Inc, Costa Mesa, Calif) to treat acne in patients. The treated half of our patient's face cleared, and she had used no other topical treatments. Of course, it is necessary to continually re-treat these patients, because acne is an ongoing process. Does anyone have experience using lasers to treat acne?

David B. Vasily, MD: Yes. A few years ago, we looked at using the Q-switched Nd:YAG laser, because the infrared wavelength does kill *Propionibacterium acnes* very effectively. If we combined microdermabrasion with the Q-switched YAG, it was an effective treatment of active acne.

Dr Dover: What class of acne did you treat?

Dr Vasily: Inflammatory acne. Class 2 or 3.

Lasers in the Treatment of Tattoos and Dermal Pigment: What's New and What's Next?

Resistance of Tattoos to the Q-switched Laser

Whitney D. Tope, MPhil, MD

The optimal laser configuration for tattoo pigment removal delivers pulsed light in the picosecond time domain.[1,2] These very brief pulses generate photoacoustic waves whose tensile strength exceeds the fracture threshold for disruption of nanoparticulate and microparticulate tattoo pigment. Unfortunately, picosecond-domain lasers at appropriate wavelengths are not commercially available at this time. Commonly performed Q-switched (QS) laser tattoo removal employing nanosecond-domain pulses causes pigment removal by fragmenting tattoo particles, inciting inflammation, converting opaque black carbon particles to a translucent state, and allowing transepidermal elimination of pigment particles. Q-switched laser treatments injure tissue immediately adjacent to pigment particles. This injury incites an acute inflammatory response. Circulating macrophages recruited in this response more easily carry fragmented particles to the lymph nodes. Treatment with high fluences and small spot sizes frequently causes ablation of epidermis, with pinpoint bleeding of treated skin observed minutes later. Anecdotal reports indicate that, much like dermabrasion, ablative laser resurfacing has been used alone and in combination with QS laser tattoo removal to lighten tattoos by removing the epidermis. This incites inflammation and allows tattoo pigment to depart the exposed dermis. Tattoo treatment methods that disrupt the epidermis may well lighten tattoos through the additional mechanism of transepidermal elimination of tattoo pigment. Bayoumi and Marks[3] demonstrated that a charcoal suspension injected intradermally in guinea pig skin caused downward growth of epidermal extensions that surrounded and expelled the particles. It is possible, but unproven, that transepidermal elimination may more efficiently remove tattoo particles than by extrusion of pigment at the surface of completely deepithelialized skin treated by dermabrasion or ablative laser resurfacing.

An excellent way to treat allergic tattoo reactions is by "overtattooing" (Fig 44-1). In this technique, a tattooing machine and normal saline solution are used to perforate the epidermis and injure the papillary dermis, allowing transepidermal elimination of pigment and inciting an episode of inflammation. After healing, much of the tattoo pigment comes out through the perforated

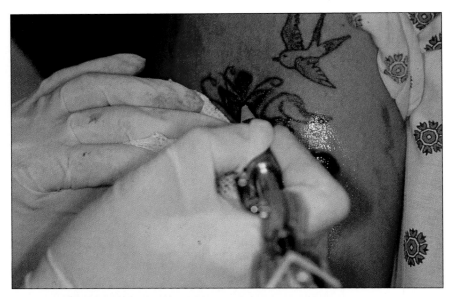

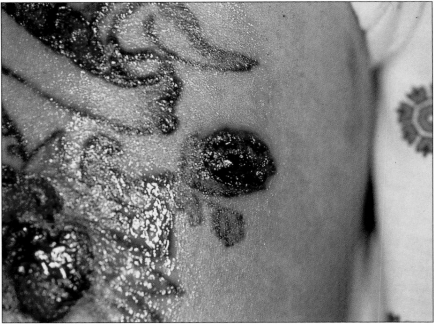

FIGURE 44.1

Top, Overtattooing red tattoo reaction using traditional tattoo machine and normal saline solution. Bottom, Immediate post-treatment appearance of overtattooed skin. Note presence of oozing hemorrhage. Papular or nodular foci of granulomatous inflammation often are lifted off in this technique.

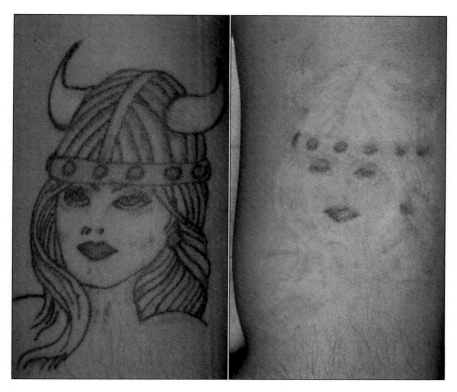

FIGURE 44.2

Tattoo of Viking maiden before (left) and after (right) multiple treatments with Q-switched ruby and neodymium:YAG (1064 nm) lasers. Note treatment resistance of blue-green and yellow tattoo pigments.

epithelium. Overtattooing should not be performed by a tattoo novice but by an experienced tattoo artist familiar with this technique.

RESISTANCE TO Q-SWITCHED LASER

Some tattoos resist treatment with the QS laser and may become dark (Fig 44-2). The typical QS laser–resistant tattoo has remaining green pigment, which fails to lighten with multiple treatments. Ross et al[4] showed that resistance of green tattoos may occur through darkening of the titanium dioxide, which is added as a brightener or enhancer of the tattoo pigments. For tattoos with yellow pigment, we need a blue-wavelength laser. Yellow tattoo treatment has been performed successfully using blue laser lines in the laboratory, but no blue-wavelength laser is commercially available yet.

I speculate that QS laser–resistant tattoos might respond better to less specific, more destructive therapies, such as the infrared coagulator, which has been used for tattoo removal. First reported for tattoo removal by Colver et al,[5] the infrared coagulator was eclipsed by the advent of QS lasers. Some physicians have just begun to reexamine its use in tattoo removal. Another alternative therapy for QS laser–resistant tattoos may be millisecond-domain light sources, such as the intense pulsed light (IPL) source. Theory and experience suggest that these more destructive modalities may well be associated with a higher risk of scarring.

CLINICALLY USEFUL TATTOO INK DARKENING

Tattoo ink darkening may be used to advantage in selected patients. Casparian and Krell[6] described a patient whose eyebrows had been tattooed with dark pigment. The pigment faded to red over time. In cosmetic tattooing, the blended pigment sometimes can lose certain components and fade to the color of the remaining pigment. The authors tested the QS neodymium:YAG laser at 1064 nm and 532 nm to treat this patient. The 1064-nm laser lightened the tattoo, but the 532-nm laser darkened it back to black. Subsequent treatment of the entire tattoo with 532-nm light resolved the cosmetic tattoo to an acceptable color.

"SMART" TATTOOS

The ability to safely localize inert foreign bodies in human skin may offer substantial benefits in medicine. Goda et al[7] showed that electron paramagnetic resonance (EPR) lines can be detected from carbon particles and that these EPR signals are sensitive to physiologic (molecular oxygen) levels but are unaffected by temperature, pH, or the presence of various reductants. The authors were able to measure an EPR signal from a human subject's black tattoo. One could also consider using tattoos to interrogate physiologic parameters we already measure, such as serum glucose levels. We need to develop "smart" tattoos.

COMPLETE TATTOO REMOVAL?

Laser surgeons should consider whether the tattoo is really gone after laser treatment. I think all of us would say no, and a recent report confirms this.[8] A computed tomographic (CT) scan was performed to rule out gastric carcinoma metastases in a patient who had no clinically obvious tattoos after successful QS laser removal. Yet the CT showed metal-density lymph nodes in the patient's axillae and chest wall, and he had high-density signals within skin at the previous tattoo sites. There was still clearly pigment in the skin and in the lymph nodes. This fact is of note for patients undergoing magnetic resonance (MR) imaging. Ferromagnetic pigments may rarely cause symptoms due to pigment heating during MR imaging.[9]

NOVEL DERMAL PIGMENTS

The next dermal pigments are likely to be laser-sensitive inks. Maybe we could find a laser-sensitive brightener, so tattoo artists would not have to use titanium dioxide, and we could more successfully lighten the tattoos with QS lasers. If one defines a pigment as something that absorbs light, then lipid-rich structures, sebaceous glands, and adipose lobules are next on the list of dermal pigments.[10] Other novel photosensitizers include those we either create or that we administer exogenously in photodynamic therapy.

REFERENCES

1. Herd RM, Alora MB, Smoller B, Arndt KA, Dover JS. A clinical and histologic prospective controlled comparative study of the picosecond titanium:sapphire (795 nm) laser versus the Q-switched alexandrite (752 nm) laser for removing tattoo pigment. *J Am Acad Dermatol*. 1999;40:603–606.
2. Ho DD, London R, Zimmerman GB, Yoong D. Laser tattoo removal: a study of the breakup mechanism and the optimal treatment strategy via computer simulations. *Lasers Surg Med*. 2001;28(S13):20.
3. Bayoumi AH, Marks R. Transepidermal elimination: studies with an animal model. *Br J Exp Pathol*. 1980;61:560–566.
4. Ross EV, Yashar S, Michaud N, et al. Tattoo darkening and nonresponse after laser treatment: a possible role for titanium dioxide. *Arch Dermatol*. 2001;137:33–37.
5. Colver GB, Cherry GW, Dawber RPR, Ryan TJ. Tattoo removal using infra-red coagulation. *Br J Dermatol*. 1985;112:481–485.
6. Casparian JM, Krell J. Using a side effect to therapeutic advantage: the darkening of red eyebrow tattoo pigment following Q-switched laser treatment. *Dermatol Surg*. 2000;26:255–258.
7. Goda F, Liu KJ, Walczak T, O'Hara JA, Jiang J, Swartz HM. In vivo oximetry using EPR and india ink. *Magn Reson Med*. 1995;33:237–245.
8. Kobayashi H, Togashi K. CT of tattoos removed with laser therapy. *Am J Roentgenol*. 2000;174:1468–1469.
9. Tope WD, Shellock FG. Magnetic resonance imaging and permanent cosmetics (tattoos): survey of complications and adverse events. *J Magn Reson Imaging*. 2002;15:180–184.
10. Manstein D, Erofeev AV, Altshuler GB, Anderson RR. Selective photothermolysis of lipid-rich tissue. *Lasers Surg Med*. 2001;28(S13):6.

chapter 45

Removal of Dermal Pigment and Tattoos: Can't We Do Better?

E. Victor Ross, Jr, MD

I believe that laser surgeons can improve removal of dermal pigment and tattoos. What we are doing so far, I think, is inadequate. We can remove epidermal pigment using Q-switched lasers and sometimes by light ablation with an erbium:YAG or carbon dioxide (CO_2) laser. The difficulty, however, is in removing dermal pigment so there is no clinical evidence that it was there.

MELASMA

Melasma, I think, is one of the most challenging skin conditions, and as we have a growing number of darker and darker patients in America, it will be an ever-increasing problem. Chemical peels can work pretty well in decreasing hyperpigmentation, but the overall efficacy of lasers in this setting has proved unsatisfactory. The challenge is how to atraumatically remove dermal pigment without stimulating new pigment production. Taylor[1] and many other authors have shown that if melasma—what I call dynamic hyperpigmentation—is treated with Q-switched lasers or even with moderate-depth CO_2 or erbium:YAG laser resurfacing, typically the results are poor. It may be necessary to perform deeper ablation with the erbium:YAG laser to truly eliminate the pigment, but then one risks hypopigmentation.

On a woman with typical severe melasma, I treated a large test site using the erbium:YAG laser, with the goal to eliminate all the pigment I could see in that area (Fig 45-1). Then I performed full-face CO_2 laser skin resurfacing several weeks later, partly because I no longer had the erbium:YAG laser and partly because I believed the CO_2 laser should achieve a similar response as the erbium:YAG laser. At the time of the full-face treatment, I noticed there was some pigment remaining, even after removal of the epidermis (Fig 45-2). I thought the pigment might go away through some sort of elimination process, but it did not. A year later, more melasma had appeared in the area treated with the CO_2 laser, but the site treated with the erbium:YAG laser was still unpig-

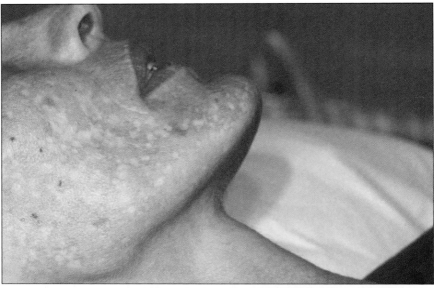

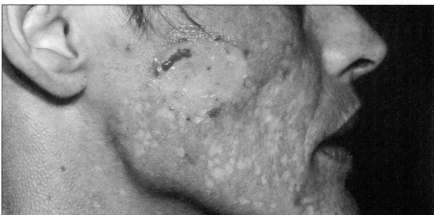

F I G U R E 45.1

Woman with typical severe melasma before (top) and just after (bottom) treatment with erbium:YAG laser.

mented (Fig 45-3). Thus, the more aggressive treatment with the erbium:YAG worked better than the moderately aggressive treatment with the CO_2 laser. A possible reason is that with the erbium:YAG laser, I actually drove the pigment out of the dermis, whereas with the CO_2, I took off just the epidermis and created some thermal damage in the papillary dermis.

In my experience, when I have used the erbium:YAG or the CO_2 laser for moderate-depth resurfacing (to the papillary dermis with the CO_2 laser or the

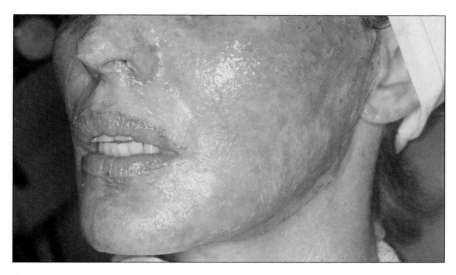

FIGURE 45.2

Just after full-face resurfacing with carbon dioxide laser.

superficial papillary dermis with the erbium:YAG laser), hyperpigmentation almost always develops in types IV and V skin. I treated 5 Filipino women with melasma over the course of 5 weeks with the erbium:YAG laser at moderate fluences and moderate depths, and a hyperpigmented test site developed in every patient. Clearly, researchers need to explore whether there is a better way to treat melasma than with Q-switched lasers or light laser skin resurfacing using the erbium:YAG or CO_2 laser.

More recently, the intense pulsed light (IPL) source and long-pulse potassium-titanyl-phosphate (KTP) lasers have been used to gently heat the melanosome with millisecond-long pulses rather than destroying a melanosome with Q-switched pulses. Bitter[2] as well as Weiss and colleagues[3] have used a broadband light source (IPL) in serial treatments to improve pigment homogeneity. Another option is to combine a light erbium:YAG laser resurfacing with glycolic acid or bleaching agents.

As an example, in a patient with melasma and postinflammatory hyperpigmentation who was treated using the long-pulse 532-nm Nd:YAG laser (Aura, Laserscope, San Jose, Calif), one can see the combinations of epidermal and dermal pigment (Fig 45-4). This condition responds quite well to serial KTP treatments with almost no risk of worsening the degree of pigmentation.

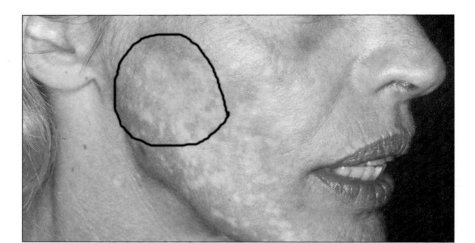

FIGURE 45.3

One year after erbium:YAG laser test site and full-face carbon dioxide laser resurfacing. Note that erbium test site remains improved (inside circle).

POSTINFLAMMATORY HYPERPIGMENTATION

Postinflammatory hyperpigmentation is a dynamic process at an early stage and a more static process late. I have had good success when waiting 1 year after the onset of postinflammatory hyperpigmentation before instituting laser treatment. Hyperpigmentation in a black woman, made worse by liquid nitrogen treatment 1 year earlier, was removed with the Q-switched alexandrite laser (Fig 45-5) on a test site. Subsequently, the rest of the lesion was removed. Early, dynamic postinflammatory hyperpigmentation, I think, responds poorly to laser treatment, but static, prolonged hyperpigmentation, whether after sclerotherapy or trauma, tends to respond quite well.

TATTOO REMOVAL

Most tattoo inks absorb light. The absorption spectrum in Figure 45-6 shows that the absorption of red light by a dark-green tattoo is very good. The subsequent laser surgery with red light produces heat. However, many tattoos, especially green tattoos, do not go away completely, as shown in Figure 44-2. One reason for this is titanium dioxide.[4] A standard electron microscopic analysis demonstrated that titanium dioxide composes approximately 58% of the most commonly used tattoo inks (Fig 45-7). Attempts to remove tattoo pigment with

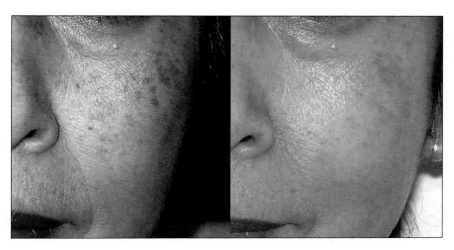

FIGURE 45.4

Before treatment (left) and 4 weeks after 3 monthly treatments with potassium-titanyl-phosphate (KTP) laser (right).

a high concentration of titanium dioxide using Q-switched lasers or the alexandrite laser causes a little darkening with reduction of the ink. However, the same laser treatment can lighten an ink with less titanium dioxide, such as a red ink with only about 27% titanium dioxide.

The second reason for resistance to lasers is the depth and amount of ink. We have noted in biopsy specimens that many resistant green tattoos showed larger numbers of granules and deeper placement of thick granules than their less resistant counterparts.

There are several potential ways to improve laser removal of tattoos. One is to use larger spots and high fluences, or to use picosecond pulses, possibly with more moderate fluences.

One way to generate higher "subsurface" energy densities is photon recycling. With photon recycling for tattoo-removal devices, it is possible to greatly improve the conservation of laser energy. Without recycling, about 70% of the energy is wasted during treatment of many of these tattoos.

Other manipulations we might try in the future include agents to improve beam penetration. Barton and colleagues[5] have shown that injection of glycerol into the skin can improve the mismatch in the refractive indexes in the skin and actually make the skin transparent by sucking water away from the area. In addition, perhaps the postoperative inflammatory process can be enhanced. Maybe we could use imiquimod (Aldara) cream or a neutrophil chemotactic factor after

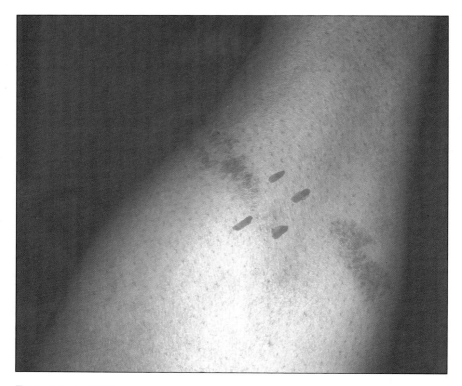

FIGURE 45.5

Eight weeks after Q-switched alexandrite laser treatment to test spot (center of photograph, 8-mm circle).

tattoo removal. For example, I applied the leukotriene LTB4 to my skin and produced erythema. Although I have not yet used this compound on a tattoo, it might be another way to modulate the postinflammatory immune response after laser treatment.

Finally, laser-removable tattoos are available. If more tattoo artists used them, there would not be as great a problem with removing tattoos.

REFERENCES

1. Taylor CR, Anderson RR. Ineffective treatment of refractory melasma and postinflammatory hyperpigmentation by Q-switched ruby laser. *J Dermatol Surg Oncol.* 1994;20:592–597.
2. Bitter PH. Noninvasive rejuvenation of photodamaged skin using serial, full-face intense pulsed light treatments. *Dermatol Surg.* 2000;26:835–842.

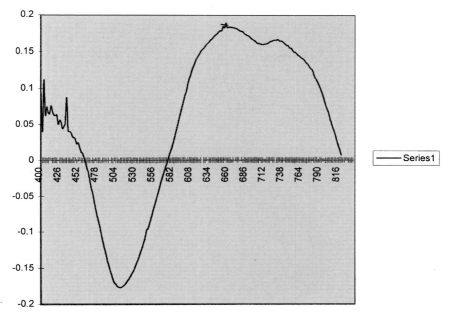

F I G U R E 45.6

Absorption spectrum of typical green tattoo. Note peak at 660 nm.

3. Weiss MA, Weiss RA, Costarangos C. Long term results 4 years using intense pulsed light for treatment of actinic changes including poikiloderma, telangiectasias and blotchy pigmentation [abstract]. *Lasers Surg Med.* 2001(suppl 13):81.
4. Ross EV, Yashar S, Michaud N, et al. Tattoo darkening and nonresponse after laser treatment: a possible role for titanium dioxide. *Arch Dermatol.* 2001;137:33–37.
5. Vargas G, Chan EK, Barton JK, et al. Use of an agent to reduce scattering in skin. *Lasers Surg Med.* 1999;24:133–141.

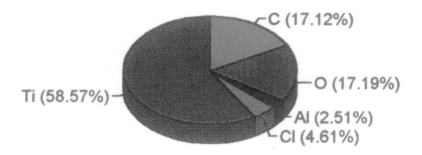

FIGURE 45.7

Composition of typical green tattoo ink. O indicates oxygen; Al, aluminum; Cl, chlorine; and Ti, titanium.

chapter 46

Tattoos

R. Rox Anderson, MD

What is new in tattoos is that the prevalence has increased. It is no longer a subculture; it is mainstream. The number of states that regulate tattoo parlors is decreasing. For example, Massachusetts recently passed legislation that includes body art under the First Amendment right to free speech. More tattoo inks are available, and they are more complex. Europe, for example, had a fluorescent tattoo ink that was visible only under ultraviolet light, which was made for people who visit discotheques, but this ink was also a potent photosensitizer. It was taken off the market after quite a few people got in trouble due to photosensitivity.

TATTOO REMOVAL TECHNIQUES

Present laser techniques to remove tattoos are still not very good. Picosecond pulses are more efficient than nanosecond pulses but are not as commercially available because of expense. We actually do not know if they are better clinically than what we do now with nanosecond Q-switched lasers, but they are not really available to us. Ort[1] conducted a study to determine whether laser resurfacing followed by Q-switched laser therapy would be more effective for tattoo removal than Q-switched laser alone, and he did not find any benefit. Dierickx reported that production of delayed-type hypersensitivity with injection of Candida antigen did nothing to help the tattoo ink removal process. To summarize, we just have not made much progress on tattoo removal.

Tattoo ink is, for the most part, not really removed from the body by Q-switched laser treatment. The ink particles, after being freed by laser treatment from phagocytic skin cells, are taken up into lymphatic vessels and transported to the regional lymph nodes. I therefore looked into what is known about increasing lymphatic transport, to identify a potential aid to tattoo "removal." Somewhat surprisingly, massage is a great stimulant for lymphatic transport. I would like to try combining massage with laser treatment for tattoo removal in the future.

DESIGNER TATTOOING

Rather than trying to improve laser parameters to make tattoo removal easier, I believe that a better solution is to change the tattoo materials. In my laboratory,

317

we are looking at 2 different ways of making tattoo inks that can be easily re-moved. One way is to make an encapsulated liquid ink particle, so that if any micron-sized insoluble particle is placed into the skin, the skin treats it like a tat-too. What we are trying to do is to synthesize an envelope and put a liquid ink drop in the middle so that the laser no longer has to do anything but rupture this package. The liquid ink would then just dissolve after laser treatment. We hope to be able to use safe materials to make tattoos that will definitely be re-moved in a single treatment.

Our other approach is to make a magnetic tattoo and then extract it with a strong external magnetic field. This method uses a completely inert substance that has no biological relevance, called Fe_3O_4. We tested this magnetic tattoo in rats and found that we can manipulate it using external magnets (M. Huzaira, MD, and R. R. Anderson, MD, unpublished data, 2001). We were hoping to fully extract the ink, but it gets stuck at the dermal-epidermal junction. We know, for example, that if we treat a magnetic tattoo with a laser and then place a magnet on the skin, we prevent the tattoo from being removed. This finding indicates that the mechanism for laser tattoo ink removal involves, as discussed, transport into the lymph nodes.

REFERENCES

1.   Ort RJ, Anderson RR, Arndt KA, Dover JS. CO_2 laser resurfacing of tattoos prior to Q-switched laser treatment. *Lasers Surg Med.* 2000:23 (suppl 12).

PART TWELVE DISCUSSION

Kenneth A. Arndt, MD, *Moderator*

E. Victor Ross, Jr, MD: What is the best wavelength to use to remove a nevus of Ota?

Henry H. Chan, MD: We published the results of a study in which we compared in vivo the use of Q-switched neodymium (Nd):YAG and Q-switched alexandrite lasers (Chan HH, Ying SY, Ho WS, Kono T, King WW. An in vivo trial comparing the clinical efficacy complications of Q-switched 755 nm alexandrite and Q-switched 1064 nm Nd:YAG lasers in the treatment of nevus of Ota. *Dermatol Surg.* 2000;26:919–922). Using both subjective and objective assessment in patients with nevus of Ota, we found that after 3 or more treatments the Q-switched Nd:YAG produced superior lightening compared with the Q-switched alexandrite laser. In a subsequent report of complications, we studied 171 patients with nevus of Ota and found that the risk of hypopigmentation was least likely when we used the Q-switched Nd:YAG laser alone. (Chan HH, Leung RS, Ying SY, et al. A retrospective analysis of complications in the treatment of nevus of Ota with the Q-switched alexandrite and Q-switched Nd:YAG lasers. *Dermatol Surg.* 2000;26:1000–1006). The highest hypopigmentation risk was using the Q-switched Nd:YAG laser 1 time and then the Q-switched alexandrite laser the other time. In a later study, we used the same protocol in patients with nevus of Ota and found that the Q-switched ruby laser had the highest hypopigmentation rate, 16.8%.

Dr Ross: I think you had an article earlier in which you had said the alexandrite laser was better, and subsequently you have another article in which you say the Nd:YAG laser is better. I am a little confused.

Dr Chan: In the first article, we reported that a patient's tolerability was better with the Q-switched alexandrite, but in terms of clinical efficacy, we could not find a difference, because we did not follow up the patients long enough. At least 3 treatments are needed before one can detect any difference in clinical efficacy. The second article reported follow-up results, so that is why the results differed.

In terms of your melasma photographs, I think there is a large difference between superficial, epidermal melasma, the kind that you resurfaced with the erbium:YAG laser, and what we call Hori macule, which has been classified more appropriately as "acquired Nevus of Ota-like macule." My group and others find that we can achieve a substantial improvement in acquired Nevus of Ota-like macule, if we use a Q-switched laser combined with a bleaching agent. Treatment sessions must be repeated much more frequently, so instead of every 2 to 3 months, we tend to repeat our treatments every 4 to 6 weeks.

Dr Ross: Is this acquired dermal pigmentation you are talking about?

Dr Chan: Yes, the so-called dermal melasma that you discussed. In 1983, the Japanese described that as Hori macule, and it was later classified as acquired Nevus of Ota-like macule. It is different from Nevus of Ota. We see it frequently in Asians. It is grayish-bluish hyperpigmentation involving both cheeks. It is very different from the epidermal melasma that you mentioned, which is a lot more resistant to treatment, even resurfacing.

Dr Arndt: Last year, I showed the photograph of a woman who had a facial tattoo, which was laser-induced chrysiasis. Dr Anderson followed up this patient and found a way of decreasing this rather unique gold-induced pigment in the skin. Would you report your follow-up results, Dr Anderson?

R. Rox Anderson, MD: This patient had been administered gold 20 years ago to treat rheumatoid arthritis. She had some facial lentigines that were treated by another laser surgeon using a Q-switched alexandrite laser, which produced immediate blue-black pigmentation on her face, called laser-induced chrysiasis. The alexandrite laser was again used in an attempt to remove the blue-black pigmentation. However, the fluence for causing the darkening reaction is lower than the fluence needed to affect the pigmentation, so any attempt to use the alexandrite laser caused more pigmentation at the margin of the treated areas. The patient was referred to me, and I used reflectance spectrometry to determine the wavelengths that are absorbed by the blue-black chrysiasis pigmentation. We found that there was a broad absorption for the pigment between wavelengths of approximately 550 nm to 950 nm, with a peak around 700 nm. That is why the pigment looks blue. Then we attempted to determine whether there was a pulse width that would remove this pigment without inducing further pigment. Testing was performed with nanosecond, microsecond, and millisecond-domain pulses. We were able to clear the pigment with 50 J/cm^2 from a long-pulse (normal-mode) ruby laser at 3 milliseconds. Other high-energy, red, long-pulse lasers probably would have worked as well.

I suspect that a similar process may be happening with laser-induced tattoo darkening, in which red or white tattoos are induced to turn black by Q-switched laser treatment. My recommendation, if you encounter a patient with laser-induced chrysiasis, which is rare, is to try treatment with a long-pulse laser. Alternatively, the lesions, if appropriate, could be ablated using a continuous-wave laser or they could be excised.

Dr Arndt: There are many articles in the literature that report that the darkening of cosmetic tattoos sometimes clears with repeated laser treatments. Indeed, in this woman, the dark pigmentation did seem to clear in the center after repeated treatment; however, it just kept going appearing similar to a halo, with increasing hyperpigmentation at the periphery.

Dr Anderson: What we found with nanosecond pulses, with the Q-switched ruby laser, was that the fluence for causing this darkening reaction was less than 1 J/cm^2, which is not enough to remove the pigmentation. In a patient whose entire body has gold deposits in it, the laser surgeon cannot find a margin. With laser-darkened tattoos, that is not the case. I think Q-switched lasers succeed in removing laser-darkened tattoos when the patient does not have a systemic problem, but with chrysiasis, another type of treatment must be used.

Suzanne L. Kilmer, MD: I remove a lot of tattoos. One of the first patients that Dr Anderson and I treated in our original Q-switched Nd:YAG study, when we proved efficacy, had 4 tattoos on various parts of her body. This woman had greatly enlarged lymph nodes in her abdomen and was worked up for ovarian cancer, I think. The results of the lymph node biopsy showed the enlargement was ink-related, so I want to reiterate Dr Tope's point that systemic allergic reactions can result from tattoos and/or laser treatment of tattoos.

Also, I've been an expert witness in several lawsuits brought by individuals treated with longer pulse width for tattoo removal, in the microsecond range and the millisecond range. With those ranges, the pulses are longer than desired for thermal relaxation, and scarring can occur. Therefore, when offering treatment with longer pulse widths, it is important to obtain informed consent from patients and tell them of the potential for scarring. Scarring is almost inevitable with the infrared coagulator.

Whitney D. Tope, MD: I think the big problem with tattoo pigment is that the density of the chromophore is high in the area of the tattoo. The key, if one is going to try millisecond-domain pulses, is to be gentle. Start very conservatively and do not overdo it. Otherwise, if one targets a fresh tattoo with millisecond-domain pulses, it will blister immediately.

Dr Kilmer: Right. I just didn't want people to think they could treat tattoos with millisecond lasers, but you are right. I still will want to use a laser with a big spot size and a high fluence.

Robert A. Weiss, MD: I want to warn laser surgeons who perform hair removal on people with tattoos in the same area, because they may inadvertently remove the tattoos.

Another comment I have is that my coworkers and I have treated more than 35 patients with recalcitrant tattoos using the erbium:YAG laser. These were cosmetic tattoos with unusual fluorescent inks or green inks that were persistent. One must understand the histologic effects of the erbium:YAG laser (tissue removal of about 5 mm removed per joule per square centimeter). Then one can easily go into the dermis, the upper reticular to midreticular dermis with magnification, focusing on the tattoo pigment, and obtain very good results in removal of these tattoos, with minimal or no scarring.

Dr Anderson: Some time ago, I conducted a study with Myrna Armstrong and others to assess the motivations of patients desiring tattoo removal (Armstrong ML, Stuppy DJ, Gabriel DC, Anderson RR. Motivation for tattoo removal. *Arch Dermatol.* 1996;132:412–416). Most of these patients went through some positive changes in their life that led them to want their tattoo removed. I am aware of some recent pediatric research that found that tattoo and body piercing is strongly correlated with risk-taking behaviors, including suicide attempts and drug use—behaviors that may change later in life. So although the prevalence of tattoos has increased, I do not think it means that people with tattoos will no longer want to have them removed. My own feeling is that when the young people currently getting tattoos reach 30 years of age, they are going to want the tattoos off by the droves.

Dr Kilmer: I am already seeing a recent increase in the number of people who want their tattoos removed. After performing approximately 40 tattoo removals per week in 1993 and 1994, we removed only about 10 tattoos a week in 1995 through 1998. In 1999, that number increased to 20 per week. In 2000, the number of tattoo removals returned to 40 per week. I can tell you that 35 of those 40 people are coming to me not because they are former members of gangs, as was the case early in my practice, but because they now are raising children and getting jobs and they regret the cosmetic tattoos they had put on 5 or 6 years earlier. I believe we will continue to have patients who want tattoos removed. There will definitely be an increase.

Arielle N. B. Kauvar, MD: I have 2 comments. Ablative lasers can be used to treat tattoos. I do not think that there is an additive effect. We routinely use successive, very superficial ablative treatments with the erbium:YAG laser or even superficial carbon dioxide (CO_2) laser to remove cosmetic types of tattoos, such as permanent lip liner, that we know we cannot treat with Q-switched lasers. These patients do very well, so laser resurfacing is an option for tattoos resistant to other lasers. Obviously, when using this treatment, one must be more careful treating skin other than the face, in terms of the reepithelialization.

The second thing I wanted to mention was the use of immunomodulators. Last summer I started treating 12 patients with imiquimod (Aldara) cream in conjunction with the Q-switched ruby laser. I split the tattoo into treatment and control halves, treated the patients with the laser, and told them to wait until they were totally healed and all the crusting was gone before applying the imiquimod cream twice a day every other day. In some of the patients, the imiquimod-treated half of the tattoo had better results. However, I think that the imiquimod affects a much greater area of skin than the application site. For instance, if the cream is applied on 2 cm of a small tattoo, it will affect the entire tattoo. Nevertheless, I definitely think there is a benefit to this combination therapy. In some patients who had professional tattoos with many vibrant colors, we achieved 80% to 90% clearing after 4 treatment sessions, and we cannot do that with the laser alone. To minimize side effects of the imiquimod, I told every patient to call me if skin irritation started to occur, and we would modify the amount they applied. As soon as some patients started getting a superficial erosion, I cut back the amount and then gently restarted it. Other patients were able to tolerate the side effects of the cream every day. I do think there is an important role for agents that will increase macrophage clearance of the tattoo pigments. I believe that is the way to go for tattoo removal.

Dr Chan: Dr Anderson, you mentioned about Hu's work in intradermal focusing. The spot size can be very small, and it could potentially take a very long time to complete a treatment, so do you think it would actually work in a practical sense?

Dr Anderson: For a 10-mm spot size inside the dermis, it will take a lot of pulses. To do that, the physician has to change laser types, to high-repetition-rate, low-pulse-energy Q-switched lasers, such as the potassium-titanyl-phosphate (KTP) laser. If the laser surgeon were to lay down 10,000 pulses per second, it would go very quickly, but such a machine has not been made yet.

I wanted to make another comment. Dr Kilmer asked whether we can make a shorter-pulse laser. I think that a laser manufacturer is coming out soon with a 2-nanosecond device. If one looks at the theoretical models for inertial confinement, and given the size of the tattoo ink particles, the best pulse duration is probably around 1 nanosecond. No one knows for sure, because, to my knowledge, there have been no clinical studies done with this new device. I don't have one of these 2-nanosecond lasers. The possibility is there, I think, to step down from 10 nanoseconds to 1, and one would probably see a large difference in the efficacy.

Dr Ross: I want to comment about the large spots and high fluences. I have reviewed many biopsy results of resistant tattoos. Clearly, there is a line deep in the dermis at which the laser stops having an effect, and there often are intact tattoo particles deep in the dermis. So I think there is room for improvement beyond just increasing the spot size and the fluence of nanosecond-domain lasers.

Jo S. Bohannon, MD: This spring I surveyed my patients to ask which services they would like us to offer that we currently do not offer. Overwhelmingly, 2 services were requested. Number 1 was belly button piercing, and the second one was tattooing; they want a safe place, a medical office, where tattoos can be discreetly administered. The tattoo requests came from women aged 35 to 49 years, and I practice in an upper-class suburb. The requests for navel piercing came from mothers of teenagers and young adults, who are going to the tattoo parlors to get this done, and they would prefer that their children come to a medical office.

Also, what is the experience with tattoo removal using intense pulsed light (IPL)?

Dr Weiss: We initially tried it in 1996 and 1997. What appears to happen if one uses a subblistering dose of IPL is that there is a urticarial response. After about 2 treatments, there is a 50% reduction in pigment, and then the lightening of pigment stops and that's it.

Dr Arndt: If the epidermis overlying a tattoo is removed with a CO_2 or Er:YAG laser and then a Q-switched laser is aimed at pigment in the dermis, one would expect the beam to get there a little more intact and have more of an effect. In studies carried out with Dr Richard Ort, we did not find that, however. In fact, some patients seemed to have more of an adverse reaction.

Richard E. Fitzpatrick, MD: I don't know why you got a different response from what our group found. We do find it works clinically. It sometimes makes dramatic differences.

Dr Arndt: Are you treating primarily the head and neck? Many of our cases of tattoos were on the trunk.

Dr Fitzpatrick: No, I have treated the arms, legs, and trunk as well as the head and neck. I treated a tattoo that covered a patient's entire lower leg, which without CO_2 laser resurfacing first, took 15 to 20 treatments to remove it, but with CO_2 resurfacing first, it took only 5 or 6 treatments.

Richard Ort, MD: We performed a study in patients with nonfacial tattoos, using 1-pass CO_2 laser resurfacing, followed by wiping to remove the debris, and then we followed that with either a Q-switched alexandrite, Nd:YAG, or ruby laser in 1 quadrant. We had 1 or 2 patients experience a subtle benefit in the quadrant that received combination treatment. Most patients, however, obtained much the same lightening in the combination quadrant and with the Q-switched laser alone. With the quadrants that received 1-pass CO_2 treatment alone, there was no lightening at all. We were hoping to see a lot of pigment in the dressings afterward, and we did not find that too often. Clabaugh, in the 1960s, performed some studies of superficial dermabrasion, in which he must have gone deeper than 1 pass with the CO_2 laser, because he found a lot of pigment in the gauze after treatment (Clabaugh W. Removal of tattoos by superficial dermabrasion. *Arch Dermatol.* 1968;98:515–521). I suspect that if one goes deeper than 1 pass, some pigment will be removed through the denuded skin, but the risk of scarring might also increase.

Dr Weiss: I think that is the difference, because when we performed only epidermal single-pass resurfacing, there was not as much of a change as we thought, but after a second pass, we did achieve greater removal of the pigment. I guess one is also taking away a little tissue that has ink in it.

I also wanted to discuss a dermal pigment that has not been mentioned, hemosiderin. In the past few months, I have seen many patients with hemosiderin in the legs after sclerotherapy, trauma, or surgery, and 1 patient had vasculitis that left her with dense hemosiderin deposits over her legs. As I remember, the absorption spectrum for hemosiderin peak is very short, below 500 nm. I did test spots with wavelengths of 532, 755, and 1064 nm, and the 755-nm laser worked best; the hemosiderin in 3 or 4 of these patients has cleared after treatment with the 755-nm Q-switched alexandrite laser. I am curious what Dr Anderson thinks about this.

Dr Anderson: I have had pretty good results with the Q-switched ruby laser in treatment of hemosiderin when it is really dense. A helpful clinical point about hemosiderin pigment is that it can only persist in a patient who is relatively well supplemented with iron. Many women, especially postmenopausal women who continue to take iron supplements, do not clear this cutaneous hemosiderin quickly. The physician can eliminate a lot of the hemosiderin just by getting the patients to stop taking their vitamin pills and waiting a few months for their ferritin level to drop. Hemosiderin has an absorption band at 630 nm, and I don't think we currently have the right laser to treat it. If I were to design a laser for treatment of hemosiderin, I would probably use a 630-nm pulse somewhere in the microsecond domain. I think Con-Bio (Palo Alto, Calif) has a red converter on their Q-switched laser for tattoo removal, and I think its output wavelength is around 650 nm.

ADDENDUM

Dr Arndt: Someone asked for words of wisdom on removing traumatic and implantation tattoos. In general, these tattoos respond well to Q-switched lasers. The same person had used Q-switched lasers in attempting to remove eyebrow tattoos and eyeliner tattoos, and the eyebrow tattoos went away, but the eyeliner tattoos did not. I have not had experience in those areas. Dr Tope, do you want to comment on that?

Dr Tope: I have treated permanent eyeliner at the lash line and have been able to remove a large amount of the pigment with Q-switched lasers, using a series treatment just like at any other body site. However, what I prefer to do now is light resurfacing, because it more uniformly removes or decreases that pigment.

Dr Arndt: Using what instrument?

Dr Tope: I have used the CO_2 laser (UltraPulse 5000C, Coherent Inc, Santa Clara, Calif), with a single pass to take off the epidermis and then 1 more pass to injure the dermis, and then I stop and let the pigment work its way out during wound healing. It works better than performing multiple treatments with Q-switched lasers.

Dr Arndt: There was also a comment about optimal ways to approach treatment of allergic granulomas in tattoos. Avoid use of a Q-switched laser, because if patients are allergic to mercury or whatever the antigen in the tattoo ink is and the laser surgeon liberates it, the patient can get an accelerated or immediate response and a rather considerable systemic reaction. Granulomatous tattoo reactions should be either ablated using a continuous-wave laser or excised. Certainly, it is not advisable to try to break the pigment up with a Q-switched laser. There have been some life-threatening complications. Dr Tope, do you want to comment on that?

Dr Tope: That is another situation for which resurfacing is a good option. After removal of the epithelium, a lot of that pigment and the granulomatous inflammation will work its way out.

Jerome M. Garden, MD: I disagree with that. I give the patients large doses of steroids the day before and during the laser procedure. I used a Q-switched laser a few times and have removed a lot of pigment. Then after a while, the pigment is gone, and the patients do very well.

Dr Kilmer: My recommendation is to perform excision or ablation when the lesions are very small, because there have been near deaths and anaphylaxis resulting from Q-switched laser treatment in these cases. I routinely give the patients large doses of antihistamines and steroids, and go ahead and try to treat them with the Q-switched laser, but I am very careful.

Cyrus Chess, MD: To make a diagnosis of such an allergic reaction in a patient with a tattoo, must there be physical signs at least periodically? I recently saw a patient who told me that her tattoo gets itchy in the sun but said there is no bumpiness, blistering, or any other physical sign, just itching. Could that be treated with a Q-switched laser, or should the tattoo be ablated? Does that patient need steroids and antihistamines, or can I just go right ahead with laser treatment?

Dr Kilmer: Mercury can be photosensitized, and mercury is a red dye that often was added into the other dyes. There also is another metal, cadmium, that can be photosensitizing. The patients who tend to suffer a major allergic reaction usually have itching in the treatment area after the first Q-switched laser treatment, and they might even get a few local urticarial plaques. After the second treatment, their lips swell. Stop treatment when the first urticarial plaques develop.

Dr Tope: In 1976, the Federal Food, Drug, and Cosmetic Act banned the use of mercury, so mercury is not currently used in tattoo pigments unless they are from abroad.

Dr Kilmer: Mercury can, however, be a problem with old tattoos.

A physician: Cadmium was not one of those banned by the act; the 3 agents were lead, mercury, and another that I cannot recall.

Dr Kilmer: I think cobalt is still available.

Lasers and Light Sources for Hair Removal

Hair Removal by Light: Accomplishments and Challenges

Christine C. Dierickx, MD

Laser hair removal began in 1993, with a prototype of the ruby laser. Today, the family of laser hair-removal systems available includes the ruby, alexandrite, diode, and neodymium:YAG lasers. In this chapter, I will not attempt to answer the question of which device is the best to use. I will instead discuss some of the accomplishments in laser hair removal.

PERMANENT HAIR REDUCTION

Before 1993, the removal of hair by lasers and light sources was not possible. Today, not only is it possible to remove hair using lasers, some epilation systems have received clearance from the Food and Drug Administration (FDA) for permanent hair reduction (Table 47-1).[1] The definition of permanent hair reduction, according to the FDA, is that each treatment must achieve a significant reduction in the number of terminal hairs, and that reduction must be stable for a period longer than the complete growth cycle of follicles at a given body site.

This accomplishment has brought with it challenges. Patients want to know how many treatments they will need for all their unwanted hair to be gone forever, and I find that a difficult question to answer. In addition, attempts at laser hair removal have instead induced new hair growth in some patients, or treatments have turned dark hair white, thereby making these patients no longer candidates for permanent hair removal.

HAIR REMOVAL ON DARK SKIN TYPES

A second accomplishment has been the FDA clearance of light-based epilation systems for hair removal in individuals with darker skin types. Two diode lasers (LightSheer, Lumenis, Santa Clara, Calif; SLP 1000, Palomar Medical Technologies Inc, Burlington, Mass) are approved for this use, as are 2 long-pulse neodymium:YAG systems (CoolGlide, Altus Medical, Burlingame, Calif; Lyra,

TABLE 47.1

Epilation Systems Approved for Permanent Hair Reduction

Year	Epilation System	Type of Device	Company
1998	E2000	Ruby laser	Palomar Medical Technologies Inc
1999	LightSheer	Diode laser	Lumenis
2000	EpiLight	Flashlamp	Lumenis
	GentleLASE	Alexandrite laser	Candela Corporation
2001	CoolGlide laser	Neodymium:YAG	Altus Medical
	LYRA laser	Neodymium:YAG	Laserscope
	SLP	Diode laser	Palomar

Laserscope, San Jose, Calif) and a flashlamp (EpiLight, Lumenis). These lasers have several things in common. First, they have longer wavelengths. Wavelengths increased from 694 nm to 800 and 1064 nm. All of these devices also have a longer pulse duration, in the range of 30 to 100, even 1000, milliseconds. Longer pulse duration, combined with effective epidermal cooling, provides increased epidermal protection and, therefore, enables hair removal in individuals with dark skin types.

Despite these accomplishments, there are still limitations in laser hair removal that need improvement. Laser surgeons want to be able to effectively treat not only dark-colored hair but also the light colors—white, gray, blond, and red. There have been attempts to dye light-colored hair before laser hair removal.

PHOTODYNAMIC THERAPY

Hair removal with photodynamic therapy (PDT) has been reported. In a pilot study by Grossman et al,[2] a topical photosensitizer, aminolevulinic acid, was applied, taken up in the follicles, and converted into protoporphyrin IX. Fluorescence from the epidermis demonstrated that the photosensitizer was concentrated in the follicular opening, and an immunofluorescence biopsy showed that the photosensitizer was accumulated in the surrounding follicular epithelium. This technique means that the ability to perform hair removal is no longer dependent on the hair color but on the concentration of the drug in the follicular epithelium. The advantage is that all hair colors can be treated, but the main disadvantage is pain. Transient hyperpigmentation often occurs after treatment as well. The procedure also is very time-consuming; conversion to protoporphyrin

IX takes a couple of hours. Another disadvantage of this procedure is that it needs very high light doses.

Also on the wish list of laser surgeons is to increase the efficacy of laser hair removal. Wouldn't it be nice if we could remove all the hairs with a single treatment? To be able to do that, laser surgeons first must know what we need to target for destruction—the stem cells, the hair bulb or matrix, or the vessels in the dermal papilla. My coworkers and I have tried to answer this question but do not yet have the answer. Once that information is available, focusing the beam at the depth of the target and delivery of a very high power at the target itself might increase the efficacy of hair removal.

Finally, laser surgeons want devices that are less expensive, and, of course, patients would like to pay less for treatment. Certainly, there is progress in technology today. Diode lasers are becoming more powerful and less expensive. Light-emitting diodes and flashlamp technology have become available.

FLASHLAMP DEVICES

Two small and less expensive flashlamp devices are now available for hair removal. One of these intense-pulsed light sources is the EsteLux from Palomar Medical Technologies; the other is the SpaTouch from Radiancy, Orangeburg, NY. Both devices have a large spot size and therefore a high coverage rate. With the EsteLux, both legs can be treated in only 7 minutes, so it has a high treatment speed also. Efficacy of these devices has not yet been established, but preliminary results look promising. If such devices prove effective long term, hair removal may evolve to home devices and laser razors.

REFERENCES

1. Dierickx CC, Grossman MC, Farinelli WA, Anderson RR. Permanent hair removal by normal-mode ruby laser. *Arch Dermatol.* 1998;134:837–842.
2. Grossman MC, Dwyer P, Wimberley J, et al. PDT for hirsutism [abstract]. *Lasers Surg Med.* 1995;7(suppl):44.

chapter 48

Laser Hair Removal: Optimal Parameters

Eliot F. Battle, Jr, MD

L aser hair removal is one of the treatments that laser surgeons have become very good at performing. New trends in laser hair removal include increasing the speed of treatment by both increasing the Hertz and increasing the treatment spot sizes, and to decrease treatment cost. As the cost of lasers decreases, hopefully laser surgeons will pass these savings on to the patients. That change should attract more patients by making the procedures more affordable. An exciting advancement in the last few years is the ability to perform laser hair removal on patients with darker skin, both ethnic and tanned patients. However, as we reduce the fluences to safely treat these patients, are we providing permanent hair removal or just hair management? More research needs to be done.

In regard to laser hair removal, the laser industry is going in 2 different directions now: (1) high-powered lasers and flashlamps for permanent hair reduction and (2) low-power light sources for temporary hair reduction. The question is, Will we confuse our patients by offering both permanent-hair-reduction lasers and temporary-hair-reduction light sources? Practitioners and people in the industry need to keep patients very clear on the differences.

OPTIMAL WAVELENGTH AND PULSE DURATION

Shorter wavelengths have worked very well. They are, by far, our best chance to treat hair that is light in color and thin in diameter. The longer wavelengths allow us to treat darker skin types more safely, but they are not as effective on light and thin hair.

There has been a dramatic change in the length of pulse durations used over the last 3 years. Short pulse durations work very well. They are based on the thermal relaxation time (TRT) of a hair shaft, whereas long pulse durations are based on the TRT of a hair follicle. Pulse durations shorter than 30 milliseconds are classified as short, and pulse durations 30 milliseconds and longer are classified as long. Short pulse durations are probably the most effective way to treat hair, and longer pulse durations are safer for darker skin types. If epidermal protection were not an issue, then short pulse durations would probably be more effective.

OPTIMAL COOLING METHOD

There should be no debate on how essential skin cooling is. The darker the skin of the patient, the greater the need for skin cooling. Cooling reduces epidermal damage, erythema, edema, and pain, and it increases tolerated fluences. I believe that when longer pulse durations are used, parallel cooling (cooling the skin during the laser pulse) is the best cooling method. For short pulse durations, precooling (cooling the skin immediately before the laser pulse) is probably as effective as parallel cooling.

OPTIMAL PATIENT CHARACTERISTICS

The optimal laser or light source depends on the patient population one plans to treat (Table 48-1). Patients have a wide variety of skin colors, based on their epidermal melanosome distribution. The darker the patient's skin, the more the epidermis will absorb light, and thus less light will get to the hair follicle. The size of hair follicles also varies widely. The larger the hair follicle, the further the heat needs to diffuse from the chromophore (hair shaft). Patients also have a wide variation of hair shaft diameter and color.

TABLE 48.1

Applications of Epilation Systems

Application	Ruby	Alexandrite	Short-pulse Diode	Long-pulse Diode	Super-long-pulse Diode	Nd:YAG	IPL
Safe on dark skin				✓	✓	✓	✓
Safe on tanned skin	✓	✓	✓				
Effective on light hair	✓	✓	✓				✓
Effective on thin hair	✓	✓	✓				✓
Effective on coarse hair	✓	✓	✓	✓	✓	✓	✓

Nd indicates neodymium; IPL, intense pulsed light; and check mark, works for that application.

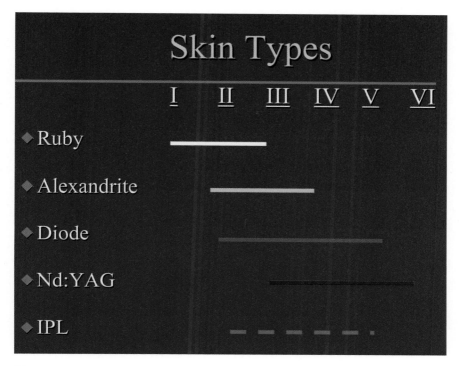

F I G U R E   48.1

Optimal hair removal lasers for various skin types.

Figure 48-1 shows that for light-skinned patients, the ruby or alexandrite laser, or even the short-pulsed diode laser, is best. To safely treat darker patients, use a long-pulse or super-long-pulse diode laser or a neodymium (Nd):YAG laser. In addition to the 4 lasers approved by the Food and Drug Administration (FDA) for darker skin types (Fig 48-2), an optically filtered light (intense-pulsed light) source (Photoderm, Lumenis, Santa Clara, Calif) is approved for this use.

I thank R. Rox Anderson, MD, Christine C. Dierickx, MD, Valerie Campos, MD, Kittisak Suthamjariya, MD, Dieter Manstein, MD, Mabet Alora, MD, Shari Hicks, MD, Gregory Altshuler, PhD, and William Farinelli for their contribution and assistance in research of lasers on darker skin, performed at Wellman Laboratories of Photomedicine, Boston, Mass.

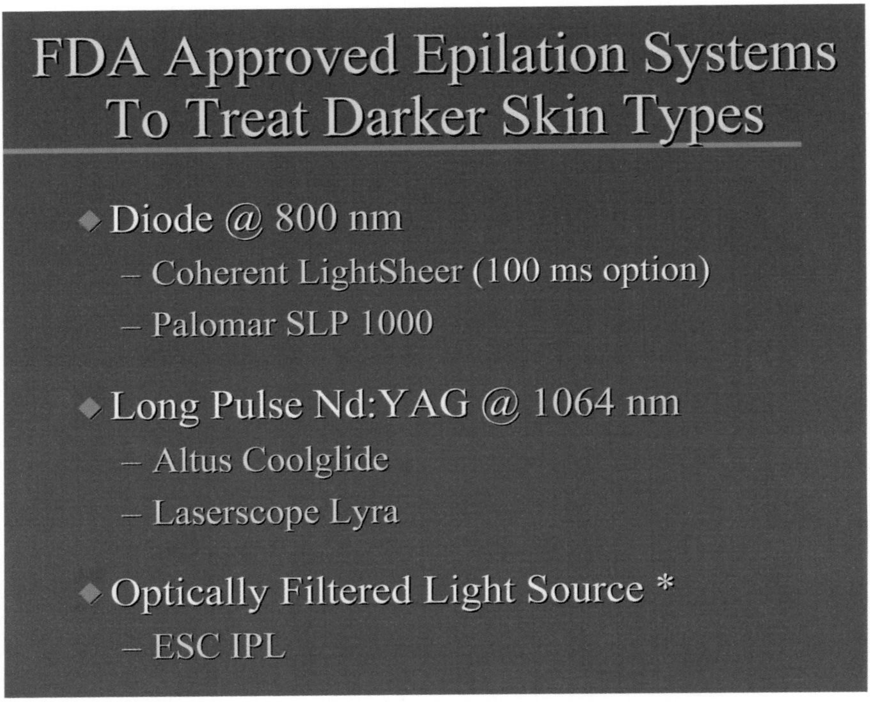

FDA Approved Epilation Systems To Treat Darker Skin Types

◆ Diode @ 800 nm
 – Coherent LightSheer (100 ms option)
 – Palomar SLP 1000

◆ Long Pulse Nd:YAG @ 1064 nm
 – Altus Coolglide
 – Laserscope Lyra

◆ Optically Filtered Light Source *
 – ESC IPL

FIGURE 48.2

Epilation systems for darker skin types.

chapter 49

Current Practice and Experience in Laser Hair Removal

Melanie C. Grossman, MD

Many lasers and light sources are used for short-term and long-term hair loss. Rather than there being a single laser system that is best for hair removal, I believe that the type of laser that works best depends on the patient being treated. In my opinion, many of the available laser systems can be used safely and effectively to achieve excellent results in most light-skinned, dark-haired individuals. Thin-haired, lighter-haired patients are a challenge to treat but benefit most from the shorter wavelengths and pulse durations. Longer pulse durations and wavelengths, combined with cooling, allow safest treatment in darker-skinned patients.

In an effort to stimulate a discussion for future improvement of clinical hair-removal techniques and technologies, I surveyed a group of dermatologists regarding their current practice and experience in performing laser hair removal.

MATERIALS AND METHODS

I developed a questionnaire with open-ended questions pertaining to laser hair-removal practices and opinions (Table 49-1). The questionnaire was sent in July 2001 to 27 physicians who are considered experts in laser surgery and who were scheduled to speak at the 2001 Controversies and Conversations in Cutaneous Laser Surgery Symposium. After the questionnaires were returned, I informally collected the responses.

RESULTS

Only 3 of the 27 people asked to fill out the questionnaire did not respond. All but 3 of the 24 respondents perform laser hair removal in their practice. Approximately 45% of the respondents reported that the physicians in their office perform the treatments. The other 55% of the respondents reported that

TABLE 49.1

Questionnaire on Laser Hair Removal

1. Does your practice offer laser hair removal?
2. Who performs the hair-removal laser surgery in your practice?
3. What percentage of your patients are female vs male?
4. Is there any area on the body you do not treat for hair removal?
5. How many treatments do you give on average?
6. What is the time interval between treatments?
7. Do you prescribe eflornithine hydrochloride (Vaniqa) cream for your patients? If so, how and where do you have your patients apply it? Do you prescribe it for both male and female patients?
8. Have you seen either of these phenomena after laser hair-removal surgery in any of your patients?
9. Black hair turning white
10. Unexpected hair growth
11. Have you seen other unexpected side effects, either favorable or unfavorable? If so, what?
12. Are you aware of local medical-legal cases against spas or other facilities pertaining to laser hair removal?
13. What improvements would you like to see in laser hair-removal technology?
14. What do you think the public awareness is regarding laser hair removal, and how can laser surgeons improve patient education?
15. Is there any other issue you wish to discuss?

the treatments were done by nurses (35%) or other people, including electrologists, physician's assistants, and technicians (65%).

Almost 90% of the respondents said that more than 90% of their patients are female. A few physicians responded that their patient population was as high as 30% male.

In reply to the question about areas not treated for hair removal, most of the respondents said that they do not treat the eyebrows or eyelashes. Two people mentioned that they did not treat the genitalia.

Almost all respondents said they give 3 to 7 treatments at 1- to 3-month intervals, depending on the area treated. Approximately 50% of the respondents prescribe eflornithine hydrochloride (Vaniqa) cream. Most of them recommend this for women to apply on the face. One person mentioned that he prescribes it in men.

Approximately 50% of the respondents said that they have seen black hair turn to white after laser hair removal. In addition, about 50% of the respondents have seen the phenomenon of an increased amount of facial hair, and they believe that laser surgery can induce hair growth. Almost always, though, this happened in women on the face.

Some unexpected benefits and adverse effects were seen after laser hair-removal surgery. Interesting benefits included less acne, folliculitis, or pseudofolliculitis barbae as well as skin rejuvenation. One person reported less axillary sweating after treatment, but somebody else noted increased axillary sweating. Among the adverse effects encountered were scarring and pigmentation, which are, I think, problems that people expect to see if the lasers are not used properly. A few people mentioned severe edema, particularly after treatment with the long-pulse neodymium:YAG laser.

An issue that has come up often in New York, where I practice, is the question of who should perform laser hair-removal. About 30% of the respondents are aware of adverse effects stemming from laser surgery performed at spas and non–physician-run facilities.

I asked people what improvements in laser technology they would like to see. The most common response was more efficient, more versatile lasers that produce less pain. Also, some people were interested in the ability to treat white hair, which currently cannot be done well. One person would like a laser to grow hair. Another person asked why we cannot tan hairs like we can tan skin.

Many of my patients were misinformed about laser hair removal, so I asked the survey respondents about public awareness and patient education. Comments included the need to clearly inform patients about the risks and benefits of laser hair removal.

COMMENT

The survey population was too small for statistical analysis, but the results of this questionnaire did provide some interesting information. The large percentage of respondents (approximately 50%) who prescribe eflornithine hydrochloride (Vaniqa) suggests that this cream may be the only way now to help in the short term for treating white or wispy blond facial hair in women. Laser surgeons need a better understanding of how patients should use Vaniqa. Should we have patients use it while we are treating with the laser, or should we wait until later? The optimal timing for treatment with Vaniqa remains to be determined.

About 50% of the respondents have seen an increased amount of facial hair after laser hair removal, a phenomenon whose cause is unknown. How many of you have done an endocrine workup in these patients experiencing a stimulation of hair growth, and of the physicians who have, are the results of the endocrine workup consistently negative? Also unclear is why black hair turns white after laser surgery or even whether it actually does. I have never been sure whether the black hair has actually turned white or whether the patient and I have just then started to notice white hair. I wonder whether this phenomenon has something to do with fluence. More study is needed about both of these post-treatment phenomena.

The results of this survey show that laser technology for hair removal is not yet fully meeting the needs of clinicians and patients. A few survey respondents and I would like to see hair-removal lasers with some sort of a device to decrease the odor. In terms of versatility and size of the machines, we would like to have machines that are smaller. Small machines are available, but they have higher outputs. I think that many laser surgeons want lasers with a bigger handpiece, but when I treat hair around the ears, I would like a smaller handpiece.

Although this survey did not specifically address the need for nonlaser sources of hair removal, I think we definitely need to look into developing photodynamic therapy (PDT) for hair reduction.

Also needed is better public education about the risks and benefits of laser hair removal. I think that the public's conception about laser hair removal spans the gamut from thinking this is the greatest thing to thinking it is awful and has been misrepresented. We need to dispel the misconceptions and clearly inform our patients about what laser hair removal can and cannot do.

PART THIRTEEN DISCUSSION

Jeffrey S. Dover, MD, FRCPC, *Moderator*

Henry H. Chan, MD: We performed a study for hair removal comparing the 810-nm diode laser (LightSheer, Lumenis, Santa Clara, Calif) and the 1064-nm neodymium (Nd):YAG laser (Lyra, Laserscope, San Jose, Calif) in terms of patient tolerability. We found that the Nd:YAG was substantially more painful. Most of my patients could not tolerate the Nd:YAG treatment. At that stage, however, we had used a cooling system with the scanning, hexagonal pattern, not the new 10-mm recycling handpiece, which I have been informed by the manufacturer substantially reduces pain. I want to ask the audience members, as well as the panelists, if they have any experience using the new handpiece and whether they find the diode to be more tolerable than the Nd:YAG laser. I am wondering whether the new handpiece from Laserscope is substantially better.

Dr Dover: I believe it is. Our group used the old scanning, hexagonal-pattern cooling system on the Nd:YAG laser. It was so painful, we could not treat any patients. Laserscope built a 10-mm photon recycling handpiece that is much easier to use, much more comfortable, very effective. Does any panelist have experience with that device?

Eliot F. Battle, Jr, MD: The Nd:YAG is a more painful device. The size of the cooling apparatus determines some of the pain threshold. The Laserscope Lyra's 10-mm handpiece is a wonderful, easy-to-use concave handpiece. It definitely causes much less pain compared with the older handpiece.

David Friedman, MD: I have 2 comments. First, I want to mention about the possibility of inducing hair growth by laser hair removal. I have done some endocrine workups, and I have not seen a tremendous increase in hair growth after laser hair removal in those people with endocrine abnormalities. This complication is very unusual, occurring in fewer than 5% of my cases. It usually happens in individuals with type IV or type V skin, and the hair usually grows on the lower part of the neck, in an area where the patients never had hair, or sometimes in the malar medial area. I think that there is some kind of scatter, and then there is maybe some kind of low-grade biostimulation of the follicle. Originally, I thought that patients, once they no longer had noticeable hair, were able to see this fine hair, but this problem happened too often, so I think it is a real phenomenon. I now mention it in my informed consent.

Second, I want to mention how I deal with dark-skinned patients, since 50% of my patients have type IV or type V skin. When dealing with very thick hairs, the laser surgeon could increase the pulse duration, using at least 30 milliseconds, with no problem. The problem is with subsequent treatments as the regrowth is thinner. In those cases, I definitely have wanted to use shorter pulse durations. Even though my laser has contact cooling, for the last few years, I have been using the cryogen system with it, and patients love it. By using a second cooling—cold air—I am able to use higher fluences and shorter pulse durations, with much greater patient comfort. Before using cold air, it behooves the laser surgeon to ask patients if they are extremely sensitive to cold. Two of my patients have had chilblain-like reactions, and a workup showed that both had cryoglobulinemia. They told me later that in the winter they are very sensitive to the cold. If you use cold air in such cold-sensitive patients, they should really move around in the cold air and not be in 1 place.

Dr Dover: Which device do you use?

Dr Friedman: I use a 810-nm diode laser, the LightSheer.

Dr Dover: And you use both contact cooling and cold air with the Zimmer cold-air device on the site?

Dr Friedman: Definitely. After the second or third treatment in patients with type IV or V skin, I can use 30 J/cm^2, or 35 J/cm^2 on the "auto" setting.

Dr Dover: So you are treating at 30 J/cm^2 at 15 milliseconds with double cooling?

Dr Friedman: Easily. And with every treatment, I increase the fluence.

Dr Battle: Those who cannot afford the cold-air device can use ice to precool before treatment or ice after treatment. Any method of removing the heat from the epidermis in addition to what the laser cooling system provides is a good way to be able to increase fluences and use shorter pulse durations. By far the hardest patient to treat is the dark-skinned patient with fine hair.

Dr Dover: My only problem with the Zimmer cold-air device is that it is quite large and very noisy. It is the size of most big lasers. We have fairly large-sized laser procedure rooms, but we frequently trip over the machine because the wheels stick out. Anyone who has used it realizes the footprint is bigger than the device because of the way the wheels are set. If the device could be shrunk in half and made into a tabletop model, I think more laser surgeons would use air cooling for many techniques, not just laser hair removal.

Kenneth A. Arndt, MD: I have read news releases from Microwave Medical that the company is working on new devices. What is the state of the microwave hair-removal device?

Jerome M. Garden, MD: I used the machine for a long time but have not used it recently. The concept of using microwaves to try to selectively destroy hair follicles does have some solid basis in science, and therefore it seems to be an interesting approach. Unfortunately, the device still needs a lot of work in development. It is difficult to control the delivery of the microwave energy within the system without affecting damage to the surrounding structures.

Maria I. Martinez, MD: I have 2 questions. First, in removing white hairs with photodynamic therapy (PDT), what kind of device and settings do you use? The other question is, When you have hair induction with laser treatment, which patients get the hair induction and why? Does anyone know if the causative factor is the kind of laser used or the skin type or the thickness of the hair? What is it?

Dr Dover: First, let's talk about white hair. Any comments?

Christine C. Dierickx, MD: The PDT work I discussed was a dose-response study, in which we tried to optimize delivery, that is, selectively deliver the photosensitizer to the follicles, and to find the optimal dose. The optimal concentration of the drug (aminolevulinic acid, or ALA) was 20%, and the optimal dose of 630 nm of laser light was 200 J/cm^2. However, it was never made into a practical PDT treatment modality for several reasons. There was accumulation of the photosensitizer in the epidermis, causing epidermal damage, pain during light delivery, and postinflammatory hyperpigmentation. Further work needs to be done to make this a practical treatment modality.

Dr Dover: While we are on this topic, are there devices that work for reducing blond hair?

Melanie C. Grossman, MD: The treatment options for removing thin, blond hair are poor.

Dr Dover: There are companies, however, that market their devices for removal of blond hair. Some of my patients have come into my office with the manufacturer's marketing information. Has anybody ever effectively removed blond hair permanently on a regular basis?

Harvey Jay, MD: I know this is controversial, so I am not going to say I can remove white hair. If you mean removal of red or blond hair, I think it has been shown to be possible. We have removed red or blond hair, and we have also found removal possible with gray hair.

Dr Dover: What is your device and technique?

Dr Jay: We use the intense pulsed light (IPL) device. I think we have usually been successful using higher power. I think it's an issue of power with IPL. The reality is that removal depends on whether the hairs are coarse or fine and on the pulse duration used. In general, these patients with light hair are light-skinned, so the laser surgeon can increase the power. I think that the density of the hair follicles is more important than the color.

Dr Dover: So on a regular basis, you are achieving pretty good results with treating blond hair?

Dr Jay: The vast majority of people coming in for hair removal are darker haired. There is not as much demand for removal of blond hair, so we do not get anywhere near the number of patients with blond hair as with dark hair.

Dr Dover: Right, but on a routine basis, are your light-haired patients doing well after treatment? We see lots of patients—young and middle-aged women—with blond hair, what I call peach fuzz, who want their excess hair removed. We turn them all away because we believe they are not good candidates for laser hair removal.

Dr Jay: I think you should try IPL in those patients.

Dr Dover: Are there other people in the audience who have had a similar experience with IPL being able to permanently reduce blond hair? Dr Jay specifically said it does not work for white hair in his experience. Obviously more needs to be done for the treatment of light hair.

I would like to ask the panelists the question raised earlier. What do you think about the induction of hair growth, which we see in our practice on a somewhat regular basis?

Kenneth A. Arndt, MD: Dr Dover and I have some patients who have been treated 6 or 8 times and who are convinced—and I think they are right—that they have more hair at the end than they did in the beginning.

Dr Dover: The hair develops on the treated site, sometimes distant sites, usually on the side of the face and the neck.

Dr Arndt: This has occurred primarily with the long-pulse alexandrite laser. If this happens, we then proceed to use the long-pulse 1064 nm-Nd:YAG laser.

Dr Battle: I hear that most of the patients affected in this way are Mediterranean women, with skin types III and IV, and the affected area is usually the face. Normally the induction of hair growth occurs outside the treatment area, so probably scattering has a play in that. The cause of hair stimulation may be lower-than-optimal treatment fluences.

Dr Dover: There is a definite increase in hair growth after 6 or 8 treatments in some individuals. It usually occurs in young women who have fairly dense hair to start with, and when treatment is done, they have even more hair. We assumed it was because we were using a suboptimal fluence, because we were using a device that was not safe for darker skin. However, when we switched to a wavelength of 1064 or 810 nm and pushed the fluence up to the maximum, we still did not get good results in this small group of patients. This phenomenon is reproducible. We can now predict when this problem will happen when the patients first come in for consultation. Other people must be encountering this problem.

A physician: Were the hairs thick and dark, or were they more thinned?

Dr Dover: They were thick and dark.

David Vasily, MD: We have a series of 16 patients treated with the ruby laser, in whom hair growth was induced. I think the skin color is actually a teleological explanation as to why it happens. There is no difference in this group of patients compared with age-matched controls and sex-matched controls. However, I think they are a group of people who may have some difference, possibly at the molecular level. I don't know about scatter stimulating hair growth; I am not sure that is what is happening. The hair growth occurs in areas of lymphatic drainage, which implies to me that there may be a soluble mediator or cytokine in that area of lymphatic drainage. According to the literature on this, there is 1 particular mediator that I think could be involved, called sonic hedgehog. People have taken sonic hedgehog and made it into a topical solution that can regrow hair. The problem is that this solution also can grow basal cell carcinoma. I think the induction of hair growth may be related to multiple hair-removal treatments. Consequently, we use the spectrophotometer, and we have built algorithms. If the patient is above a certain BL ratio, we use the diode laser (SLP 810, Palomar Medical Technologies Inc, Burlington, Mass) instead of the ruby laser. The key thing is to use the maximally tolerated tissue fluence. When we do that, we do not see biostimulation of hair.

Dr Dover: Your description, I think, is exactly what happened. We probably undertreated these patients, because they tend to have skin type III, and we probably stimulated hair as opposed to removing it. The big concern, of course, with aggressive treatment, is that hyperpigmentation often develops.

A physician: On my 532-nm frequency-doubled Nd:YAG laser (VersaPulse, Lumenis, Santa Clara, Calif) I have reduced the temperature of the cooling device to 1°C, and I wonder why the other lasers cannot do the same thing. I sent it to the manufacturer, and it has been set so that I can reduce the temperature on my Versa-Pulse to even 0.5°C.

Dr Dover: That can be done. It is the way the machine is set, because I think the same device comes with the long-pulse Nd:YAG laser (Lyra).

A physician: When I asked the manufacturer of the Lyra whether it is possible to lower the temperature, the representative said no.

Dr Dover: What is yours set at with the Lyra? What is the lowest temperature it goes to?

A physician: The lowest temperature I can get is 4°C.

Dr Dover: Ours goes to 1°C, so I think it actually depends on how it is set.

R. Rox Anderson, MD: I think the VersaPulse has a separate temperature control on the cooler. Maybe other manufacturers could consider doing that. There are lasers that go quite a bit lower with contact cooling. Of course, the temperatures of the spray-cooling devices are far below that. The E2000 ruby laser (Palomar Medical Technologies Inc, Burlington, Mass) has a supercold version, which runs down to −10°C. When I use that laser, I almost always use it in supercold mode, and I get much less epidermal injury and so forth. You raise a good point, which is that cooling systems can be at or below 0°C. The trouble is you get some frosting. I think one of the flashlamp devices has some −0°C cooling to it.

A physician: I have another question. Using a diode laser, I treated a woman with skin type II or perhaps slightly darker. There were no complications during the first, second, and third treatments, but after the fourth treatment, hyperpigmentation developed, and she supposedly had not been exposed to the sun. How can I prevent that?

Dr Grossman: That happened to a patient of mine who did not live in the United States after I treated her arms and her legs. Fortunately, the hyperpigmentation faded. I believe it happened because I had used an upgraded laser at the time and was treating her at the same fluence but it was faster. I think that she did not receive the same cooling by having the faster treatment.

Dr Anderson: I want to make a comment about hair-growth stimulation. It is a very real problem. I think the sonic hedgehog concept may be great, but we really don't know that this is, in fact, the mechanism. There is a clinical condition of porphyria in which hypertrichosis results from long-term sun exposure. The same process, PDT driven with porphyrins, can kill the hair follicles at high doses. One sees this over and over again in nature. A noxious stimulus at a low injury level that is survivable or repairable will frequently lead to a stimulation process, whereas high doses will kill. The problem is that, although laser pulses can treat the terminal hairs, there is an approximately 4:1 ratio of vellus to terminal hairs, and laser therapy is, to some extent, stimulating these hairs. My impression is that the short pulses tend to do this a little more than the long pulses. I have seen a number of these cases in my practice, and my suggestion is to recognize these patients, be honest with them, and put the risk of hair-growth stimulation in the consent form. If the problem occurs, my suggestion is to treat it with the longest pulses available. Because the vellus hairs are small, they tend to ignore the heating cycle from a very long pulse. It is this business about thermokinetic selectivity, or size-sensitive heating. I think the very long pulses of the diode lasers, for example, are much less prone to this problem. Try one of those lasers if this problem of hair-growth stimulation occurs.

Dr Friedman: We have no problem believing that we could stimulate collagen with low doses and low fluences, so I don't see it being farfetched that we could also stimulate hair. To prevent hair-growth stimulation, I advise using the highest fluence and the shortest pulse duration to do as much damage as possible in the first treatment, I think that is crucial, because if you do not do that, if you start off with a low fluence, all you do is thin the hairs, and then subsequent treatments are going to become much more difficult. In the areas where there is extreme density of hair, such as on the chin or on a man's beard, it is better to do a little less aggressive treatment. Otherwise, there is the risk of causing a lot of damage.

As far as dealing with these patients once hair-growth stimulation happens, I take a little different tack. I continue to increase the fluence. I always work with the shortest pulse duration, and these patients tend to improve if they can tolerate the higher fluence. I rarely will laser treat the arms or trunk of a man without first applying a eutectic mixture of lidocaine and prilocaine (EMLA), not only for pain but also for hydration, especially on the arms. The use of EMLA allows me to use 40 J/cm^2 on type I and type II skin with the LightSheer diode laser. Then I am able to really obtain reproducible results. I use the EMLA just to give me a little more maneuverability and fewer side effects when using the higher fluences.

INDEX

Ablation of the skin, 9
Accutane, 21
Acne scar subtypes, 275–276
Acne scars, 10, 23, 88, 108, 275–280, 290, 295–299
Acquired Nevus of Ota-like macule, 319
Actinic keratoses, 234
Acyclovir, 35
Adrian, Robert M., 25, 84, 181, 193
Adverse reactions, 10–11, 14
African Americans. *See* Dark-skinned patients
Aggressive cooling, 225
Air cooling, 220, 222
ALA, 330, 342
Alabaster-white hypopigmentation, 225
Alam M, 49
Aldara, 313, 322
Alexandrite laser
    facial lentigines, 320
    hair removal, 330, 334, 335, 344
    hemosiderin, 324
    hyperpigmentation, 312, 314
    hypertrophic scars, 281
    leg veins, 166, 181, 184
    nevus of Ota, 319
    vascular anomalies, 160
Algorithmic treatment approach, 175
Allergic granulomas, 324
Allergic tattoo reactions, 303
Alora, Mabet, 335
Alster, Tina, 50
Altshuler, Gregory, 335
Ambulatory phlebectomy, 171
Aminolevulinic acid (ALA), 330, 342
Anderson, R. Rox, 53, 83, 89, 114, 159, 161, 207,
    208, 223, 231, 232, 249, 253, 270, 271, 272,
    297, 317, 320, 321, 322, 324, 335, 345
Antihistamines, 324
Antioxidants, 10, 45, 46, 49
Aquaphor Healing Ointment, 31–33, 40, 41, 43
Arborizing telangiectasia, 121
Argon laser, 157, 158
Argon laser damage, 138
Armstrong, Myrna, 321
Arndt, Kenneth A., 21, 23, 49, 50, 52, 53, 82, 83, 88,
    113, 157, 158, 231, 233, 253, 319, 323, 324,
    342, 343, 344
Artecoll, 88
Arteriovenous (AV) anastomosis, 192
Artificial cooling. *See* Skin cooling
Atrophic scarring, 23
Atrophic scars, 291
Authors. *See* Contributors
AV anastomosis, 192
Axillary sweating, 339
Azithromycin, 35

Bacitracin, 32
Bacterial colonization, 44

Basal cell carcinoma, 245, 344
Battle, Eliot F., Jr., 333, 341, 342, 344
Beauty salons, 84
Belly button piercing, 323
Biesman, Brian S., 84, 197, 227
Bio-occlusive dressings, 29
Biochemical effects, 61–63
Biomechanical skin characterization, 58
Bjerring, Peter, 61, 82, 83, 87, 213
Black patients. *See* Dark-skinned patients
Bleaching cream, 37
Blepharoplasty scar, 292
Blistering
    psoriasis, 270, 272
    skin cooling, 234
Blue-black pigmentation, 320
Blushing, 183
Body art. *See* Tattoos
Bohannon, Jo S., 22, 89, 323
Boixeda, Pablo, 125, 158, 161, 234
Botulinum toxin (BOTOX) injections, 88, 254
Boxcar scars, 275, 276, 278, 295
Breast lift and contouring, 106
Bulk cooling, 214
Bulk precooling, 223–225
Burn scars, 291
Burns, A. Jay, 24, 50, 51

Cadmium, 324
Calcipotriene, 269, 272
Campos, Valerie, 335
Canfield photographic device, 86, 88
Carbon dioxide (CO_2) laser, 13, 25
    acne scars, 279
    complications, 291
    hypertrophic scars, 295
    incision, 197–198, 202, 203
    keloidal scars, 287
    melasma, 309–312
    permanent eyeliner, 324
    permanent lip liner, 322
    psoriasis, 265–266
    scars, 279, 287, 291, 295, 298
    single pass, 8
    skin coding, 227
    skin resurfacing, 3, 4
    tactile feedback, 208
    tattoos, 322
CD-31 stain, 257, 258
Chan, Henry H., 22, 87, 319, 322, 341
Chemical cautery, 295
Chemical peels
    acne scars, 278
    melasma, 309
    photorejuvenation/subsurface resurfacing, 77
Chess, Cyrus, 49, 87, 234, 324
Chilblain-like reactions, 341
Child abuse, 254

Chlortetracycline hydrochloride, 37
Circulating macrophages, 303
Clabaugh W., 323
Clement, Marc, 215
Cluster reangiogenesis, 121
CO_2 laser. See Carbon dioxide (CO_2) laser
Cobalt, 324
Cold-air cooling, 227–229
Cold contact cooling, 213
Cold gliding handpiece, 224
Cold-window handpieces, 224
Collagen-alginate dressing, 39, 41
Collagen contraction, 9
Collagen production, 63
Combination therapy, 88
    acne scars, 279
    psoriasis, 270
    tattoos, 322
    vascular anomalies, 151
Complete thermocoagulation, 171–172
Conductive cooling, 231
Confocal scanning laser microscopy, 237–244, 254
Contact cooling, 73, 173, 213, 220, 221
Continuous air cooling systems, 73
Continuous-wave laser
    laser-induced chrysiasis, 320
    tattoos, 325
    vascular anomalies, 157
Contributors
    Adrian, 181
    Anderson, 223, 249, 317
    Battle, 333
    Biesman, 197, 227
    Bjerring, 61, 213
    Boixeda, 125
    Burns, 43
    Dierickx, 329
    Fitzgerald, 9, 265
    Garden, 111, 153
    Geronemus, 57, 263, 291
    Goldberg, 73
    Goldman, 39, 171
    Grossman, 337
    Hruza, 29, 285
    Kaminer, 93, 275
    Kaufmann, 201
    Kauvar, 119, 165
    Kilmer, 13, 95
    list of, ix–xi
    Nelson, 219, 247
    Nestor, 149
    Raulin, 37, 145
    Rohrer, 237
    Ross, 309
    Ruiz-Esparza, 7, 101
    Tope, 281, 303
    Waner, 205
    Weiss, 77, 175
    Zachary, 3
    Zelickson, 65, 257
Cooling. See Skin cooling
Cooling gels, 224
CoolTouch II, 84, 291
Corticosteroids, 35
Cryogen injury, 225
Cryogen plus laser treatment, 75
Cryogen spray cooling. See Skin cooling

Cryogen spray (dynamic) cooling, 220–222
Cryogen spurt duration, 232–234
Cryogen system, 341
Cryoglobulinemia, 341
Custom Color, 51
Cutting instruments. See Incisional laser surgery

Darier disease, 254
Dark-skinned patients
    hair removal, 329–330, 336, 341
    hyperpigmentation, 5, 312
    hypopigmentation, 5, 22
    scarring, 298
Darvocet, 24
DCD, 224
Delayed-onset permanent hypopigmentation, 5
Dermabond glue, 276
Dermabrasion, 278
Dermal-epidermal junction, 89
Dermal fillers, 278
Dermal melasma, 309–311, 319
Dermal pigments. See also Tattoos
    hemosiderin, 324
    Hori macule, 319
    melasma, 309–311, 319
    nevus of Ota, 319
    novel, 307
    postinflammatory hyperpigmentation, 312
Dermal tethers, 276, 277
Designer tattooing, 317
Diagnostic tools, 235–254
    confocal scanning laser microscopy, 237–244, 254
    diffuse optical tomography, 250
    discussion, 253–254
    electro-optic imaging tools, 249–251
    fiberoptic skin fluorometer, 253
    laser-induced fluorescence, 249–250
    laser raman spectroscopy, 251
    Mohs micrographic surgery, 237–239
    nuclear scattering spectroscopy, 250
    optical coherence tomography, 244, 248
    port-wine stains, 247–248
    pulsed photothermal radiometry, 248
Diamond knife, 198, 201, 203, 207–209
Diazepam, 24
Dierickx, Christine C., 23, 160, 207, 208, 329, 335, 342
Diffuse optical tomography, 250
Diflucan, 51, 52
Diode laser, 53, 84
    hair removal, 329, 330, 334, 335, 336, 341, 342, 344, 346
    hypertrophic scars, 281
    leg veins, 166, 181, 192
    skin cooling, 228
Discussion
    diagnostic tools, 253–254
    hair removal, 341–346
    incisional laser surgery, 207–209
    laser skin resurfacing, 20–25
    leg veins, 191–194
    moderators. See Moderators
    photorejuvenation/subsurface resurfacing, 82–89
    post operative care, 49–53
    psoriasis, 269–272
    radiofrequency (RF) technology, 113–115
    scars/hypopigmentation/depigmentation, 295–299
    skin cooling, 231–234

tattoos/dermal pigment, 319–325
  vascular anomalies/ectasias, 157–162
Disposable scalpel blades, 203
Dog bite-related hypertrophic scars, 286
Dover, Jeffrey S., 20, 21, 23, 24, 52, 82, 85, 158, 160, 191, 269, 270, 295, 297, 298, 299, 341–345
Dressings, 29, 39–45
Dynamic cooling, 173, 213, 233
Dynamic cooling device (DCD), 161, 224
Dynamic hyperpigmentation, 309
Dynamic precooling, 223, 224

E2000 ruby laser, 345
Early, dynamic postinflammatory hyperpigmentation, 312
Eczema herpeticum, 38
Efficacy, 13–14
Eflornithine hydrochloride, 338, 339
Electro-optic imaging tools, 249–251
Electron paramagnetic resonance (EPR) lines, 306
ELM, 249
EMLA, 6, 113, 346
Encapsulated liquid ink particle, 318
Endovenous techniques, 178
Epidermal melanin, 291
Epidermal necrosis, 158
Epiluminescence microscopy (ELM), 249
EPR signal, 306
Erbium (Er): YAG laser, 25, 30
  acne scars, 279, 290
  atrophic scars, 291
  hypertrophic scars, 281
  incision, 198, 202, 203
  melasma, 309–312
  nonhypertrophic surgical scars, 288
  permanent lip liner, 322
  skin resurfacing, 3–5
  tactile feedback, 208
  tattoos, 321, 322
  three stages, 8
Erythema, 4, 10, 20, 51
  beneficial nature, 4
  keloidal scar, 288
  leukodermal, 292
  tattoo removal, 314
  treatment, 35, 41, 43
Erythematous scars, 291
EsteLux, 331
Evaporative cooling, 231
Ex vivo confocal microscopic images, 260
Ex vivo confocal scanning laser microscope, 254, 257
Excimer laser
  carcinogenicity, 270, 272
  psoriasis, 263–264, 266, 269–272
  safety of doctor, 272
  scarring, 291–294, 296, 297
Expanded polytetrafluoroethylene (Gore-Tex), 23
Eyebrow lift, 103
Eyebrow tattoos, 324
Eyeliner tattoos, 324

Facial ectasias, 154. See also Vascular anomalies/ectasias
Famciclovir, 35
Famvir, 35
Farinelli, William, 335
Farm piglet model, 227

Fatty acids, 45
Fe_3O_4, 318
Femtosecond laser-induced multiphoton fluorescence, 249
Ferritin, 324
Ferromagnetic pigments, 306
Fiberoptic-coupled skin fluorometer, 253
Fibracol, 39
Filler substances, 23
Fitzpatrick, Richard E., 9, 21, 22, 23, 49, 50, 85, 115, 157, 161, 193, 265, 269, 295, 296, 323
Flashlamp devices, 330, 331
Flashlamp-pumped pulsed dye laser, 248
Flexzan, 29, 43, 44, 45
Fluconazole, 35, 51, 52
Fluocinolone acetonide, 41
Fluorescence, 249
Fluorescent tattoo ink, 317
Fluorophores, 250
Folliculitis, 338
Fontana-Masson stain, 292
Forensic medicine, 254
Freud, Sigmund, 7
Friedman, David, 341, 342, 345
Fritz, Klaus, 269, 272
Frost formation, 231
Full-face laser abrasions, 6
Full-face radiodermoplasty, 105
Full-thickness necrosis, 192

Garden, Jerome M., 22, 51, 111, 153, 160, 295, 324, 342
Gasiorowski, Henry C., 52
GentleLASE long-pulse alexandrite laser, 160
Geronemus, Roy, 20, 23, 57, 83–87, 89, 254, 263, 270, 271, 291, 295, 297, 298
Goldberg, David J., 20, 73, 82, 87
Goldman, Mitchel P., 39, 50, 52, 82, 171, 191, 192, 207, 208
Gomez, Julio Manuel Barba, 101
Gore-Tex, 23
Granulomatous inflammation, 304
Granulomatous tattoo reactions, 324
Green tattoos, 305, 312, 313, 315, 316
Greve, Baerbel, 38
Grossman, Melanie C., 83, 253, 297, 337, 343, 345
Group discussion, Discussion
Growth factors, 10, 50

Hair removal, 327–346
  adverse effects, 338, 339
  beneficial effects, 338–339
  blond hair, 343
  chilblain-like reactions, 341
  cooling method, 334, 341, 342
  cryogen system, 341
  dark-skinned people, 329–330, 336, 341
  desired improvements, 339
  discussion, 341–346
  epilation systems, 330, 334
  flashlamp devices, 331
  hair growth, 343–346
  hyperpigmentation, 344, 345
  materials/methods, 337
  microwave, 342
  optimal parameters, 333–336
  patient characteristics, 334–335, 337

peach fuzz, 343
photodynamic therapy, 330–331, 342
public awareness/education, 339, 340
pulse duration, 333–334
questionnaire, 338
red hair, 343
skin types, 335
sonic hedgehog, 344, 345
tattoos, and, 321
wavelength, 333
white hair, 342
Handheld mercury lamps, 270
Harmonic scalpel, 207
Harton AM, 49
H&E staining, 237, 238
Hematoxylin-easin (H&E) staining, 237, 238
Hemosiderin, 324
Herpes labialis, 34
Hicks, Shari, 335
Hori macule, 319
Hruza, George J., 29, 285, 295, 298
Humidity, 233
Hydration, 15–17
Hydrocodone bitartrate, 24
Hydrogel, 39
Hydroquinone medications, 35
Hyperpigmentation, 10, 14
    hair removal, 344, 345
    leg veins, 169, 183, 186
    melasma, 311
    PDT, 330
    postinflammatory, 312
    therapy, 35
Hyperplastic epidermis, 295
Hypertrichosis, 345
Hypertrophic scars, 281–287, 291, 295–299
Hypopigmentation, 10, 14, 20, 22
    laser resurfacing, 291
    scarring, 291, 298
    skin type, 4, 5
Hypopigmented face-lift scar, 293

Ice formation, 231–233
Ice-pick scars, 107, 275, 276, 295
Ideal tissue effects, 9
Imaging techniques. See Diagnostic tools
Imiquimod, 313, 322
Immunomodulators, 322
Impedance, 94
In vivo confocal scanning laser microscope, 243
Incipient hypertrophic scars, 287
Incisional laser surgery, 195–209
    CO$_2$ laser, 197–198, 202, 203
    comparative evaluation, 201
    diamond knife, 198, 201, 203, 207–209
    discussion, 207–209
    histologic study, 198
    indications for laser, 199
    laser, 199, 201–202
    metal blade knives, 203
    scalpel, 201, 202, 205, 207
Infection, 44, 53
Inflammation
    postoperative care, and, 50, 51, 53
    tattoo removal, 303, 304
Infrared coagulator, 321
Infrared visualizing system, 253

Intense pulsed light (IPL)
    hair removal, 331, 334, 335, 336, 343
    hypertrophic scars, 298
    leg veins, 176
    melasma, 311
    nonablative dermal remodeling, 65–69
    nonablative laser resurfacing, 73
    photorejuvenation/subsurface resurfacing, 77
    QS-laser resistant tattoos, 306
    tattoos, 306, 323
    vascular anomalies, 121, 147, 150
Intralesional steroids, 282
Intraluminal lasers, 171
Intravascular purpura, 157, 160
Isotretinoin, 21

Jacob, Carolyn, 299
Jay, Harvey H., 113, 114, 208, 269, 270, 295, 343

Kaminer, Michael S., 93, 113, 114, 275, 295, 296
Kaufmann, Roland, 85, 113, 157, 201, 253
Kauvar, Arielle N. B., 119, 157, 165, 193, 297,
    298, 322
Kellett, Lisa, 85, 271
Keloidal chest scars, 283
Keloidal scars, 287–288
Ketorolac tromethamine, 24
Kiernan, Mike, 215
Kilmer, Suzanne L., 13, 24, 49, 51, 95, 113, 320,
    321, 325
Kirchoff laws, 115
Koebnerization, 271
Koop, Dale, 233
KTP laser
    leg veins, 181
    melasma, 311, 313
    nonablative dermal remodeling, 65
    tattoos, 322
    vascular anomalies, 121, 150

Laryngeal papillomatosis, 207
Laser-based imaging devices. See Diagnostic tools
Laser incisional surgery. See Incisional laser surgery
Laser-induced chrysiasis, 320
Laser-induced fluorescence, 249–250
Laser-induced tattoo darkening, 320
Laser raman spectroscopy, 251
Laser-removable tattoos, 314, 318
Laser skin resurfacing, 1–53
    adverse reactions, 10–11, 14
    discussion, 20–25
    efficacy, 13–14
    hydration, 15–17
    ideal tissue effects, 9
    improvements, 7–8
    postoperative care, 27–53. See also
        Postoperative care
    side effects, 10–11, 14, 84
    three-stage resurfacing, 8
    unmet expectations, 7
Laserscope Lyra's 10-mm handpiece, 341
Lead, 324
Lecithin, 45
Leg veins, 147, 163–194
    alexandrite laser, 166, 181, 184
    algorithmic treatment approach, 175
    AV anastomosis, 192

avoidance of epidermal damage, 173
clinical/histologic findings, 181–189
complete thermocoagulation, 171–172
complications, 183, 191
cooling, 165, 173
diode laser, 166, 181, 186, 192, 193
discussion, 191–194
endovenous techniques, 178
full-thickness necrosis, 192
future considerations, 174
indications, 168–169
IPL, 176
KTP laser, 181
laser parameters, 173
Nd: YAG laser, 166–167, 172, 173, 177, 181–183,
    185, 186, 188, 193
photothermal treatment, 171–174
pulmonary embolism, 191
pulse stacking, 192, 193
pulsed dye laser, 165–166, 176, 181
sclerotherapy, 171, 183, 191, 192
side effects, 169
thrombus formation, 166, 168
ulceration, 192
Leukoderma, 291, 292
Leukotriene LTB4, 314
Leyden, James, 21
Lichen simplex chronicus, 272
Lidocaine, 24
Lidocaine and prilocaine (EMLA), 6, 15–17, 19,
    113, 346
LightSheer diode laser, 346
Lipid, 114
Long-pulse laser
    hair removal, 329, 334, 336, 339, 344
    hypertrophic scars, 281
    laser-induced chrysiasis, 320
    melasma, 311
Low-level light therapy, 53
Lymphatic transport, 317
Lymphocyte trafficking, 254

Magnetic resonance (MR) imaging, 306
Magnetic tattoo, 318
Majaron, Boris, 234
Manstein, Dieter, 335
Manuskiatti, W., 50
Martinez, Maria I., 271, 342
Massage, 317
Maximum tolerated fluence (MTF), 228
MED, 263
Melanin, 22, 158, 291
Melanocytic lesions, 254
Melasma, 309–311, 319
Mepitel, 44
Mercury, 324
Metal-blade knives, 203
Microdermabrasion, 77, 278
Microwave, 111
Microwave hair-removal device, 342
Mie scattering, 250
Mihm, Martin H., Jr., 234, 254
Milia, 10, 35
Minimal erythema dose (MED), 263
Moderators. See also Contributors, Discussion
    Anderson, 207
    Arndt, 49, 113, 157, 231, 253, 319

Dover, 20, 82, 191, 269, 295, 341
Mohs defects, 298
Mohs micrographic surgery, 237
Molecular beacons, 250
Monsel's (ferric subsulfate) solution, 295
MR imaging, 306
MTF, 228
Multiple passes, 158–162. See also Pulse stacking
Mupirocin, 44
Mycostatin, 51

NADH, 250
Narrow-spectrum antibiotic, 35
Near-infrared diode lasers, 53
Necrosis, 129
Nelson, J. Stuart, 219, 231–234, 247
Neodymium (Nd): YAG laser, 57, 58, 59, 77, 78, 83,
    88, 89
    acne scars, 299
    hair removal, 329, 330, 334, 335, 336, 339,
        341, 344
    hypertrophic scars, 281
    leg veins, 166–167, 172, 173, 177, 181–183, 185,
        186, 188, 193
    Mohs defects, 298
    nevus of Ota, 319
    nonablative laser resurfacing, 73
    psoriasis, 266
    scars, 281, 297, 298, 299
    skin cooling, 224, 233
    tattoos, 305, 306
    vascular anomalies, 122, 147, 150, 154, 157, 160
Neosporin, 32
Nestor, Mark S., 85, 149
Neutrophil chemotactic factor, 313
Nevus of Ota, 319
Nitroblue tetrazolium chloride stain, 138
NLite pulsed dye laser, 83
Noe, Joel, 82
Nonablative dermal remodeling, 65–71
Nonablative laser resurfacing, 73–75
Nonablative radiofrequency on submental area, 104
Noncontact cooling, 213
Nonhypertrophic surgical scars, 288
Nose, 133–136
Novel dermal pigments, 307
Novel photosensitizers, 307
Nuclear scattering spectroscopy, 250
Nystatin, 51

Occlusive dressings, 45
Occlusive lipid-containing ointments, 38
Ohm's law, 94
Oozing hemorrhage, 304
Optical coherence tomography, 244, 248
Optical Doppler tomography, 248
Optimal cryogenic temperature (OCT), 239
Oral dicloxacillin sodium, 35
Ort, Richard, 233, 323
Overlapping pulses, 127–131
Overtattooing, 303–305
Oxycodone, 24

Panel discussion, Discussion
Pantanowitz L, 49
Parallel cooling, 223, 224, 334
PASI score, 269

PDT
  hair removal, 330–331, 342
  psoriasis, 271
Peach fuzz, 343
Percocet, 24
Permanent dermal fillers, 23
Permanent eyeliner, 324
Permanent lip liner, 322
Persistent redness. *See* Erythema
Petrolatum, 33
Petrolatum ointment, 39
PG-9.5 stain, 257, 258
Phlebosurgery, 253
Photodynamic therapy (PDT)
  hair removal, 330–331, 342
  psoriasis, 271
PhotoGenica V-Star, 83
Photon recycling, 313
Photons, 53
Photorejuvenation and subsurface resurfacing, 55–89
  biochemical effects, 61–63
  combined therapy, 88
  discussion, 82–89
  IPL, 65–69
  nonablative dermal remodeling, 65–71
  nonablative laser resurfacing, 73–75
  pulsed dye laser, 61–71
  treatment algorithm, 77–78
Phototherapy, 265
Photothermal light-skin interaction, 213
Photothermal treatment of leg telangiectasia, 171–174
Photothermolysis, 139
Picosecond-domain lasers, 303
Pigmentary change improvement, 18
Pitted scars, 83–84
Poikiloderma of Civatte, 121–122, 150
Polymyxin B sulfate-bacitracin zinc, 32
Polymyxin B sulfate-bacitracin zinc-neomycin, 32
Polysporin, 32
Porphyria, 345
Port-wine stain, 120–121, 125–146, 160–162
  geometry, 247
  infants/young children, 233
  noninvasive diagnostic tools, 248
  pulse duration, 154
  pulsed dye laser, 150
  repigmentation of scars, 292
Postcooling, 223–225
Postinflammatory hyperpigmentation, 312
Postoperative care, 27–53
  antioxidants, 45, 46
  cooling, 49, 51. *See also* Skin cooling
  discussion, 49–53
  dressings, 29, 39–45
  erythema, 51. *See also* Erythema
  infection, 44, 53
  inflammation, 50, 51, 53
  prophylaxis, 29–34
  review of literature, 43–45
  wound care, 29–34
Postoperative scars, 287
Postresurfacing hypopigmentation, 296–297
Potassium-titanyl-phosphate laser. *See* KTP laser
Preauricular scar, 292
Precooling, 334
Primos 3-D imaging, 86
Problem-oriented treatment algorithm, 77–78

Prophylaxis, 34–35
Propoxyphene napsylate-acetaminophen, 24
Protoporphyrin IX, 330
Pseudofolliculitis barbae, 339
Psoralen-UV-A (PUVA) therapy, 291–292
Psoriasis, 255–272
  blistering, 270, 272
  children, 271–272
  CO_2 laser, 265–266
  combination therapy, 270
  cost, 272
  discussion, 269–272
  excimer laser, 263–264, 266, 269–272
  Nd: YAG laser, 266
  optimal dose, 271
  PASI score, 269
  PDT, 271
  pulse duration, 259
  pulsed dye laser, 257, 258, 266
  review of literature, 257–259
  UV-B treatment, 265, 269
Psoriasis area severity index (PASI) score, 269
Pulmonary embolus, 191
Pulse stacking, 128–130, 140–142, 158–162, 192, 193
Pulsed dye laser
  acne scars, 299
  erythematous scars, 291
  hypertrophic scars, 282, 290, 291, 296, 297, 298
  keloidal scars, 287
  laryngeal papillomatosis, 207
  leg veins, 165–166, 176, 181
  nonablative dermal remodeling, 65–71
  nonablative laser resurfacing, 73
  photorejuvenation, 61–64, 77, 82
  psoriasis, 257, 258, 266
  skin cooling, 214–216
  sternotomy scars, 295
  vascular anomalies, 121, 125, 132, 139, 146, 147, 158, 160
Pulsed photothermal radiometry, 248
Punch elevation, 276
Punch excision, 276, 295
Punch grafting, 276
Punch knives, 203
Purpura
  acceptability, 150
  defined, 125–126
  fascial vascular lesions, 119–120, 121, 131, 158
  intravascular, 157, 160
  long-pulse laser, 157
  psoriasis, 259
PUVA therapy, 291–292
Pyruvic acid sodium salt, 45

Q-switched laser, 59, 83
  allergic granulomas, 324, 325
  facial lentigines, 320
  hemosiderin, 324
  hyperpigmentation, 312, 314
  leukoderma, 292
  near death/anaphylaxis, 325
  nevus of Ota, 319
  nonablative laser resurfacing, 73
  scars, 297, 299
  tattoos, 303, 305, 306, 320, 324, 325
QS laser-resistant tattoo, 305–306

Radiodermoplasty, 108, 109
Radiofrequency (RF) technology, 91–114
    animal studies, 95–96
    cautionary note, 111–112
    clinical trials, 96–100
    cooling, 95
    discussion, 113–115
    microwave, compared, 111
    potential clinical targets, 94
    volumetric tissue heating, 93–94, 101, 115
Ramelet, Albert, 173
Raulin, Christian, 49, 86, 145, 157, 272
Raulin, Christina, 37
Razor blades, 203
Reangiogenesis, 121
Red striae distensae, 109
Reepithelialization, 14
Reflectance spectrometry, 320
Refrigerated air systems, 51
Reinisch, L., 227, 229
Rejuvenation of the neck, 6
Renova, 35
Repetitive pulsing, 161. See also Pulse stacking
Residual epidermal melanocytes, 291
Retin-A, 35
RevitaDerm, 44
RF technology. See Radiofrequency (RF) technology
Ring knives, 203
Robotic surgery, 208
Rohrer, Thomas E., 158, 159, 237, 253
Rolling scars, 276–278
Rosacea, 150
Ross, E. Victor, Jr., 89, 193, 309, 319, 322
Round table discussion, Discussion
Rubeosis, 146
Ruby laser
    hair removal, 330, 334, 335, 344, 345
    hemosiderin, 324
    nevus of Ota, 319
    skin cooling, 244
    tattoos, 305, 320
Ruiz-Esparza, Javier, 7, 22, 24, 51, 101, 113, 208, 266

Saucer-shaped acne scars, 290
Scalpel, 201, 202, 205, 207
Scarring, 10, 273–299
    acne scars, 10, 23, 88, 108, 275–280, 290,
        295–299
    cooling, 298
    dark-skinned patients, 298
    discussion, 295–299
    dog bite, 286
    excimer laser, 291–294, 296, 297
    hypertrophic scars, 281–287, 291, 295–299
    infrared coagulation, 321
    keloidal scars, 287–288
    nonhypertrophic surgical scars, 288
    pitted scars, 83–84
    prophylaxis, 287
    repigmentation of scars, 292–293
    shininess, 285
    tattoos, 323
    varicella scars, 288
Sclerotherapy (leg veins), 171, 175, 83, 191, 192
Second Skin, 44
Selective photothermolysis, 149
Shaw scalpel, 205

Short-pulse lasers, 150–151
Side effects, 10–11, 14, 84
Silicone filler, 23
Silicone gel, 43
Silicone-polytetrafluoroethylene (Silon-TSR) dressing,
        29, 31, 40, 43, 49
Single-chip, TE-cooled handpiece, 227
6-0 plain gut suture, 276
Skin cooling, 38, 49, 51, 73, 211–234
    basic concepts, 219
    blistering, 234
    comparison of devices, 224–225
    cryogen injury, 225
    cryogen spurt duration, 232–234
    discussion, 231–234
    efficacy/safety, 227–229
    frost formation, 231
    hair removal, 334, 341, 342
    humidity, 233
    ice formation, 231–233
    leg veins, 165, 173
    measuring skin surface temperatures, 214–215
    methods of cooling, 220–222
    objectives/purposes, 213, 223
    scarring, 298
    timing, 219
    types, 213–214, 223–224
    vascular anomalies, 161
    whiteness, 232
Skin redness. See Erythema
Skin resurfacing. See Laser skin resurfacing; Leg veins
Skin tightening, 17
Smart tattoos, 306
Smoothing of the skin crinkling, 18
Solar elastosis, 89
Sonic hedgehog, 344, 345
SpaTouch, 331
Spectrophotometer, 344
Stacking pulses, 128–130, 140–142, 158–162
Star Wars, 7
Static, prolonged hyperpigmentation, 312
Sternotomy scars, 285, 295
Steroids, 324
Striae distensae, 109, 113
Subcision, 276, 279, 295, 296
Subcutaneous fillers, 278
Subdermal undermining, 276, 295
Subsurface bruising, 254
Subsurface resurfacing. See Photorejuvenation and
        subsurface resurfacing
Sun-induced hyperpigmentation, 10
Sunblock, 37
Sunscreen, 34
Superficial acne scars, 290. See also Acne scars
Superficial dermabrasion, 323
Superficial dermal fibrosis, 234
Superficial focal burn on tail of eyebrow, 110
Superficial Mohs defects, 298
Superficial targeted chromophores, 222
Suthamjariya, Kittisak, 335
Synalar, 41, 50
Systemic allergic reactions, 320

Tacrolimus, 297
Tactile feedback, 208
Tactile sensation, 208
Tanghetti, Emil A., 83, 157, 231, 270, 271, 297

Tattoo ink darkening, 306
Tattoos, 301–325. *See also* Dermal pigments
  allergic granulomas, 324–325
  allergic reactions, 303
  anaphylaxis/near deaths, 325
  antihistamines/steroids, 325
  beneficial uses of removal technique, 306
  designer tattooing, 317–318
  encapsulated liquid ink particle, 318
  erythema, 314
  fluorescent ink, 317
  green, 305, 312, 313, 315, 316
  hair removal, 321
  itching, 325
  laser-induced chrysiasis, 320
  laser-removable, 314, 318
  lymphatic transport, 317
  magnetic, 318
  materials used in tattoo pigments, 325
  motivation for removal, 321
  number of people who want removal, 321
  overtattooing, 303–305
  panel discussion, 319–325
  remnants after removal, 306
  removal, generally, 312–314, 317
  resistance to Q-switched laser, 305–306, 313
  scarring, 321, 323
  smart, 306
  tattoo ink darkening, 306
  yellow, 305
TE-cooled sapphire window, 227, 228
Telangiectatic matting, 183
Temperature jump, 248
Tetracaine, 25
ThermaCool RF device, 96. *See also* Radiofrequency
    (RF) technology
Thermal conduction of heat out of skin, 231
Thermal imaging, 214
Thermal relaxation time (TRT), 333
Thermal scalpel, 205
Thermocoagulation, 171–172
Thermoelectrically (TE) cooled sapphire window,
    227, 228
3-D imaging system, 86, 87
Thrombus formation, 166, 168
Tide mark, 6
Tissue effects, 9
Tissue tightening, 9
Titanium dioxide, 305, 312
Tocopherol acetate, 45
Tocotrienol, 49, 50
Tomographic reconstruction algorithm techniques, 248
Tope, Whitney D., 23, 50, 86, 87, 271, 281, 295, 297,
    303, 321, 324, 325
Topical retinoid, 270
Topical vitamin D, 270
Toradol, 24
Transient hyperpigmentation, 330
Transient postoperative hyperpigmentation, 5
Transparent zinc oxide sunscreens, 35
Trapdoor deformity, 289
Treatment algorithm, 77–78
Tretinoin, 35
Tretinoin cream, 37
Tretinoin emollient cream, 35
Triamcinolone acetonide, 282, 283
TRT, 333

True-positives, 242
Tryptophan fluorescence, 250
Tumor necrosis factor, 270
Type II skin rejuvenation, 61–64
Type V acne-scarred skin, 88

Ultraviolet B. *See* UV-B treatment
Ultraviolet light phototherapy, 263
Urticarial plaques, 324
UV-B treatment
    psoriasis, 265, 269
    scars, 292, 296

Vacuolization, 129
Valacyclovir hydrochloride, 35, 44
Valium, 24
Valtrex, 35, 44
Vaniqa, 338, 339
Varicella scars, 288
Vascular anomalies/ectasias, 117–162
    choice of device, 150
    combination therapies, 151
    DCD, 161
    discussion, 157–162
    facial telangiectasia, 121–122, 125–143
    hemangioma treatment, 120–121, 146
    leg veins, 147. *See also* Leg veins
    multiple pulses, 158–162
    nose, 133–136
    overlapping pulses, 127–131
    purpura, 119–120, 121, 131, 157, 158, 160
    poikiloderma of Civatte, 122
    port-wine stains. *See* Port-wine stain
    pulse duration, 121, 153–155
    rubeosis, 146
    short-pulse lasers, 150–151
Vasily, David B., 51, 299, 344
Vasodilatation, 159
Vbeam pulsed dye laser, 69–71, 83
Venous lakes, 150
Venulectasia, 123
VersaPulse, 344, 345
Vessel collapse phenomenon, 159
Vicodin, 24
Viking maiden (tattoo), 305
Vitamin C, 41, 49
Vitiligo, 292, 296–297

Waner, Milton, 22, 23, 160, 191, 192, 205, 207,
    209, 254
Water-in-oil emulsions, 37
Weiss, Robert A., 77, 85, 88, 175, 191, 192, 233, 298,
    321, 323
White cryogen ball, 232
Wood, Robert Williams, 249
Wood's light, 249
Wound care, 29–34

Xenon chloride lasing medium, 263

Yellow tattoo, 305

Zachary, Christopher B., 3, 20, 22, 160
Zelickson, Brian D., 65, 82, 257, 270
Zimmer cold-air device, 227, 342
Zinc oxide, 34
Zovirax, 35